History of Nephrology

Reports from the
First International Conference on
the History of Nephrology
Naples/Montecassino, Italy,
October 28–30, 1993

Guest Editors
Garabed Eknoyan, Houston, Tex.
Natale G. De Santo, Naples
Giovambattista Capasso, Naples
Shaul G. Massry, Los Angeles, Calif.

138 figures, 24 tables, 1994

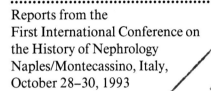
KARGER

Reprint of **American Journal of Nephrology**
Vol. 14, No. 4–6, 1994

S. Karger
Medical and Scientific Publishers
Basel · Freiburg · Paris · London
New York · New Delhi · Bangkok
Singapore · Tokyo · Sydney

Drug Dosage
The authors and the publisher have exerted every effort to ensure that drug selection and dosage set forth in this text are in accord with current recommendations and practice at the time of publication. However, in view of ongoing research, changes in government regulations, and the constant flow of information relating to drug therapy and drug reactions, the reader is urged to check the package insert for each drug for any change in indications and dosage and for added warnings and precautions. This is particularly important when the recommended agent is a new and/or infrequently employed drug.

Contents

Beginnings of Renal Pharmacology and Early Conceptualization of Diseases of the Kidney

Beginnings of Renal Pharmacology

History of Hypertension

Early Conceptualization of Diseases of the Kidney

The Salerno School of Medicine

Am J Nephrol 1994;14:255–256

Garabed Eknoyan
Natale G. De Santo
Shaul G. Massry

On the Future of the History of Nephrology

This special issue of the *American Journal of Nephrology* presents the transactions of an International Conference on the History of Nephrology held in Naples, Italy, on 28–30 October 1993 under the sponsorship of the Seconda Università di Napoli, Baylor College of Medicine and the Istituto Italiano Studi Filosofici. These institutions were represented by D. Mancino, W.T. Butler and G. Marotta, respectively.

The notion of organizing a conference on the history of nephrology was first conceived in July 1991, in a bus on the highways of Poland, by Natale G. De Santo, Shaul G. Massry and Garabed Eknoyan. The fact that these preliminary notions became a reality is primarily due to the initiative and efforts of Natale G. De Santo, who organized and arranged the venue of what is hoped will be the first of several conferences on the history of nephrology. This conference would not have attained its level of success, however, without the support of several individuals and institutions; to name but a few: A. Gargano, L. Iorio, M. DeCunzo, L. Cioffi, F. Smurra, L. Bellini, V. Zappia, L. Melillo and the National Research Council of Italy.

Initial concerns about the degree of interest in such a conference were quickly dissipated by the number of individuals who expressed an interest in attending, the stature of those who participated in it and the caliber of the presentations that were made. In fact, only the available time, space and resources limited the size and content of this first conference. As subtly stated by one of the eminent participants of the conference: 'Who would have thought that there are so many dormant historians of nephrology awaiting an opportunity to come out of the closet?'

In the few decades since nephrology became a recognized specialty of medicine, interest in its historical origins has sustained a gradual and steady growth. This is perhaps best reflected in the number of articles on the history of nephrology that have begun to appear with some regularity in most of the scientific journals devoted to nephrology. The *American Journal of Nephrology* was the first of these publications to recognize the relevance of the issue by establishing an Associate Editorship for the History of Nephrology, and by encouraging the publication of manuscripts on the topic. It is, therefore, only befitting that the *American Journal of Nephrology* should publish the proceedings of this First International Conference on the History of Nephrology.

The conference began with general presentations on the origins of nephrology followed by a series of papers on some of the early contributors to nephrology. Four papers focusing on the beginnings of renal pharmacology were then followed by 10 papers discussing the early conceptualization of diseases of the kidney. Three presentations on the history of hypertension formed a special subset of this last series.

A highlight of the conference was a visit to the Benedictine Monastery of Montecassino, which was instrumental in the evolution of the Salerno School of Medicine, and where some of the extant original manuscripts of this school are preserved. It was a touching experience to walk the hallowed hallways of this venerable historical institution and be welcomed by Abbot Bernardo D'Onorio, whose brief remarks on the links between the Salerno School of Medicine and the Montecassino Monastery are published in this issue together with the scholarly presen-

Garabed Eknoyan, MD
Baylor College of Medicine
Houston, TX 77030 (USA)

© 1994 S. Karger AG, Basel
0250–8095/94/0146–0255
$8.00/0

tations made by Father Faustino Avagliano, Maria Pasca and Massimo Oldoni on nephrology in the Salerno School of Medicine.

A special feature of the visit to the monastery was a display of the Codices on the Art of Medicine preserved in the archives of the monastery, which were presented with a specially prepared catalog for this meeting, and a display prepared by Orto Botanico di Napoli, University of Naples, of plants described by Pliny the Elder and Dioscorides for the treatment of diseases of the kidney. Additionally, an exhibit of original botanic manuscripts dating from the 15th–17th century was presented by the Department of Plant Biology of the University Federico II of Naples.

In response to the enthusiasm with which the conference was received and the interest expressed by its participants, it was decided by unanimous agreement at the close of the final session that a formal structure should be developed to organize future similar meetings. Nominations for membership in a Nominating Committee were solicited at the conference and are requested herewith. The founding officers of this organization – Natale G. De Santo, Shaul G. Massry and Garabed Eknoyan – will appoint a Nominating Committee from the proposed candidates and charge them with nominating the first slate of officers and councillors of the organization. In the appointment of the Nominating Committee and choice of officers and councillors due regard will be paid to geographic representation, reflecting the international func-

tions of the new organization. A business meeting will be held in conjunction with the next International Conference on the History of Nephrology to elect officers and adopt the constitution of the organization. A copy of the slate of proposed officers and the constitution will be made available to all interested parties at least 60 days before the meeting, by writing to G. Eknoyan, MD, Department of Medicine, Baylor College of Medicine, 1 Baylor Plaza, Houston, TX 77030–3498, USA. The site and date of the next conference will be announced 1 year before its anticipated occurrence in 1996.

It is expected that by providing a structure for existing interests, this new organization will foster, stimulate, encourage and promote research and studies in the history of medicine as it pertains to all aspects related to the kidney and urinary tract. In so doing, it should allow a better determination of the position of nephrology in the mosaic of medical history. This is an important endeavor, for the history of medicine is an essential branch of the general history of culture, and hence an indispensable component of the history of civilization.

Acknowledgement

We wish to thank Dr. Georgina Hutber for her help in editing the manuscripts, Pamela Koppay-Pinto for her guidance in editing the text, and Rosella Padulano and Charlia Due for their secreterial assistance.

Am J Nephrol 1994;14:257–258

Giuseppe Conte

Chair of Nephrology, Seconda Università di Napoli, Naples, Italy

Empiricism versus Science in the Teaching of Nephrology

Key Words
Empiricism
History of medicine
Medical education

Abstract

Recent changes in medical courses in Italy reflect a recognition that both theoretical education and clinical practice are essential components of a doctor's training. These two parallel branches of medical education find their origins in the beliefs of Galen, mentor of medicine as a pure science, and of Alexander of Aphrodisias, promoter of the predominant role of empiricism. Neither a dogmatic nor an empiric approach to the study of medicine, however, is sufficient on its own.

Medical Education in Modern Italy

Until a few years ago, Italian medical students were not required either to attend classes or, more importantly, to work in research laboratories, or engage in clinical activity. This was despite the fact that most training programs in schools of medicine elsewhere in Europe and in the rest of the world required such participation. Furthermore, for the purpose of awarding degrees, medicine was arbitrarily divided into mandatory and complementary disciplines, thus contributing to the presence of important shortcomings in the educational background of the students.

In recent years, attending theoretical courses, laboratory classes and clinical sessions has become mandatory, and the earlier division into first- and second-level knowledge has been removed by compiling a list of disciplines with which the student must be familiar in order to complete the medical course. In addition, an entry examination for medical schools has been introduced in order to select a smaller but more motivated population of medical students.

As far as diseases of the kidney and the urinary tract are concerned, the group of teaching faculties to which the Department of Nephrology in Naples belongs has selected a program of topics on the basis of their relevance to general practitioners. The topics have been the object of discussion not only in classes, but more importantly, also among small groups of students on clinical ward rounds. The outcome has been impressive: at the end of the course, student evaluations have demonstrated a radical improvement in their knowledge, and the promotion rate and score have risen considerably compared with the old system. Despite this recent reorganization of medical studies, which has allowed a positive interaction between faculty and students, some problems have emerged in its application. The main one is the disproportionate amount of time devoted to theory in comparison with clinical training, in direct contrast with the aim of this recent educational project.

Professor G. Conte, MD
Chair of Nephrology
Seconda Università di Napoli
Ospedale Incurabili, Via M. Longo
I–80100 Naples (Italy)

Classical Roots

The issue of the relationship between theoretical education and clinical practice is not recent, having been the object of discussion since the time of the ancient Greeks. As reported in a recent paper [1], the two teaching procedures find their rational basis in two different approaches to the study of medicine, namely science and empiricism. In the 2nd century AD, the occurrence of unpredictable outcomes in medicine led Greek philosophers into two different branches of thinking, headed on the one hand by Galen, mentor of medicine as pure science, and on the other hand by Alexander of Aphrodisias, promoter of the predominant role of empiricism. Galen believed that medicine in itself is as impeccable as any other science, but its practical application is fallible because of variations in individual patients. According to this view, the diagnosis and treatment of a patient finds its rational basis in the disease mechanism alone. Advances in knowledge, e.g. of pathophysiology, genetics and immunology, will eventually produce the answer to any problem. In contrast, Alexander, mentor of empiric evaluation, believed that medical practice should not proceed by syllogisms and cannot rely on universal reasoning, because unpredictability is an inherent property of medicine.

To conclude, it is perhaps pertinent to recall the lecture of William Cullen at the opening ceremony of the medical course at the University of Edinburgh in 1768. On that occasion, he proclaimed that although it is hard to choose between the dogmatic and the empiric approach to the study of medicine, teachers should always remember that either of them is, by itself, insufficient.

Reference 1 Ierodiakonou K, Vanderbroucke JP: Medicine as a stochastic art. Lancet 1993;341:542.

Am J Nephrol 1994;14:259–263

R. Joseph Petrucelli II

Department of Nephrology, New Rochelle Hospital Medical Center and Department of Medicine, New York Medical College, Valhalla, N.Y., USA

Monastic Incorporation of Classical Botanic Medicines into the Renaissance Pharmacopeia

Key Words
Botany
Medicinal herbs
Dioscorides
Classical medicine
Benedictine monasteries
Salerno School of Medicine

Abstract
Ancient Greek physicians believed that health resulted from a balance of natural forces. Many, including Dioscorides, made compilations of plants and medicines derived from them, giving prominence to diuretics, cathartics and emetics. During the Roman Empire, although Greek physicians were highly valued, the Roman matron performed many medical functions and magic and astrology were increasingly used. In Judaic and later Christian societies disease was equated with divine disfavor. After the fall of Rome, the classical Greek medical texts were mainly preserved in Latin translation by the Benedictine monasteries, which were based around a patient infirmary, a herb garden and a library. Local plants were often substituted for the classical ones, however, and the compilations became confused and inaccurate. Greek medicine survived better in the remains of the Eastern Roman Empire, and benefitted from the influence of Arab medicine. Intellectual revival, when it came to Europe, did so on the fringes of the Moslem world, and Montpellier and Salerno were among the first of the new medical centers. Rather than relying on ancient experts, the new experimental method reported the tested effects of substances from identified plants. This advance was fostered by the foundation of universities and greatly aided by the later invention of the printing press, which also allowed wider dissemination of the classical texts.

Introduction

From the earliest times and throughout the world, medicines made from plants have been utilized to treat human ailments. Plants contain a vast array of components with biologic activity and about two-thirds of medications released by the US Food and Drug Administration have their origins in plants. Folk medicine has used plants to treat illness, and herbs are particularly likely to be tried as medicines if they appeal to one of the senses, especially smell and taste. This is why most herbs are today best known for their use in the preparation of food.

The area of the Mediterranean Sea and its environs provides a large number and diverse array of plants whose use as medications was established by ancient peoples. At first, the remedies were passed on by oral tradition. Early on, plants were used in a simple straightforward fashion, but with time they were elaborately prepared or combined with other plants or substances. Two rationales can be

R. Joseph Petrucelli II, MD
Chief of Nephrology
New Rochelle Hospital Medical Center
16 Guion Place
New Rochelle, NY 10802 (USA)

applied to the use of medicinal plants. The first is the empiric or utilitarian: some medicines have an obvious and repeatable effect, e.g. hemlock which kills and opium poppies which induce anesthesia and sleep. The second rationale was called the philosophic. All health science systems have overriding thoughts of the causality of disease: does disease result from a deterioration of something within the body or from attack of things outside the body?

Classical Greek Medicine

Classical medicine in Greece dealt with both the utilitarian and philosophic aspects of botany. Aristotle and his successor Theophrastus developed a system of natural philosophy, of which botany was a major part. Pliny the Elder continued this tradition in his *Naturalis Historia* written in the 1st century AD. Medicines were written about, and many earlier sources were cited, but the major concern remained the natural world. Over several centuries, Greek physicians developed systems whereby health was thought to result from a balance of natural forces, and disease to result from an imbalance of these same forces. A cascade system was established whereby the 4 substances (earth, fire, air and water) were reflected in the 4 bodily humors (blood, phlegm, black bile and yellow bile), which in turn were reflected in 4 personality types (sanguine, phlegmatic, choleric and melancholic). Disease could result from an imbalance at any of a variety of levels. The medicine of Galen (from the 2nd century AD) fully incorporated this system into the everyday practice of medicine. Even today, many people in societies influenced by Galenic thought would scoff at taking a 'hot' medicine for a 'hot' disease.

The ancient Greek physicians made many compilations of plants and medicines made from them. The most significant, the *De Materia Medica* of Dioscorides (a contemporary of Pliny), remained the major source for the next 1,500 years after its completion in the 1st century AD. About 700 plants were included. After a brief description of their appearance and where they could be found, Dioscorides wrote of the methods by which they could be transformed into medicines and for what they could be used. Diuretics, cathartics and emetics were given prominence, possibly because an increase in urine volume over time is an easily monitored physiologic phenomenon. Removal of body fluids is often a therapeutic goal, then and now. To a modern-day nephrologist, the classical sense of balance is apt.

Roman Medicine

In the Roman world, Greek medicine remained 'foreign' even though its practitioners were highly valued and well paid. In the home, the Roman matron was entrusted with many medical functions, assisted by appropriate combinations of diet, medications, and family and local deities. The *medicus* had a strictly military role – to return troops rapidly to active duty. Neither in the army nor for the general population were there facilities for long-term care.

After the establishment of the Roman Empire, and before the acceptance of Christianity, Roman medicine was drawn to an antirational, though pragmatic, focus. Magic and astrology were increasingly used. The acceptance of Christianity further changed thoughts about health and disease. Disease in Judaic and later Christian tradition posited man as being outside nature, which he was instructed to conquer or at least control. Disease was equated with divine disfavor. Balance lost meaning.

Hence, in an age where there was a loss of belief in the constancy of cause and effect in a natural world not subject to events and phenomena from the supernatural world, medicine rapidly became a lost science. After the fall of Rome in 476 AD, a few institutions were maintained for a short while in Italy, Gaul and Spain. Germans and Celts to the north had had only limited contact with the Roman Empire and its everyday life. For reasons still obscure today, the Roman institutions of lawyer and physician were abandoned 1–2 centuries after the fall of the Roman Empire. As the conquerors of the western empire were assimilated into the society of the natives, they lost their ties with their fellow conquerors. This led to rivalry and petty wars. People left the cities. Trade and social interaction ceased. Progressively, the Rome with which people identified was that of the Church, not of the Empire.

Early Christian Medicine

After the fall of Rome, the Church maintained contact with Byzantium until the schism in the 11th century, even after governments lost contact. Monastic orders were started in the eastern desert to allow escape from society. St. Benedict of Nursia established a monastery at Monte Cassino in 529 AD at a site previously occupied by a temple of Apollo. The order was strict: eating meat was forbidden, and the monastery was required to grow and make everything it needed. Salvation was sought through prayer, good deeds, charitable acts and hard work. As had been the case with earlier eastern groups, Benedict encouraged the care of the sick. For the first time in the western world, extended care was provided, though only the Grace of God could provide cure. To think otherwise was blasphemy.

Aurelius Cassiodorus (480–573 AD) joined the Benedictines after leaving service as private secretary to the Gothic king, Theodoric the Great. He encouraged the study of Latin works, among which were translations of the Greek medical texts. Libraries and copying scribes became a part of the Benedictine monastery. An infirmary allowed the long-term housing of the sick. Although cure outside the Grace of God was thought impossible, from the start Benedictine monasteries possessed a garden of herbs. Thus, the model Benedictine monastery had a patient infirmary, a herb garden and a library. The Benedictines kept and copied Latin translations of Dioscorides and Galen.

Christianization of central and northern Europe lagged behind that of the provinces of the former Roman Empire. Even the Celtic peoples of Britain and Ireland did not become Christianized until after the fall of the Roman Empire in 476 AD. The Benedictines were heavily involved in the Christianization of the Celts. Their monasteries maintained close contact with their brothers in Hellenistic lands. They were influential in the later Christianization of people north of the Alps. As at the monastery of St. Gall in Switzerland, the non-Italian monasteries maintained the tripartite structure of patient infirmary, herb garden and library. During the medieval era, the Benedictines maintained greater contact with other regions than did either other people or towns. Plants, however, varied by regions, and plant illustrations in the Middle Ages became progressively more symbolic and inaccurate as they were only schematic diagrams. They were based on earlier illustrations and not on the plant itself. Although many examples of copies of earlier illustrations exist, it is difficult to determine independently what each illustration was meant to signify. When standard (classical) botanic specimens were unavailable, local varieties were substituted. Many different plants were thereby given the same names. In addition, although the Benedictine monasteries maintained Latin translations of the classical Greek medical texts, most of the medical techniques described in them were lost. This is particularly true for surgical procedures, which were abandoned in favor of a simplified pharmacology and herbalism characteristic of many types of folk medicine.

As Greek medicine was increasingly lost to the successors of the Western Roman Empire, it survived in the Eastern Roman Empire, though in a form that was non-experimental and lacked innovation. The Nestonians were Christian heretics who were expelled first to the south-eastern empire and then to Persia. In Persia they established a teaching medical school which incorporated classical Greek medicines. The Arabs also adopted Greek medicine. After the rise of Islam, they permitted Jews and Christians to participate in academic matters. The Arabs took their medical understanding with them as they crossed northern Africa and spread their authority to Spain, Sicily and a part of France. Hellenistic medical tracts were translated into Arabic. Arabists also introduced new techologies, e.g. distillation, which led to a quest for more potent medications.

Medieval Medicine

More than 500 years after the fall of Rome, the decline of medicine was slowly reversed. During that period, medicine had been given over to the Church in western Europe, and academic interests fared badly. When intellectual life was restored, medicine was revived first on the edges of the Moslem world. Montpellier in France and Salerno near Naples in Italy were the first among established teaching medical centers. At Salerno it was realized that much of the ancient medical knowledge that had been maintained in the monastic libraries had lost meaning. Many classical plants could not be grown in distant lands, though exactly what might be substituted was not certain. It was even uncertain which plants had been described by Dioscorides. Trade with the Near and Middle East (home of the plants mentioned by Dioscorides) had ceased. As even the monasteries were now out of touch with other plant centers, the identity of many plants described had been lost.

The Salerno School of Medicine attempted to deal with this problem soon after it was established. Early in the 12th century, a book entitled *Circa Instans* was published by a group of scholars under the direction of Mattaeus Platearius. Rather than relying on ancient experts for opinion, it reported the effects (as shown by testing) of substances from identified plants. The development of the scientific method had begun. Accurate and useful information was being recorded: specifically, all plants were identified and it was assured that they could be obtained, even from the Moslems if there existed no other source. The evaluation of the effectiveness of the drugs described was quantitative, even if not precisely so. *Circa Instans* was quickly circulated across Europe, where its

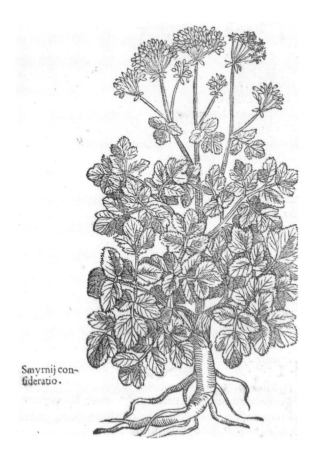

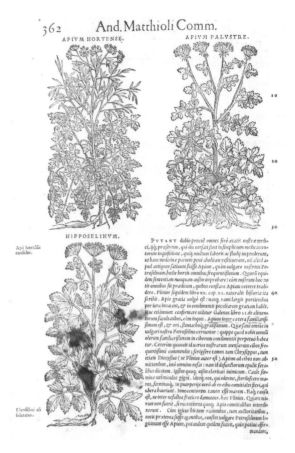

Fig. 1. Dioscorides of Anazarbos, Pedanius (1st century) *Petri Andreae Matthioli ... Commentarii, in libros sex Fedacii Dioscoridis Anazarbei, de materia medica.* Venice, Vincentius Valarisius, 1564, p. 364. Smyrnia. With permission from the New York Academy of Medicine.

Fig. 2. Dioscorides of Anazarbos, Pedanius (1st century) *Petri Andreae Matthioli ... Commentarii, in libros sex Fedacii Dioscoridis Anazarbei, de materia medica.* Venice, Vincentius Valarisius, 1564, p. 362. With permission from the New York Academy of Medicine.

impact was great, though its renown was short-lived. Its successors, however, were quickly to rise to the level of world authority. The classical concept had been greatly altered by the approach of *Circa Instans*, in which the primary considerations were availability and efficacy of the various botanic medicines.

Europe's period of isolation and social, intellectual and economic decline was rapidly reversed. The Crusaders not only reached the Holy Land but also created a demand for products available only there. This demand could only be met by commerce. The economic situation improved as a result of the new technologies that became available from the East. This in turn led to a growing desire for further technologic improvement. It was the newly founded universities, however, and not the Church who were assigned to satisfying these desires. It was the universities who accelerated the reawakening of Europe,

and medicine ceased to be an exclusively religious concern. Benedictine monasteries, however, remained a store of knowledge through their patient infirmaries, herb gardens and libraries. These monasteries had been established throughout Europe, and when the universities were founded, each was located not far from a Benedictine monastery, which served as a source of information. More importantly, though, the process by which problems were analyzed and solutions proposed was a significant step in the development of the experimental method, even though much of the magic, mysticism and astrology of the medieval mind had been retained.

The next significant movement in the advancement of ideas after the development of the universities was the invention of the printing press using movable type. To start with, medieval manuscripts were printed without change, and the ease and low cost were rapidly appre-

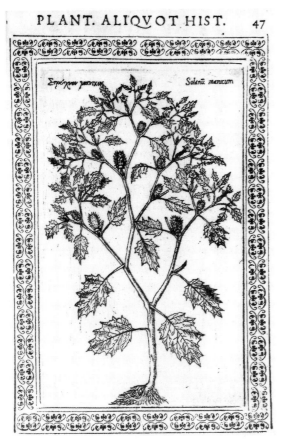

Fig. 3. Fabio Colonna, *Plantarvm Aliqvot Historia.* Naples, 1592, p. 77. With permission from the New York Academy of Medicine.

ciated. Gradually, however, printing led to a change in the composition of books. Systems of indexing allowed a more valuable way of presenting material. Dioscorides himself, in *De Materia Medica*, wrote that his tract was not in an alphabetical sequence, in order that plants from different parts of the alphabet but with similar properties could be grouped together for a common discussion. Sadly his original has not survived, and the oldest copies extant were given an alphabetical presentation.

In 1453 Constantinople, the capital of the Eastern Roman Empire, fell to the Turks. Many Greek scholars fled to the West, bringing with them copies of much of the most laudable in the ancient Greek and Hellenistic civilizations, which were the medical texts. The newly invented printing press allowed these classical works to be printed for the first time, generally in Latin or Greek. 'Modern' language versions quickly replaced them. The work of Dioscorides was printed in many editions in Latin translation. After an early period in which illustrations remained schematic, realistic presentation was used (fig. 1 and 2). In these editions the plants are clearly defined and could be readily identified, even if not known. Later works involved new experimentation with a consideration of its significance (fig. 3). The newly regained experimental method rapidly gained importance: new material was being inspected with new conclusions drawn. The Renaissance was truly a rebirth of thinking, even if the ancient classics were overthrown.

Further Reading

Arber A: Herbals, their Origin and Evolution. Cambridge, 1938.
Anderson FJ: An Illustrated History of the Herbals. New York, Columbia, 1977.
Lyons AS, Petrucelli RJ: Medicine: an Illustrated History. New York, Abrams, 1978.

Am J Nephrol 1994;14:264–269

Spyros G. Marketos

Department of History of Medicine, Athens
University Medical School and
International Hippocratic Foundation,
Athens, Greece

Hippocratic Medicine and Nephrology

Key Words

Hippocrates
Ethics
Prognosis
Nephrology

Abstract

The history of nephrology is a part of culture in general and should be treated not as a hobby or an isolated specialty of medical science, but as closely connected with medical education and everyday clinical practice. In the age of the apotheosis of renal biotechnology, medicine more than ever needs to combine Hippocratic messages with renal technologic achievements, in order both to restore quality of life in patients with renal disease and to bring harmony and balance to individuals impaired in body and soul. Indeed, Hippocratic medicine lies at the root of the development of clinical nephrology. Hippocratic writings have not lost their nephrologic interest, despite the enormous recent advances in renal technology. Today's practising nephrologist can still learn not only from Hippocratic clinical observations, but also from the prognostic thoughts, the ethical principles, the philosophic concepts and the humane messages of the 'father of clinical nephrology'.

Introduction

In the past, interest in literature relating to the history of nephrology was rather limited compared with interest in the history of other fields of medicine, e.g. neurology, ophthalmology, cardiology and urology [1, 2]. This is due to the fact that only in recent decades has nephrology begun to be recognized as a separate medical specialty [3], including various subspecialties, whereas previously it was considered as part of urology, physiology and/or clinical medicine.

Before 1950 the bulk of what is now called nephrology was considered as renal physiology, histology of the nephron and renal radiography. Up to 1950 little progress in terms of achieving any effective therapeutic result had occurred. After 1950, the rapid growth of scientific and technologic knowledge led to an enormous number of revolutionary discoveries with life-saving clinical applications. Ancient and modern nephrology are thus far removed from one another and the Hippocratic notion that a physician could embrace all of the medical information available belong to the distant past. Despite this, the concepts and principles of the 'father of medicine' have not been deprived of their great significance.

Today, the history of nephrology is fast becoming one of the most exciting and fascinating chapters in the whole of medical history. More than any other subspecialty, this history broadens medical thought and urges practising nephrologists to understand better the origins and the evolution of their specialty.

The most ancient object of nephrologic interest is a votive bronze replica of kidney (fig. 1). This important

Spyros G. Marketos, MD
Department of History of Medicine
Athens University Medical School
20 Patr. Ioakeim St.
GR–106 75 Athens (Greece)

archeologic find is approximately 3000 years old and was discovered during excavations at the temples of Kition in Cyprus [4]. Ancient Greek medicine derived its knowledge from many older sources. Because of their geographic location, the Greeks were exposed to the influence of Egyptian, Babylonian, Mesopotamian, Phoenician and Minoan (Cretan) civilizations. The Greeks also learned much from ancient Jewish medicine, particularly in the field of hygiene [5].

As today, alternative medicine was nothing new in either Hippocratic or post-Hippocratic times. Any of the sick who were not satisfied by the Hippocratic physicians could visit the temple of Asclepius of Cos (fig. 2) or other centers of faith healing around the Mediterranean sea (the so-called Asclepieia) hoping that they would be cured by alternative treatments.

The philosopher-physicians of ancient Greece were a bridge between the medicine of the Homeric age and that of the Hippocratic age, which developed in close company with philosophy. The philosopher-scientists opened the luminous path that led Greece to its Periclean golden age. According to Hippocrates, the philosopher-physician 'is equal to the Gods' [6]. The most important difference between Homeric and Hippocratic physicians was that the former were solely respected craftsmen, whereas the latter were both craftsmen and philosopher-physicians [7, 8].

Hippocratic medicine is based on the rationality of human existence. It is entirely justified, therefore, to divide Greek medicine into the pre-Hippocratic (non-rational) and post-Hippocratic (rational) eras. Hippocrates observed diseases with the eye of a naturalist, and the Hippocratic diagnostic system was based on logical reasoning and clinical observation. The 3 elements on which Hippocrates based his diagnostic interacting system are: (1) the patient, who is a psychosomatic entity; (2) the disease, which is governed by rules; and (3) the physician, who is nature's helper and the servant of the medical art.

Clinical Observations

A thorough study of the Greek text of *Corpus Hippocraticum* [6] shows that Hippocrates (fig. 3) was well aware of the cardinal problems related to renal and urologic lesions, despite the fact that the urinary system had previously suffered more than any other functional system from neglect and/or misunderstanding. According to Hippocrates [5], no other system or organ of the human

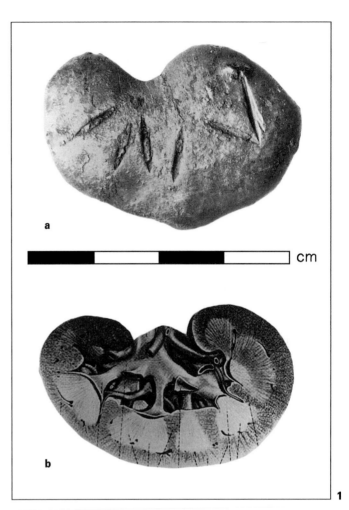

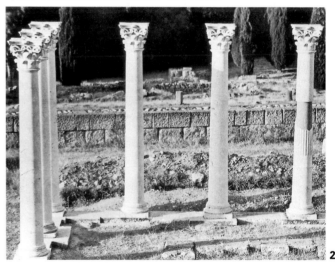

Fig. 1. a Votive bronze replica of a kidney dating from the 13th century BC. With permission from V Karageorghis [4]. **b** Gross appearance of the human kidney.

Fig. 2. Remnants of the ancient Asclepieion of Cos (4th century BC). With permission from the International Hippocratic Foundation.

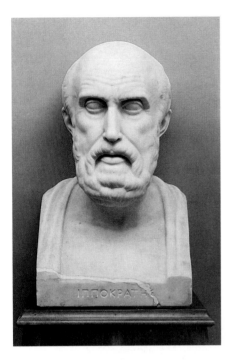

Fig. 3. Bust of Hippocrates by the Greek sculptor Cossos (1862). With permission from the International Hippocratic Foundation.

body gives so much diagnostic information by its excretion than does the urinary system with the kidney. His theory of renal stone formation and his diagnostic interpretation from macroscopic examination of the patient's urine (Hippocratic uroscopy) are still respected. One of the most typical examples refers to the need for differentiating upper from lower urinary tract infection.'

When the urine is thick and small pieces of flesh-like hairs pass with it, it means a secretion from the kidney.'
Aphorisms IV, 76 [6, 9].

'When blood and clots in the urine are accompanied by strangury, abdominal and perineal pain, it is the parts about the bladder which are affected.' *Aphorisms* IV, 80 [6, 9].

Space does not permit the quotation of numerous other examples from the Hippocratic collection (about 60 treatises), many of which are discussed in a review article by Eknoyan [10] who concludes that: 'Hippocrates is the father of clinical nephrology'. It is apt, however, to recall and briefly comment on 6 Hippocratic aphorisms which are still useful even to today's practising nephrologists.

(1) *Aphorisms* IV, 72 [6] 'colourless urine is bad' indicates a reduced ability to concentrate the urine and may refer to chronic renal failure or to diabetes insipidus.

(2) Aphorisms IV, 77 [6] 'sudden appearance of blood in the urine indicates the rupture of a small renal vessel' signifies necrotizing renal papillitis due to ischemic necrosis and may be consistent with the term renal papillary necrosis [10].

(3) *Aphorisms* VII, 34 [6] 'bubbles appearing on the surface of the urine indicate renal disease and a prolonged illness' discloses chronic inflammatory activity in the glomeruli and may be identified with the term chronic glomerulonephritis.

(4) *Aphorisms* VI, 6 [6] 'diseases of the kidney and of the bladder are difficult to cure in the aged' reveals the truism that in the elderly the response to treatment is more variable than in younger patients. The fact that the aging kidney is often associated with several concomitant pathoanatomic changes and the concomitant occurrence of diseases other than renal and/or urologic ones, and the non-specific nature (or even the complete absence) of the classic symptoms are three of the main verifications for this still contemporary aphorism.

(5) *Aphorisms* VI, 1 [6] 'the physician must not only be prepared to do what is right himself, but also to make the patient, the attendants and the externals cooperate' reflects the wisdom of an experienced modern practitioner, e.g. a practising nephrologist.

(6) The Hippocratic axion 'no longer the disease but the diseased' and *Aphorisms* VI, 87 [6] 'what drugs will not cure the knife will' serve as reminders of the triumph of modern therapeutic procedures in nephrology (the artificial kidney and renal transplantation) and recall a line from the English poet William Shakespeare: 'What's past is prologue'.

Prognostic Thoughts

Hippocratic thoughts concerning the meaning and the value of medical prognosis can be summarized as follows:

'The best physician, in my opinion, is the one who can predict; the one who is able to foretell and forestall the patients' past, their present and their future.' *Prognosticon* II, 110 [6].

What is the importance and significance of prognosis for modern nephrology? The answer is that a practising nephrologist is pressed more than any other specialist to make prognoses. He must be able to interpret promptly all the diagnostic signs and symptoms of patients with renal disease in order to foretell the course and to prepare the future management of their diseases, e.g. by preparation of a fistula or ordering compatibility tests. This situation arises because today's technologic miracles (modern dialysis and kidney transplantation) may be beneficial and are of potential value in a great variety of formerly 'end-stage' kidney diseases or 'terminal' renal failure, particularly when conservative treatment is either ineffective or deleterious. Moreover, a practising nephrologist must tell a patient with chronic renal disease which treatment is the best. It is not necessary, therefore, to explain why Hippocrates believes that: 'it seems to be highly desirable that a physician should pay much attention to prognosis' [6].

According to Hippocratic texts, prognosis is of particular importance [11–16] not only to answer the question of what the future will bring, but also for planning treatment, particularly when it applies to rapidly progressive diseases that lead to death. Therefore, prognostic knowledge of renal diseases is of great practical value. A typical example is necrotizing glomerulonephritis, in which the practising nephrologist is pressed to provide a prognosis and to make rapid therapeutic decisions. In the present age, the central slogan 'from preventive to predictive medicine' is beginning to be confirmed and hence justify Hippocrates, who believed that prognosis is primarily prediction [17].

Ethical Principles

The term 'ethics' is derived from the Greek *ethos,* which means 'character' in a broad sense [17]. Ethics in medical practice is the science of what can acceptably be done. Codes of behavior are considered essential to any profession, and throughout history have been designed to increase respect and prestige. This was certainly the case in the period of the Golden Age of Greece, during which the oath ascribed to Hippocrates was written. According to the Hippocratic ethical heritage, the medical profession was struggling to maintain a profile of respectability, confidentiality and responsibility and was not held in the same regard as religion, law and philosophy. Hippocratic medicine was completely individualized and expresses the absolute, without exception, maintenance of confidentiality by the physician.

Until the last 2 decades of the 20th century, the Hippocratic Oath was the reference point for all international medical declarations concerning medical ethics [18], e.g. the Declaration of Geneva (1949), the Nuremberg Charter (1967) and the Declaration of Helsinki (1975). It was,

and it still is, a monumental code of ethics and an ethical guide for the practice of medicine, a 1-page text about which hundreds of thousands of pages have been written down the ages and throughout the world. In the Western world, the medical profession is identified with the Hippocratic Oath. Nevertheless, in recent years the profound changes in social patterns, revised health policies and modern medical technology have given rise to many questions and some criticism of certain points of the Hippocratic Oath [18].

Today, a practising nephrologist more than any other specialist confronts many ethical and moral dilemmas and receives numerous ethical pressures during terminal renal failure (end-stage kidney disease). Only 2 practical questions related to modern nephrology are mentioned here.

Professional Secrecy (Medical Confidentiality)
One of the most difficult examples is whether anonymity can exist between a transplanted patient and the donor's family. This is rather difficult or impossible to maintain, as it may have a great impact on the postoperative social and emotional life of a kidney-transplanted patient in relation to the family of the kidney donor.

Right to Treatment
Renal terminal care requires another ethical guideline and another kind of behavior than would normally apply to the right to know, as well as to the rights of the relatives and to the rights to a better quality of life. For example, should an elderly patient be offered a type of treatment that is merely an extremely expensive prolongation of suffering? The ethical rule: 'whatever I see or hear ... I will keep secret and tell no one' [6] could surely be broken in cases of 'terminal' care by telling the truth to relatives before doing so to the patient. It must be emphasized that the first Hippocratic aphorism posits that: 'It is not enough for the physician to do what is necessary, but the patient and the attendants must do their part as well' [6]. A practising nephrologist can appreciate the meaning of this Hippocratic paragraph perhaps more than any other physician.

Philosophical Concepts

The underestimation of Hippocratic philosophy at the end of the 20th century is unfortunate. Medicine and philosophy would both benefit from Hippocratic philosophy [5]. On the other hand, for a practising nephrologist, the most important concern is not the philosophy of medicine but the need to philosophize medicine and its aggressive therapeutic applications.

'Desperate cases need the most desperate remedies.'
Aphorisms I, 6 [6]

The combination of philosophy and medicine is the most distinctly Hellenic characteristic of the ancients' attitude towards medicine [14]. Greek medicine cannot be separated from Greek philosophy. According to Hippocrates: 'The philosopher-physician is equal to the Gods' [6, 9], and according to Galen [19], the greatest Greek physician after Hippocrates: 'The best physician is also a philosopher'. The first Hippocratic aphorism [6, 9] probably contains the essence of medical philosophy:

'Life is short; and the art long; and the right time an instant; and treatment precarious; and the judgement difficult.'

Hippocratic philosophy combined the concepts of the Ionian philosophers of Asia Minor with Pythagoras' and Alkmaeon's theories from southern Italy regarding the equilibrium of dissimilar elements and of opposing quantities, thus establishing the humoral theory for human physiology and pathophysiology [15, 16]. According to this theory, human beings are made of soul and body, which contains the 4 humors: blood, phlegm, black bile and yellow bile. These humors are in continuous motion through the circulation, which anatomically Hippocrates had not understood.

The equilibrium of the 4 humors (eucrasia) is identified with health, while the disequilibrium (dyscrasia) produces disease. Motion of the humors ensures unity of the body and soul, so that even a small disorder in any part of the body is reflected in the whole. Quality of life and its variables, a term often mentioned recently particularly in modern nephrology, is based on the Hippocratic principle of whole-person (holistic) medicine. It could be proposed, therefore, that health is a state of harmonic mixture (balance) of the four humors (eucrasia), and with the same logic that disease is a state of faulty mixture (imbalance) of the four humors (dyscrasia). Hippocrates was concerned with the body as a whole, rather than with lesions of parts. Hippocrates also suggested that an excess of 1 of the 4 humors would result in various disorders in human elements [10, 16].

The humoral theory of Hippocrates reminds nephrologists of the main function of the kidney, which is the maintenance of the normal volume and composition of the body fluid (water, acid-base and electrolyte balance).

Furthermore, it can be suggested that Claude Bernard's theory concerning the *milieu intérieur* had its roots within Hippocratic philosophy [17].

Humane Messages

A humane education is nowhere so important and so necessary as in scientific medicine [5, 20]. In our present times, the medical profession possibly needs much more humanism than in the past. Clinical nephrology is an illustrative example. Humane medicine is both an antidote to overconcentration on kidney technical minutiae and a stimulus to even more humane technical accomplishments. In the age of triumphant medical technology history of medicine is necessary to correlate humanities with the natural sciences, to enlarge the physician's horizon, and to protect the nephrologist from the risks of overspecialisation.

Hippocratic writings include many highly valuable humanistic messages [17], of which 5 are mentioned here because they are far in advance of the Hippocratic age in which they were written.

'Benefit or do not harm.' *Epidemics* (Book 2) II, 636 [6, 7]

'For where there is love of man, there is also love of the (medical) art.' *Precepts* IX, 238 [6, 7]

'Knowledge of medicine is not possible without the knowledge of man: this is necessary for anyone wishing to treat correctly men.'
Tradition in Medicine I, 620 [6, 7]

'I will keep pure and holy both my life and art.'
The Oath IV, 630 [6, 7]

'I will use my power to help the sick to the best of my ability and judgement; I will abstain from harming or wrong-doing any man by it.' *The Oath* IV, 630 [6, 7]

References

1 Murphy LJT: The History of Urology. Springfield, Illinois, C Thomas, 1972.

2 Dimopoulos K, Gialas A, Androutsos G, Lykourinas M, Kostakopoulos A: Hippocrates: founder and pioneer of urology. Br J Urol 1980; 52:73–74.

3 Black D: The story of nephrology. J R Soc Med 1980;73:514–518.

4 Karageorghis V: Excavations at Kition. The pre-Phoenician levels (part 2). Nicosia, Department of Antiquities, 1985, vol 5, 93.

5 Marketos SG, Papaeconomou C: Medicine, magic and religion in ancient Greece. Humane Med 1992;8:41–44.

6 Littre E: Œuvres Complètes d'Hippocrate. Paris, JB Baillière, 1841.

7 Miller GL: Literacy and the Hippocratic art: reading, writing and epistemology. J Hist Med Appl Sci 1990;45:11–40.

8 Horstmanshoff HFJ: The ancient physician: craftsman or scientist? J Hist Med Appl Sci 1990;45:176–197.

9 Coar T: The Aphorisms of Hippocrates. London, Valpy, 1822.

10 Eknoyan G: Origins of nephrology: Hippocrates the father of clinical nephrology. Am J Nephrol 1988;8:498–507.

11 Marketos SG, Eftychiadis AG, Diamandopoulos A: Acute renal failure according to ancient Greek and Byzantine medical writers. J R Soc Med 1993;86:290–293.

12 Patersen WF: Hippocratic Wisdom. A Modern Appreciation of Ancient Scientific Achievement. Springfield, Illinois, C Thomas, 1946.

13 Edelstein L: The genuine works of Hippocrates. Bull Inst Hist Med 1939;7:236–248.

14 Edelstein L: The distinctive Hellenism of Greek Medicine. Bull Hist Med 1966;40:197–255.

15 Sigerist HE: On Hippocrates. Bull Inst Hist Med 1934;2:190–213.

16 Smith WD: The Hippocratic Tradition. Ithaca, New York, Cornell University Press, 1979.

17 Marketos SG: The prophetic messages of Hippocratic medicine, in Proceedings of the First International Congress on History, Knowledge and Quality of Life in Urology, Fiuggi, Italy, 1992. Pavia, Fondazione 'A Scarpa', 1993, 78–80.

18 Marketos SG: Le serment hippocratique est-il anachronique? Athens, International Hippocratic Foundation of Cos, 1993.

19 Kuhn G: Claudii Galeni. Operal Omnia. Lipsiae, Cnoblochii, 1828.

20 Marketos SG: Medicine is an aspect of civilization: lessons from the Hippocratic medicine. Microsurgery 1993;14:4–5.

Am J Nephrol 1994;14:270–278

Garabed Eknoyan

Section of Nephrology, Department of
Medicine, Baylor College of Medicine,
Houston, Tex., USA

Arabic Medicine and Nephrology

Key Words
Islam
Avicenna
Rhazes
Nephrology
Anatomy
Arabic medicine

Abstract

During the Dark Ages following the fall of the Roman Empire, the Arabic world was instrumental in fostering the development of the sciences, including medicine. The quest for original manuscripts and their translation into Arabic reached its climax in the House of Wisdom in Baghdad, and the dissemination of the compiled texts was facilitated by the introduction of paper from the East. Foremost among the Arabic physicians were Rhazes, Avicenna, Haly Abbas and Albucasis, who lived during the period 950–1050 AD. Their writings not only followed Hippocrates and Galen, but also greatly extended the analytical approach of these earlier writers. The urine was studied and the function and diseases of the kidneys described. Despite the fact that experimentation on the human body was prohibited by religion, some anatomic dissection and observation seems to have been undertaken, and the pulmonary circulation was described by Ibn Nafis. Anatomic illustrations began to appear in Arabic texts, though they did not have the detail and artistic merit of those of Vesalius.

Introduction

The decline in civilization that immediately followed the fall of the Roman Empire has been aptly termed the Dark Ages. The host of external and internal circumstances that contributed to this general degeneration of culture has and continues to be a source of fertile study, perhaps best summarized in Gibbon's voluminous classic *The Decline and Fall of the Roman Empire*. While somewhat more favorable conditions in the Eastern Roman Empire allowed preservation of the rudiments of ancient knowledge and survival of isolated beacons of enlightenment, all of the sciences underwent a steady deterioration which threatened the very roots of civilization.

Neither Byzantium nor its zealous version of Christianity, however, provided a fertile ground for nurture of the natural sciences. This is perhaps best exemplified by the fate of some of the early centers of erudition, e.g. the Schools of Edessa and Nisibis in Syria, established under the influence of Christianity in the 3rd century. It is in these institutions that a concerted effort was made to preserve and translate the classical manuscripts of Greece and Rome. Unfortunately, the Nestonians operating these centers were declared heretics by the Council of Ephesus and expelled by imperial edict in 489 AD. The Nestonians of Edessa fled, taking with them their manuscripts. They sought refuge in the Persian Empire where, under the auspices of the ruling Sassanids, they established a center of

G. Eknoyan, MD
Section of Nephrology
Department of Medicine
Baylor College of Medicine
Houston, TX 77030 (USA)

culture and a medical school in Jondishapur [1]. This center of translation, and particularly its medical school, was to play a prominent role in the subsequent evolution of medicine [2], for with the decline and fall of the Roman Empire medicine, which had culminated in the works of Galen, sustained the same fate as the other sciences. Not only was it in a state of steady decline but also in one of actual decimation, despite the isolated attempts by physicians of the Byzantine era, e.g. Oribasius of Pergamon (326–403 AD), Aetius of Amida (502–575 AD), Alexander of Tralles (525–605 AD) and Paul of Aegina (625–690 AD), or even the miraculous works of the brothers Cosmos and Damian (about 303 AD) [1].

The favorable turn of events in this otherwise sorry state of events was provided by the emergence of Islam. Within less than a century from the Hegira (622 AD), the Islamic Empire had swept from Arabia through the Middle East, Persia, Egypt, North Africa, Sicily and Spain, and made inroads into India and the Asian plains [3]. This was a phenomenal achievement by any criteria and was obviously not accomplished without bloodshed, some destruction and episodes of cruelty. In the main, however, it provided a structure that not only salvaged the sciences but also provided a fertile environment for the evolution of a new golden age in their development [4, 5].

The medicine that flourished during this era has been variously termed Islamic, Arabian and Arabic medicine [1, 6–8]. The last is the one used in this article, for although there is no question that the zeal, drive and energy were religious and that the Pax Islamica that was established provided the resources necessary for its development, not all the principal contributors were Moslems (Islamic) or ethnic Arabs (Arabian) [1, 9]. Indeed, the early contributors to and translators of Arabic medicine were the recruited Nestonians from Jondishapur, and its later and most prominent figures were Persians. What can more justifiably be considered a unifying factor was language (Arabic), which as the language of the Qur'an became the lingua franca of the empire and allowed the interchange and integration of medical knowledge not only from Greece and Rome but also from Persia, India and China [3, 10]. This is an important consideration, for where Western sources have received due credit for their contribution to the development of Arabic medicine, that of Far Eastern sources has been underestimated or neglected.

So far as medical progress is concerned, religious dogma did provide some obstacles to its development, in areas such as anatomy and physiology, but in the main it allowed and encouraged the growth of the medical

Table 1. Chronology of Arabian dynasties

Dynasty	Period	Capital
Caliphs	630–656 AD	Medina
Umayyads	661–750 AD	Damascus
Abassid	750–850 AD	Baghdad
Umayyads (West)	711–1492 AD	Cordoba
Fatimites	969–1171 AD	Cairo
Mamelukes	1250–1517 AD	Cairo

sciences [4]. To quote from the Hadith, the compiled sayings of the Prophet:

'The quest of knowledge is obligatory for every Muslim.'
'Verily the men of knowledge are the inheritors of the prophets.'
'Seek knowledge from the cradle to the grave.'
'He who leaves his home in search of knowledge walks the path of God to Paradise.'
'The ink of the scholar is holier than the blood of the martyr.'

Thus, at a time when the triumph of Christianity allowed monastic medicine to hold sway in Europe, emerging Islam allowed new vigor and resources to be injected in the progress of scientific medicine, an energy and source of support that was maintained throughout several periods of instability and changes of rulers and dynasties (table 1). Even when the central power of the initial dynasties passed on to the fighting rulers of small local fiefdoms, the quest for knowledge remained a measure of the success of each ruler. This competition was to ensure the continued availability of national resources for the support of the sciences [4].

The work of Leclerc summarizes this era:

'The world has but once witnessed so marvelous a spectacle as that presented by the Arabs in the ninth century. This pastoral people, whose fanaticism had suddenly made them masters of half of the world, having once founded their empire, immediately set themselves to acquire that knowledge of sciences which alone was lacking to their greatness. Of all the invaders for the last remains of the Roman Empire they alone pursued such studies; while the Germanic hordes, glorifying in their brutality and ignorance, took a thousand years to reunite the broken chain of tradition, the Arabs accomplished this in less than a century' [11].

Development of Arabic Medicine

The century referred to by Leclerc is the century following the establishment of the empire, when the quest for original manuscripts and their translation into Arabic

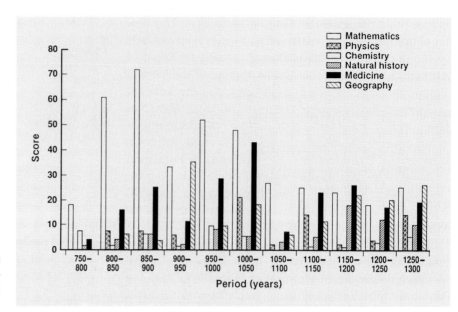

Fig. 1. Course of comparative scientific intellectual development of Arabic civilization, based on data presented by Sorokin and Merton [13]. See text for explanation.

was undertaken in earnest, reaching its climax in Baghdad when the Bayt al Hikma (the House of Wisdom) was established by the Khalif Ma'amun (813–833 AD), the son of Harun el Rashid, the Khalif of the 'thousand and one nights', commonly called the 'Arabian nights'. Here, in one building, were gathered translators, manuscripts and all the necessary resources for translation into Arabic of the original works collected from all corners of the empire. An important facilitator for the dissemination of the compiled texts was paper, which had been introduced from the East during the 8th century. For this effort, Arabic medicine has been duly credited with the conscious preservation of classical medicine and its incorporation into its culture.

The process initiated during the 8th century and expanded in the 9th century was not merely one of compilation and integration, but one which laid the foundations for a new maturity and cycle of discoveries that were to change the face of medicine. Not only teaching hospitals, pharmacies and chemistry were to find their origins in Arabic medicine, but the whole discipline of clinical medicine was to advance to a level of refinement never attained before [5, 6, 12]. These advances in medicine did not occur in isolation, but evolved in a setting of parallel advances in the sciences in general. The course of this progress is illustrated in figures 1 and 2, which are based on data presented by Sorokin and Merton in an attempt to provide an objective basis for the course of Arabic intellectual development [13]. Using the classic *Introduction to*

the History of Science by Sarton [14], these authors rated, by 50-year periods, the comparative importance of the contributions of Arabic-writing scientists for the given period. Three different scales were employed to convert Sarton's qualitative estimates of various intellectual contributions: in the 1st scale each individual mentioned was given a value of 1 in the field of contributions; in the 2nd scale a value of 1–3 points was given depending on the importance of the work mentioned; and in the 3rd scale a range of 1–15 was used depending on the importance of the work in the evolution of the discipline. Fig. 1 is based on the 3rd scale and shows the evolution of medicine compared with that of the other sciences. Fig. 2 shows the evolution of medicine using all 3 scales. A peak period is evident during the span of 950–1050 AD, which is about a century after the establishment of the House of Wisdom and corresponds to the period when Arabic medicine matured and attained a stage of investigation and novel observations that were to contribute to the actual progress of medicine [15].

In summary, Campbell says of Arabic science: 'In the beginning (it) received, accepted and even developed the classical legacy. For some five or six rich centuries there is an impressive [Arabic] record of scientific thought experiment, and research, particularly in medicine' [16]. Sarton, in his commentary about the Middle Ages, says: 'The most valuable, the most original and the most pregnant [texts] were written in Arabic'. Finally, to continue the quote of Leclerc from the previous section:

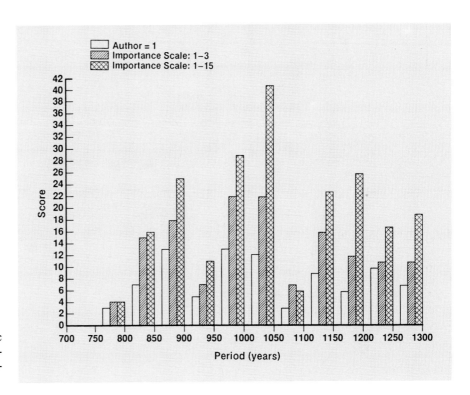

Fig. 2. Course of development of Arabic medicine, based on data presented by Sorokin and Merton [13]. See text for explanation.

'At the end of the eighth century, their [Arabic] whole scientific possessions consisted of a translation of one medical treatise and some books on alchemy. Before the ninth century had run to its close, the Arabs were in possession of all the science of the Greeks; they had produced from their own ranks students of the first order, or had raised among their initiators men who, without them, would have been groping in the dark; and they showed from this time an aptitude for the exact sciences, which was lacking in their instructors, whom they hence-forward surpassed' [11].

Nephrology in Arabic Medicine

A time course of medicine during the period covered in figures 1 and 2 is given in figure 3, showing some of the prominent physicians of the time. The principal figures in Arabic medicine, whose works were to have the greatest influence in the subsequent evolution of medicine in Europe, were Rhazes, Avicenna, Haly Abbas and Albucasis (table 2). All four lived and worked during the period 950–1050 AD (fig. 1 and 2), which can be easily be described as the golden age of Arabic medicine. Of the four, Avicenna (Abu Ali Husayn ibn Abdullah ibn Sina, 980–1037 AD) attained the most renown and exerted the greatest influence on Western medicine. A child prodigy who was an ambitious politician, a *bon vivant* and entre-

preneur, he learned medicine at the age of 16 years from Abusheikh El-Massihi (massihi = Christian). He was a prolific author, an empiricist, but primarily a classifier. The last quality is probably the principal feature of his voluminous *Al Quanun fit Tibb (Canon of Medicine)* that contributed to its popularity [17, 18]. The more astute and meticulous clinician, however, was his predecessor, Rhazes (Abu Bakr Muhammad ibn Zakariya Al-Razi, about 865–925 AD). A musician by vocation, he was taught medicine later in life by an apothecary, but soon developed a clinical judgement that led to his being labeled the 'Galen of Islam' [19]. His clinical acumen is best displayed in his classic *Treatise on the Small-Pox and Measles (Kitab fi al Jadari wa Alhusbeh)* [20]. He never had the time to bring the same meticulousness to his *Kitab al Hawi fit Tibb (Content of Medicine),* which although lacking the detailed classification of the *Canon* of Avicenna, is the more astute clinical work of the two. For while Avicenna was undoubtedly a *hakim* (wise man), Rhazes was the *tabib* (doctor) *par excellence.*

Writings of Rhazes
A good insight into the aptitudes of Rhazes and into the notions of diseases of the kidney at the time can be gleaned from some of his writings [19]. The approach fol-

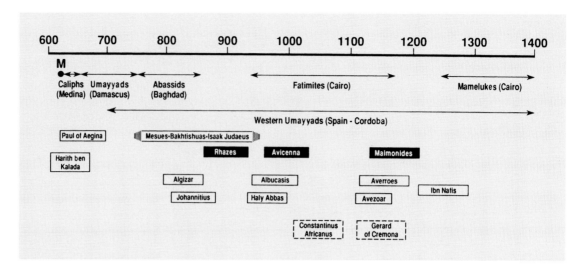

Fig. 3. Time course of Arabic medicine.

lowed is similar to that of Hippocrates and relies on case presentations. The analytic superiority of the clinical material, however, becomes evident in any comparative reading of the two authors. Rhazes' descriptions of a renal abscess or severe pyelonephritis follows:

'Case I: Abdallah ubn Sawada used to suffer from attacks of mixed fever which overtook him some times every 6 days, sometimes like a tertian, quartan or quotidian. They were preceded by a slight rigor, and micturition was very frequent. I gave it as my opinion that either these accesses of fever would turn into quartan, or that there was an abscess *(khuraj)* of the kidneys. Only a short while elapsed before the patient passed pus in his urine; I informed him that these feverish attacks would not recur, and so it was.

The only thing that prevented me at first from giving it as my definite opinion that the patient was suffering from an abscess of the kidneys was that he had previously suffered from tertian and other types of fevers, and in this the [my] opinion that this mixed fever might be due to inflammatory processes, which would tend to become quartan, was strongly supported. Moreover, the patient did not complain to me that he felt in his loins, when standing, as it were a weight hanging from him; and I neglected to ask him about this. The frequency of micturition should have strengthened my suspicion about an abscess in the kidneys, except that I was unaware of the fact that his father suffered from weakness of the bladder and was subject to this complaint, and that he, himself, had suffered from it when he was healthy. It is, therefore, our duty to avoid lack of solicitude with the utmost care – if Allah will!

That the abscess was small, was indicated to me by the fact that he did not complain to me at the first of a weight in his loins. After he had passed pus, however, I inquired of him whether he had experienced this symptom, and he replied in the affirmative. Had the abscess been extensive, he would of his own accord have complained of this symptom; and the rapid evacuation of the pus showed the

Table 2. The golden age of Arabic medicine and its classic texts

Author	Text	Latin version
Rhazes (865–925 AD)	Kitab al Hawi	Continens
Avicenna (980–1037 AD)	Al Quanun fit Tibb	Canon
Haly Abbas (90?–994 AD)	Kitab al Maliki	Liber Regius
Albucasis (936–1014 AD)	Kitab al Tasrif	Liber Servitoris

small volume of the abscess. Other physicians, however, (whom he consulted beside myself) did not understand his case at all, even after the patient had passed pus in his urine.'

Another example is his description of what was most likely a case of Schönlein-Henoch purpura:

'Case XXIV: The little son of Ibn Sawada had a yellow bile fever from his throat. On the fourth day in the morning he began to urinate blood and to pass with the stool green and bloody bile, resembling water in which fresh meat had been washed; his strength decreased suddenly. We were baffled because his malady had been slight and benign and then had changed in one night to this acuteness and severity; we supposed that he had drunk something [harmful]. When the afternoon came, he had a quite black micturition and equally black stools. He died in the early morning of the sixth day. He had from the beginning a malign form of measles, prone to attack the internal organs.'

Yet another example is a probable case of hepatorenal syndrome:

'*Case XXXIII:* The son of Amr ibn Wahb became feverish and a very intense jaundice made its appearance on him, so that his eye looked on the fifth day like a piece of cartham [safflower or bastard saffron]. On the ninth day he had a retention of urine, and he passed only very little, three drops [colored] like the contents of the gallbladder. He passed blackbiled stools, and his urine on the sixth day was black, then red with yellow froth on it. Then ... [a gap in the Arabic text]. On the eleventh night he had a severe hemorrhage from the right nostril; then he died on the thirteenth night without having lost his sound mental capacity and consciousness. He was attacked by a gasp (death rattle) and coryza, and the swelling of his liver was manifest.'

Further insight into Rhazes' clinical judgement is provided in his differential diagnosis for kidney stones from his *Alkinnash al-Fakhir (Glorious Compendium)*:

'The kidney can have stones and their pain resembles the pain of the colon and these two must be differentiated. Pain in the loin, sediment in the urine or the passage of stone, black urine passed with pain several months before, denote stone pain. If there is nausea or the pain follows a meal or is located in the abdomen and more to the front than the back, then it is more likely to be colonic pain. The site of the pain is important: in abdominal colic the pain is more generalized and tends to be anterior, while in kidney stones the pain is more limited and tends to be in the back.'

Rhazes' recommendations for the prevention of stones is quite relevant, for in their empiric derivation they are no different from current recommendations to avoid hypercalciuria and increased saturation of the urine:

'By avoiding heavy food which we have mentioned. Do not lie long on your back. Avoid cheese, milk derivatives, especially fresh cheese, hard-boiled eggs, unleavened bread, wines, especially dark ones. Use diuretics – cucumbers, melons, figs, grapes, light wines, crystal- clear water from natural sources.'

Writings of Avicenna

The multifaceted Avicenna was also a famous poet. He summarized his medical knowledge in a series of poems called *Arjuzat fit Tibb* (*Poem on Medicine*, the *Canticum Avicennae* of the Middle Ages and the Renaissance). His description of the urine [20] foretells the science of uroscopy, which was to flourish in centuries to come:

'It is in the liver that the humors are born; from there they are spread throughout the body. Every organ functions because of it and it alone has no need of the others. The vital spirit is born in the vapor of the liver; the body is healthy according to its state. Water carries food to it and the water is mixed with the predominant humor and, with its expulsion in the urine, shows that it contained residues. Urine has different colors and everything that the humors have left in it appears to us as a sediment. It is apparent, from what I have stated and wise men witness, that urine is a faithful guide for the knowledge of the illness.

Of urine and first about the color – While urine witnesses the quantity of ingested food and drink, it is a sign of bad digestion, phlegm, cold, restlessness, or of hepatic obstruction. Somewhat yellow, it indicates the presence of a certain quantity of bile. The color of fire, that means the presence of a great deal of yellow bile. Very yellow and tinted with red, it proves a superabundance of yellow bile. Dark red urine of the one who has not ingested saffron and who has had neither fever nor colic contains blood. When found black after having been dark, it signifies that the patient has suffered a great chill. Black after having been very red indicates a poor combustion of humors. Judge the illness according to the odor of urine on the condition that the patient has not ingested a coloring food, certain vegetables, cassia fistula and that which may tint like murri.

On the density of urine – The tenuity of the urine indicates inadequacy of digestion. Sometimes it is fluid after digestion or obstruction of the liver or because of a tumor. The thickness of the urine indicates good digestion or the abundance of phlegm in the body.

On the sediments of urine – The white sediment indicates recovery: yellow, it marks acuteness of the bile; if it is red like the bloodwort, it is a question of disease of the blood. If a similar sediment continues without modification, that indicates an abscess of the liver. Black after having been dark red and that after loss of strength, going to the bottom after floated, that means the soul is about to escape; the patient can no longer benefit from the prayers of the sorcerer; death is at hand through the excess of humoral combustion. If the sediment appears black after having been dark and if it does not occur in the course of acute illness, especially if this appearance coincides with a favorable sign, and if the origin of the illness is in black bile, it indicates the end of the illness.

On the location of the sediment – If a cloud appears floating in the upper portion of the vial, it indicates crudeness of the illness. If a certain maturity exists in the urine, wind (gas) is causing the sediment to reascend to the surface. If the sediment is halfway up, be aware that the wind is in a small quantity. If it is white, after having been yellow, coherent without being thick, falls to the bottom, appears with a changeable color, it marks the maturity of the illness.

On the consistency of the sediment – An ephemeral sediment indicates the weakness of the patient. If there are elements similar to barley meal in the urine, one is dealing with scrapings of the vessels. If the sediment looks like bran and has a bad odor it indicates ulceration within the ducts; like metal filings, it proves the elimination of portions of organs. If pus appears in the vial, it marks the opening of a collection. If the sediment has decomposed blood, there is a phlegmonous tumor. If it goes to the bottom, resembles sperm, it comes from an immature lymph swelling. If one sees sand in it, be aware that there is a calculus.

Of the odor of urine – If the urine has no odor, it is that the food has not been digested or has been ingested raw. The degree of decomposition agrees with the intensity of the odor of the urine. If this odor is dreadful, be aware that the illness is in the bladder. Thus, I have reported on the different kinds of urine; guide yourself by what I have stated about their composition.'

The second part of the *Poem on Medicine* on the practice of medicine focuses on the conservation of health through diets and drugs and is probably a predecessor of the *Regimen Sanitatis Salerni* which was to contribute so much to the fame of the Salerno School of Medicine.

Overall, the medical writings of Avicenna lack the meticulous clinical detail provided by Rhazes. He is more a classifier and integrator. His description of the kidney and its function follows:

'The kidneys were created to clear the blood of aqueous humor. The aqueous humor does not reach the kidney separated from the blood but mixed with it. Removal of the aqueous humor occurs by sieving into the collecting system. Since the humor was abundant, there was a need to create either a single large organ or two small organs. A single organ would have caused crowding ... the benefit of two small organs is that if either is diseased the other would compensate for its function ... The right kidney was created higher than the left because of the need to be close to the liver in order to attract aqueous humor.'

Writings of Haly Abbas

The above description by Avicenna can be compared with the more careful description of the kidneys by Haly Abbas (died 994 AD), a contemporary of Rhazes and another one of the luminaries of the golden age of Arabic medicine (table 2). In his *Kitab al Maliki (Liber Regius* or *Royal Book)* he writes:

'As to the two kidneys they are located on each side of the vertebrae of the back near the liver. The right kidney is higher than the left in position so much so that it could be the lower edge of the liver. As to the left kidney its location is lower. The two concave sides of the kidneys face each other. The two convex sides face the side of the body of the animal on which the kidneys are located. Each one is connected to the vena cava when it comes out of the liver, two large branches, each of which divides the substance of the kidney; and bring to it blood for the nourishment of the kidney. And the other draws fluid of the blood which is in the urine. And joining them from the aorta a branch of adequate caliber brings them the force of life and exits from each one at the site of insertion of these vessels, a long neck with a large cavity, covered by a layer, and joins the neck of the bladder. In them passes the urine from the kidneys to the bladder. These two necks are called ureters. And for this purpose are the kidneys created. I mean to pull the blood fluid from the liver and to clear the blood from its (residues) (refuse) (waste) and this is the description of the two kidneys and their function. Learn this!'

Although more detailed than that of Rhazes, both descriptions are quite similar, if not identical, to the description of the kidney and its function by Galen [21]. They both perpetuate the notion, derived from animal dissection, that the right kidney is located higher than the left. This is not unexpected, given the religious taboos for human dissection.

Writings of Albucasis

Knowledge of the therapy of disease continued to advance, as is illustrated in the writings of the fourth of the leaders of Arabic medicine in its golden age (table 2). Albucasis (936–1014 AD), in Chapter 58 of his *Kitab al Tasrif (Liber Servitoris)* writes on the treatment of urine retention:

'Retention of the urine is caused by an obstruction, from a stone or a clot of blood or pus or a fleshy tumour, or similar cause. When you have carried out treatment in the ways we have prescribed in their place and the urine is not released; and when you see that it is held back by a stone sticking in the neck of the bladder, then you should attempt to bring it out with the instrument called a catheter. It is made of silver, slender and smooth and hollow like the quill of a bird's feather; as slender as a probe; about a span and a half in length; and with a tiny funnel at the end. This is the manner in which you draw the urine through it: take a double thread and with a strong knot tie a little wool or cotton on the end, introduce the end of the thread into the lower end of the catheter, and trim off with scissors any superfluous wool, so that it will go into the tube and close it like a tassel. Then smear the catheter with oil or butter or egg-white. Make the patient sit down; then anoint the bladder and the meatus of the penis with humid oils or with olive oil and warm water. Then gently introduce the catheter into the urethra until it reaches nearly to the seat. Then turn the penis down, with the catheter in it, and push until it reaches the bladder, and the patient now feels that it has entered a hollow. The reason why the operation is done in this manner is that the passage by which the urine is excreted is curved. Then withdraw rather firmly the thread with the wool plug attached, for the urine follows the wool; then pull it right out and the urine will pour out. Apply the catheter again and again until the bladder is emptied and the patient finds relief.'

The attention to detail and refinements on the writings of Galen in the management of obstruction is evident in any comparative reading of the two authors [21].

Other Writings

Some insight into the perception of the kidney can be obtained from a later text by Al Taflisi in his *Taqwim al Adwiyah (Listing of Drugs)* written in 1155 AD:

'Kidney – Changes its humor according to the constitution of the animal. The best kind: the kidney of the kid [young goat]. Its nature: according to Dioscorides moderate. Indications: for wrestlers and athletes and those with liver problems. Its side-effects: difficult to digest. Improve its usefulness: seasoned with salt. Dose: as needed.
Quotation from the Opinion of Physicians – Said Massajunih: it is bad nutrition. Said Rhazes: its humor is bad because it is the receptacle of the residues which it has cleared. It is difficult to digest. Said Hunain: it is not recommended on account of its poor digestion, because of the thickness of its nature; nor is it recommended for nutrition; nor as a laxative because of the thickness of its nature. Said Massawyah [Mesoue]: it is bad, cold, dry and the blood formed in it is very little because it is far from the heart. Must be seasoned with vinegar and hot spices.'

Anatomy in Arabic Medicine

Although experimentation on the human body was prohibited by religion, some dissection and anatomic observation seems to have been undertaken, particularly during the later part of the prime of medicine, as evidenced by some of the extant texts on anatomy, e.g. *Mukhtasai dai ilm il Tashrih (A Brief Manual of Anatomy), Tashrih el Badan (Anatomy of the Body)* and *Tashrihil Mansuri (Mansur's Anatomy)* [4, 5, 7, 11]. It is of interest that long before Vesalius achieved renown for his illustrated text on the anatomy of the human body, anatomic illustrations began to appear in Arabic texts, though clearly not of the detail and artistic merit of the anatomic drawings of Vesalius (fig. 4). The best evidence that some undeclared anatomic observation and experimentation may have been undertaken comes from the writings of Ibn Nafis (Ala ad din ibn Nafis al Qurashi al Dimashqui, 1210–1288 AD) in his description of the circulation:

'We say, however – Allah knows better – as the production of the [vital] spirit is one of the functions of the heart, and as this spirit consists of much-refined blood with a large admixture of airy substance, it is necessary that the heart should contain both refined blood and air so that the spirit may be generated out of the substance produced by their mixture; this takes place where the spirit is generated, viz. in the left cavity of the heart. It is, moreover, indispensable for the heart of man and of such animals as have lungs like him, to possess another cavity in which the blood is refined in order to become apt for the mixture with the air; for, if air is mixed with thick blood, it is not possible to form a homogeneous substance out of them. This cavity is the right cavity of the heart. The blood, after it has been refined in this cavity, must be transmitted to the left cavity where the [vital] spirit is generated. *But there is no passage between these two cavities;* for the substance of the heart is solid in this region and has neither a visible passage, as was thought by some persons, nor an invisible one which could have permitted the transmission of blood, as was alleged by Galen. The pores of the heart there are closed and its substance is thick. Therefore, *the blood,* after having been refined, *must rise in the arterious vein to the lung in order to expand in its volume and to be mixed with air* so that its finest part may be clarified *and may reach the venous artery in which it is transmitted to the left cavity of the heart.* This, after having been mixed with the air and having attained the aptitude to generate the [vital] spirit. That part [of the blood] which is less refined, is used by the lung for its nutrition.'

For this description, Ibn Nafis has been credited with the discovery of the pulmonary circulation [22, 23]. It is unfortunate that his focus on the kidney was more limited. In the same text his commentary on the kidney is only a repetition of that of others:

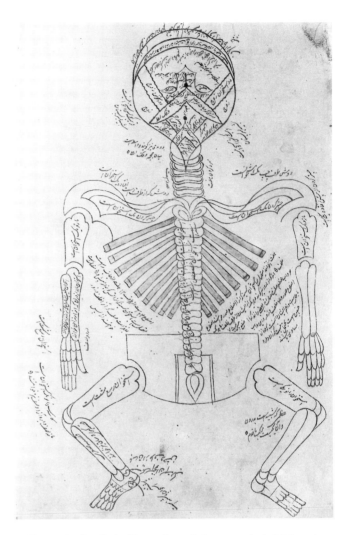

Fig. 4. A simplistic illustration of the musculoskeletal system from a 13th century Arabic manuscript on human anatomy in the collection of Farid S. Haddad.

'It is impossible for the body to persist without food or nourishment. Nourishment is possible by the function of the liver. Nourishment contains excess water which must be extracted. That is why it [the kidney] is closer to the liver to extract water. It has to be to extract water from the liver for their energy needs to pull the water.'

Acknowledgements

The author would like to express his special gratitude to Dr Farid S. Haddad for sharing his insights into Arabic medicine, for allowing access to his collection of Arabic medical manuscripts, for his help in selecting and translating some of the sections quoted in this article, and for providing the illustration reproduced here as figure 4.

References

1 Neuberger M: History of Medicine. Oxford, Oxford University Press, 1910, pp 344–394.
2 Brody IA: The School of Medicine at Jondishapur. The Birthplace of Arabic Medicine. Trans Stud Coll Physicians Phila 1955;23:29–37.
3 Lewis B: The Arabs in History. Oxford, Oxford University Press, 1993.
4 Nasr SH: Islamic Science. An Illustrated Study. World of Islam Festival Publishing Company, Kent, England, 1976.
5 Hamarneh SK: The life sciences, in Hays JR, (ed): The Genius of Arab Civilization. Source of Renaissance. New York, New York University Press, 1975.
6 Khan MS: Islamic Medicine. London, Routledge and Kegan Paul, 1986.
7 Browne EG: Arabian Medicine. Cambridge, Cambridge University Press, 1962.
8 Ullman M: Islamic Medicine. Edinburgh, Edinburgh University Press, 1978.
9 Bayon HP: Arabic philosopher-physicians and Christian doctors of medicine. Proc R Soc Med 1952;45:310–314.
10 O'Leary D: How Greek Science Passed to the Arabs. Chicago, Ares, 1951.
11 Leclerc L: Histoire de la Médecine Arabe. New York, Burt Franklin, vols 1 and 2, 1876.
12 Hamarneh SK: Health Sciences in Early Islam – Collected Papers. Edited by Anees MA. Blanco, Zahra Publications, vols 1 and 2, 1983.
13 Sorokin PA, Merton RK: The course of Arabian intellectual development, 700–1300 AD. A study in method. Isis 1934–5;22:516–524.
14 Sarton G: Introduction to the History of Science. Baltimore, Williams and Wilkins, 1927–1931.
15 Haddad FS: Arab contribution to medicine. Leb Med J 1973;26:331–346.
16 Campbell J: Myths to Live By. New York, Arkana (Penguin Group), 1993.
17 Mujais SK: Nephrologic beginnings. The kidney in the age of Ibn Sina (980–1037 AD). Am J Nephrol 1987;7:133–136.
18 Afnan SM: Avicenna. His Life and Works. Westport, Greenwood Press, 1980.
19 Meyerhof M: Thirty-three clinical observations by Rhazes (circa 900 AD). Isis 1935;23:321–372.
20 Krueger HC: Avicenna's Poem on Medicine. Springfield, Illinois, C Thomas, 1963.
21 Eknoyan G: The origins of nephrology. Galen, the founding father of experimental renal physiology. Am J Nephrol 1989;9:66–82.
22 Meyerhof M: Ibn al-Nafis (XIIth century) and his theory of the lesser circulation. Isis 1935;23:100–120.
23 Khairallah AA, Haddad SI: A forgotten chapter in the history of circulation of the blood. Ann Surg 1936;104:1–8.

Am J Nephrol 1994;14:279–281

The Biblical View of the Kidney

Joel D. Kopple

Division of Nephrology and Hypertension, Department of Medicine, Harbor-UCLA Medical Center, Torrance, Calif., and the Schools of Medicine and Public Health, University of California, Los Angeles, Calif., USA

Key Words
Bible
Kidney
Morality

Abstract

The biblical view of the kidney differs radically from the modern perception. For example, there is no reference in the Bible to the fact that the kidneys make urine. The kidneys were viewed as the seat of conscience and of ethical feelings and yearnings, and the source of morality and ethical activity. The kidneys were believed to be associated with the innermost parts of the personality. There are references to God examining the ethical nature of man through the kidneys or punishing man by injuring the kidneys. The fat around the kidneys was considered to be of special value for sacrifice and may have symbolized luxury or opulence. Much of the biblical understanding of the anatomy of the kidneys and the anatomic relationships between the kidneys, perirenal fat and the liver appears to be derived from observations made in domestic animals.

Introduction

The kidney was a well-recognized organ in the biblical world. There appear to be 13 references to the kidney in the Old Testament [1] and 1 reference in the New Testament [2]. (All quotations from the Old Testament are taken from reference 1. Italics have been added by the present author.) Present day knowledge of the biblical view of the kidney is inferred from the context of the allusions to the kidney, as the function or role of the kidney is not explicitly defined in the Bible. The fact that the authors of the Bible did not explicitly define the role of the kidney probably indicates that the biblical perception of the kidney was rather widely shared, at least among the Jews and Christians of that time.

Knowledge of the kidney was largely derived from animal anatomy, presumably from animals killed for food or for sacrifice. There is no mention in either the Old or New Testament, however, of the excretory functions of the kidney. Indeed, it seems that it was not recognized that the kidneys made urine, and it was probably Galen (130–201 CE) who first reported that the kidney excreted urine [3]. Instead, in both the Old Testament and the New Testament (*Revelations* 2:23) [2], the kidneys were associated with moral life, conscience, guilt and satisfaction over morally correct actions.

The Kidneys and Morality

In the Bible, the kidneys were considered to be associated with the innermost part of the personality. They were viewed as central to the soul and to morality. The kidneys were perceived as the source or impetus for moral yearning, a force for moral or righteous action, and as capable of engendering feelings of guilt or moral approval. The kidney was also represented as a vehicle or medium through which God examined the moral nature or worth

Joel D. Kopple, MD
Division of Nephrology and Hypertension
Harbor-UCLA Medical Center
1000 West Carson Street
Torrance, CA 90509 (USA)

of man and as a target organ for God's punishment of humans for immoral behavior [2]. The extent to which the allusions to the kidneys in the Old and New Testaments were written to be metaphorical rather than literal is not known. The following passages from the Old Testament give examples of these views of the kidney.

When God assessed the moral character or moral worth of an individual, this was perceived as being carried out through an examination of the heart and the kidneys [1, 2]:

'O Lord who ministerest judgment to the peoples,
Judge me, O Lord,
According to my righteousness, and according to mine integrity
    that is in me.
Oh that a full measure of evil might come upon the wicked,
And that thou wouldest establish the righteous;
For the righteous God trieth the heart and reins' [4].

In another psalm:

'Examine me, O Lord, and try me;
Test my reins and my heart' [5].

The kidneys are viewed as exerting moral leadership or moral force:

'I will bless the Lord, who hath given me counsel;
Yea in the night seasons *my reins instruct me'* [6].

The kidneys are also viewed as a seat of desire, particularly of a moral nature. Because of yearning for God, Job's kidneys withered within him:

'And when after my skin is destroyed,
Then without flesh I shall see God;
Whom I, even I, shall see for myself,
And mine eyes shall behold, and not another's.
My reins are consumed within me' [7].

The above passage indicates that the kidneys can sense or engender joy over morally correct actions, the kidneys also can cause feelings of guilt:

'As a dream when one awaketh,
So, O Lord, when Thou arousest Thyself,
Thou wilt despise their semblance.
For my heart was in a ferment,
And I was pricked in my reins' [8].

When God is punishing man physically, the injury to the kidney is an indication of the severe and overwhelming nature of the punishment:

'His archers compass me round about,
He cleaveth my reins asunder, and doth not spare;
He poureth out my gall upon the ground' [9].

Anatomy in the Bible

Animal sacrifice played a central role in the religious life of Jewish people during biblical history. The kidneys, and particularly the fat surrounding them, were believed to be of special value for animal sacrifice. The fat around the kidneys appears to have represented special luxuriousness or opulence:

'He made him ride on the high places of the earth,
And he did eat the fruitage of the field;
And He made him to suck honey out of the crag,
And oil out of the flinty rock;
Curd of kine, and milk of sheep,
With fat of lambs,
And rams of the breed of Bashan, and he-goats,
With the kidney-fat of wheat;
And of the blood of the grape thou drankest foaming wine' [10].

It should be noted that most of the biblical knowledge of the anatomy of the kidney and surrounding tissues was probably derived from animals. These organs were observed when the animals were prepared for cooking or were eaten. This is borne out by some of the descriptions of the anatomy of the abdominal viscera, which more closely resembles that of domestic animals than of humans. Thus, in *Leviticus* there are references to a hepatic lobe that is physically adjacent to the kidney [11–13]. In fact, in cows, goats and sheep, the caudate lobe of the liver may only be connected to the liver by a stalk. This lobe overlies the right kidney, and the kidney actually may form an impression on the caudate lobe where the two organs are in contact [14].

The Kidneys in Modern Translations of the Bible

In modern translations of the Bible or ancient prayers, the allusions to the kidneys pose a problem for the writer. The biblical view of the kidney differs markedly from the modern view of the function or role of the kidney. Moreover, almost all modern readers of the Bible are unaware of the biblical perceptions of the kidney, unless these readers are specially trained or biblical scholars. To address these issues, many of the modern versions of the Bible and prayers in which the kidney or perinephric fat is mentioned translate these passages loosely. The kidney and perinephric fat are not mentioned and the gist of the passage, as interpreted by the translator, is paraphrased.

References

1 The Holy Scriptures According to the Masoretic Text. Philadelphia, The Jewish Publication Society of America, 1955.
2 The Holy Bible containing the Old and New Testaments, King James Version. New York, American Bible Society.
3 Ackerknecht EH: A Short History of Medicine. Baltimore, Johns Hopkins University Press, 1982, p 74.
4 Psalm 7: 9, 10. The Holy Scriptures According to the Masoretic Text. Philadelphia, The Jewish Publication Society of America, 1955.
5 Psalm 26: 2 (Ibid).
6 Psalm 16: 7 (Ibid).
7 Job 19: 26, 27 (Ibid).
8 Psalm 73: 20, 21 (Ibid).
9 Job 16: 13 (Ibid).
10 Deuteronomy 32: 13, 14 (Ibid).
11 Leviticus 3: 3, 4 (Ibid).
12 Leviticus 3: 10 (Ibid).
13 Leviticus 3: 15 (Ibid).
14 Getty R: The Anatomy of the Domestic Animals, 5th ed. Philadelphia, WB Saunders, 1975.

Am J Nephrol 1994;14:282–289

Luciana Rita Angeletti
Berenice Cavarra

Department of Philology and History,
Section of History of Medicine,
University of Cassino, Cassino, Italy

Critical and Historical Approach to Theophilus' *De Urinis*

Urine as Blood's Percolation Made by the Kidney and Uroscopy in the Middle Ages

Key Words
Theophilus
Uroscopy
Middle Ages
History of medicine

Abstract

In classical Greek medicine, neither Hippocrates nor Galen considered the condition of the urine to be an important sign of systemic diseases, and they did not relate its characteristics to definite illnesses, except in obvious cases of urinary tract disease. In their teaching, urine was used together with other physical signs as a prognostic indicator. With Theophilus, however, uroscopy gained an important role, and the appearance of the urine became pathognomonic of specific diseases. *De Urinis* owed its popularity to this new approach and to its didactic character, as it was written as a practical handbook. After the 12th century, *De Urinis* occupied an assured position among the few ancient medical treatises that in Latin translation formed a worldwide teaching canon for medieval and Renaissance medical schools.

Introduction

In the long transition from theurgic and priestly medicine to rational medicine, a very important role was played by the efforts directed to correlating signs to individual pathologies. The literary models *(moduli)* recurring in the transmitted medical texts illustrate this process. For example, in the Hammurabi Codex (18th century BC), the model is simple, with an observational and didactic pattern, i.e. directly therapeutic: 'if someone has this, you will do ...'. The references to specific diseases, including urinary diseases, are very sparse [1]. In the Egyptian medical papyri (19th–15th centuries BC), however, a rise of medical methodology may be found, with a first reference to the inspection of the body undertaken to identify pathologic signs: 'If a man has stomach ache ... put a hand on the abdomen ... and give the following

remedy ...'. There also appears in some cases a prognostic judgment, with formulae of this kind: 'It is a disease I will treat'; or 'It is a disease I will fight against'; or finally, and only in the Smith papyrus: 'It is found incurable'. Thus, the treatment is oriented to the single organs and systems, including the urinary system [2, 3].

It is possible that this development of medical methodology influenced the rise of rational medicine in Greek culture, particularly at Cnidus and later at Cos, as is suggested by some written evidence [4]. For example, the Egyptian physician Ninyas was active in Cnidus [5]. In the *Anonymus Londinensis* papyrus, which reports the writings of Nero, pupil of Aristotle, and provides information on Alexandrine medicine from the 2nd century BC to the 1st century AD, research on signs is developed and includes a quantitative dimension for the phenomena. This is illustrated by the estimation of *perspiratio insensi-*

Luciana R. Angeletti
Via R. Fusco 107,
I-00136 Rome (Italy)

bilis, obtained by weighing an animal and then weighing it anew with its feces after it had been segregated in a large vessel for a short period of time.

Signs Related to Diseases in Greek Medicine

It was with Hippocratic medicine that research on signs and prognostic judgment acquired great importance, because they allowed a rational theory of medicine which included all diseases, even the so-called 'sacred' one (*De Morbo Sacro*, 1). Urine, pulse and temperature became the three main signs to be considered in the patient. Therefore, in *Prognosticon* II, 12, 110–191 and in *Coacae Praenotiones* V, 588–733) color, appearance and presence of urinary sediment are related to prognosis (long-term illness, acute illness; propitious or inauspicious sediment). Thus, fetid urine brings a fatal prognosis, greenish urine means a deposit in the hepatic subdiaphragmatic region and cloudy urine reveals a bladder disease [6]. It is clear that the reported symptomatology is related to specific pathologies, e.g. hepatic, renal, or bladder pathology.

Deriving from the quotations of urology and uroscopy, urologists are right to claim the existence of their professional specialty in Hippocratic medicine and probably from the days of Homer [7]; they believe as proof that they have been mentioned in the Oath attributed to Hippocrates:

'I shall not operate those suffering of the gravel stone, even if suffering, and I will let the expert to do this.'

The urologists' pride of primogeniture corresponds, with no less important reasons, to that of nephrologists. The physical assessment of the distinctive features of the pulse and urine marks the development of a medicine for which semiotics represents the borderline between the scientific and the irrational. Consequently, this medicine makes general use of signs related to a 'special' part of the body. These signs include facies, respiration, perspiration, vomiting, expectoration, stools; they indicate the composition of the unbalanced humors.

Following the death of the master, the Hippocratic tradition developed in Alexandria, where Herophilus of Chalcedon (4th century BC) and Erasistratus of Cos (3rd century BC) are thought to have tried to estimate physiologic functions. It is said that Erasistratus went round with a sand-glass in order to measure pulse rate. Galen (2nd century AD) refers to the Alexandrine tradition when he recommends a stay at a medical school studying anatomy and physiology as a guaranteed way to become a good physician. In Galen (edited by Kühn (K)) the role of urine is directly treated in a passage of *De Crisibus* (K IX, 550–768). The argument is well explained in many pseudo-Galenic books, e.g. *De Urinis Liber* (K XIX, 574–601) and *De Urinis Compendium* (K XIX, 602–608). A commentary to many authors is contained in a pseudo-Galenic *De Urinis ex Hippocrate, Galeno et Aliis Quibusdam* (K XIX, 609–628). To the pulse and pulsology are dedicated other pseudo-Galenic books, including *De Usa Pulsuum (K V, 149–180), De Pulsibus Libellus ad Tirones* (K VIII, 453–492), *De Differentia Pulsuum* 1–4 (K VIII, 493–765), *De Cognoscendis Pulsibus* 1–4 (K VIII, 766–961), *De Causis Pulsuum* 1–4 (K IX, 1–204), *De Praesagitione ex Pulsibus* 1–4 (K IX, 205–430) and the *Synopsis Librorum Suorum De Pulsibus* (K IX, 431–549). In this connection, it is worth noting the comment of Baader and Keil that all the traits of urine included by Chartier and Kühn in their editions of Galen are spurious [9].

The importance of the character of urine was discussed by many medical authors living about the 2nd century AD: Caelius Aurelianus in the *Tardae Passiones* V, 3; Aulus Cornelius Celsus in *De Medicina* 4, 17; Aretaeus in the books *De Causis et Signis Acutorum Morborum* 2, 9 and *De Causis et Signis Diuturnorum Morborum* 2, 3. In *De Causis et Signis Acutorum Morborum* 2, 9, Aretaeus describes the function of the kidney, which is devoted to the separation of urine from blood. Finally, Rufus of Ephesus, in his *De Renum et Vesicae Affectionibus*, described many kidney and bladder diseases and also diabetes, which is 'a massive passage of urines'. Eknoyan has recently discussed this subject [10].

In the 4th–6th centuries AD, when it was clear that Galen had exhausted the possibilities of acquiring new medical knowledge, some authors devoted themselves to summarizing Hippocratic and Galenic treatises into handbooks to be used both as critical and, especially, as practical guidebooks. Among the epitomists may be mentioned Oribasius of Pergamon (5th century), Aetius of Amida (6th century), Alexander of Tralles (6th century) and Paul of Aegina (7th century). Aetius of Amida studied at Alexandria, became first physician at the Court of Constantinople at the time of Justinian I and wrote an extensive epitome (8 books in the Aldina edition, Venice, 1534), in the 5th book of which he devotes 15 chapters to urine.

The most outstanding physicians of the period were more concerned with Alexandria than directly with Galen, e.g. Palladius (5th century AD) and Stephanus of Athens (2nd half of the 6th century/7th century AD). The latter was an extraordinary exponent of the medical and

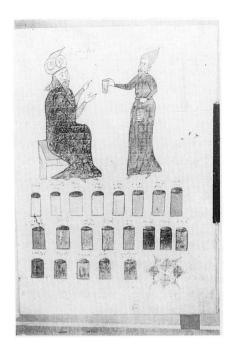

Fig. 1. Theophilus of Byzantium (about 7th century AD) being handed a flask of urine by his assistant Posos (right). Below them are uroscopy flasks, arranged according to texture and color as described in *De Urinis*. Manuscript from Byzantium (15th century), Bononiensis ms 3632, folio 51.

philosophic school flourishing at Alexandria between the 5th and 7th centuries AD, where medicine and philosophy were included in a single dimension. This concept spread in the Mediterranean basin, in Ravenna and in southern Italy, as well as in Constantinople and in the Arabic world [11–13]. Stephanus completed many comments on the classical medical texts, including Galen's *Therapeutica ad Glauconem* and Hippocrates' *Prognosticon* and *Aphorismi*. Theophilus, an eminent physician of Byzantium (fig. 1), produced scholia on hippocratic aphorisms, in which he showed his conceptual and lexical dependence on Stephanus' commentary. Moreover, Theophilus' *scholia* are based on the Galenic commentary on Hippocratic aphorisms and reveal the high respect of the Byzantine scholar towards Hippocrates, more than once quoted textually. Some of the most important works of Theophilus include *De Humani Corporis Fabrica Libri V, De Urinis, De Excrementis, De Pulsibus* and *De Hippocratis Aphorismorum Commentario. De Arte Medica ex Hippocrate et Galeno* is as yet unpublished.

As far as urine is concerned, however, it must be considered that Theophilus enriches the subject with notions and comments drawn from his own medical knowledge.

Stephanus' commentary reflects the didactic form of a course of lessons, whereas Theophilus' work starts from the Alexandrine commentator's sources and becomes a fluent and comprehensible text in a clear lexicon, free from any theoretic, philosophic and cultural ambitions. Theophilus' commentary reveals the influence of Stephanus, but it also sometimes shows a scientific independence when dealing with urologic matters. Theophilus' urologic doctrine expressed in his commentary originates, therefore, from an acquaintance with the classical tradition mediated through Stephanus of Athens, and from a deep personal knowledge of the subject; these two strands were joined in the treatise *De Urinis*. It is worth noting that the *De Urinis* of Stephanus was known in Arabic medicine, as indicated by the quotation in the *Kitab al Hawi* XI,102 *(Continens)* of Rhazes (865–923 AD).

The urologic tradition reached Byzantium through the work of the Alexandrine medical circules in late antiquity. Byzantine medicine strengthened the inheritance of the ancient tradition by means of a medical practice that emphasized semiotics. Study of the pulse also had a considerable role in diagnostics and was developed by the Byzantine heirs of Galen, who expanded this field considerably. In his treatise *De Pulsibus*, Theophilus shows traces of Galen, but with an easier literary style and greater clarity of diagrams.

The Centrality of Uroscopy: Theophilus of Byzantium

The role of uroscopy and of urine, conceived of as the result of *'percolation* of the humors', is found in both original and spurious treatises, and in commentaries and compendia of the ancient physicians' works and thoughts [14, 15], from Hippocrates to Galen – the marvellous physician – to the learned Byzantine physician Magnus and to Aetius' epitome. Referring to these authorities, Theophilus begins going deeper into the subject.

The closest to him is Magnus (about 5th–6th century AD), who was said to have had such a reasoning skill as to be able to prove a patient was still sick when the other physicians maintained the opposite, and vice versa. In that way of thinking, the objectivity of the clinical survey has little weight. Therefore, Theophilus' work becomes relevant: in fact, urine examination becomes pre-eminent, apart from the importance of pulse measurement, and is conceived of as a hematic percolation, a definition employed in the past only once by Aretheus of Cappadocia (1st century AD). The subject of the urine per se began to be considered by the Byzantine physicians and was developed through many specialized texts, which were different from the ones dealing with the pulse and other signs. Rufus of Ephesus (2nd century AD), an outstanding physician, is the only earlier author to attach so much importance to urine. He wrote *De Renum et Vesicae Affectionibus*, taking into consideration both urology and nephrology. It is important, however, to emphasize that uroscopy marks the empiric trend typical of Byzantine medicine: a trend above all addressed to praxis and destined to form the basis of Arabic medicine.

Theophilus' identity is very uncertain: it is almost impossible to outline his biography and difficult to place him in a precise historical period. Conventionally, Theophilus has been placed in the 7th century AD, but he could equally have lived in the 9th–10th centuries AD. He is mentioned in the manuscript tradition by the titles of *protospathàrios, archìatros, monachòs* and *philòsophos*. Until the problem of Theophilus' chronologic placing is resolved, it will be impossible to determine for certain his historical identity. In the Byzantine world, a 7th century philosopher was very different from a 9th century one. According to Hunger [16], an ideal career of the *De Urinis* writer can be imagined, drawing his figure as that of a 9th century imperial officer, then retired in a cloister to ponder mystical theology; the possibility should not be omitted, however, that 2 centuries earlier Theophilus could have been a scholar learned in medical science *(archìatros).*

The Christian faith of Theophilus comes out clearly from his *De Corporis Humani Fabrica Libri V*, in which, despite his dependence on Galen, the author glorifies God and ascribes to Him the marvels of the human body. In addition, in the Preface and Conclusion of *De Urinis*, appear divine invocation and glorification.

Theophilus' *De Urinis*

The most important doctrinal contribution of Theophilus concerns the role of uroscopy. According to his introduction, Theophilus viewed *De Urinis* as an attempt to interpret consistently the meaning of the different types of urine and the role of uroscopy (fig. 2) [17]. This latter was never exhaustively demonstrated by the ancient masters such as Hippocrates, Galen and Magnus of Nisibis. It is not really their doctrine that Theophilus criticizes, however; in fact, he says in the Preface to *De Urinis* that it is possible that Galen and Magnus knew the subject, though neither of them examined it closely.

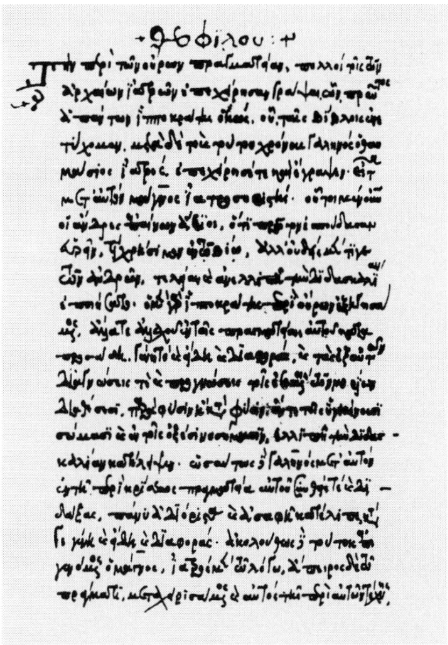

Fig. 2. Frontispiece of the *De Urinis* of Theophilus. Ms. Mutinensis gr. 61 (15th century), Modena, Estense Library (manuscript chart, 21.8 × 16 cm, ff 1ᵛ–99; *Theophili Protospatharii Liber De Urinis* 2ʳ–13ᵛ).

In the Preface, Theophilus considers as inadequate the interpretations and the didactic work of Hippocrates, Galen and Magnus of Nisibis. This last was celebrated as an orator and a philosopher more than as a physician (see, e.g. Eunapius, *Vitae Sophistarum* 497 ff; Philostorgius, *Historia Ecclesiae* VIII, 10; Libanius, *Epistulae* 497, 1208, 1358) [18]. The treatise *De Urinis* of Magnus of Nisibis is conserved in the Arabic version and only in part in the *Physici et Medici Graeci* [19]. Magnus might still have been famous at the time of Theophilus, for the author of *De Urinis* mentions him together with the two most outstanding masters of ancient medicine. Theophilus says that, in comparison with them, it is necessary: 'to look for a different doctrine and not to examine in vain the things taught by them, and not to take into consideration facts and opinions which are doubtful' *(De Urinis Prooemium)*. In order to undertake such an enterprise of doctrinal renewal, Theophilus concludes by invoking God's help and proposing to teach his own knowledge.

The treatise has the characteristics of a handbook with practical aims, which explains its large circulation. It is didactically divided into 3 parts: (1) what urine is; (2) the place where urine originates and the place where urine separates; and (3) the *genus* (kind), aspect and differences of urines. The whole doctrine is framed within this

Table 1. Conventional chromatic scale for describing the color of urine

a   White; milk-white; light grey camel's wool; grey
b   Pale yellow; yellow; celtic gold reddish; yellowish red;
       lightish brown; saffron-colored yellow
c   Flame-colored reddish or purple-red; red; wine-colored
d   Dark blue; dry fig grey
e   Grass or cabbage pale green; verdigris; emerald green; turquoise;
       livid green
f   Black

Table 2. Chromatic scales for light (*De Urinis* 92) and thick (*De Urinis* 100) urine

'Light'	'Thick'
Light and white	Thick and white
Light and milk-white	Thick and milk-white
Light and grey	Thick and light grey
Light and light grey	Thick and reddish
Light and yellow	Thick and red
Light and pale yellow	Thick and wine-colored
Light and reddish	Thick and dark blue
Light and yellowish-red	Thick and pale green
Light and yellowish	Thick and livid green
Light and saffron yellow	Thick and black

scheme, beginning from the enunciation of the theory of urine formation, which arises – as stated in the Preface – by a 'bending' of the hematopoietic force according to nature. Urine, Theophilus soon afterwards explains, is not the result of an expulsion process related to the compound of humors, for it is essentially the percolation of the blood – he says – and this aspect is different according to the coction. Some Latin translators, interpolating the original text with the opinion of Isaac Judaeus, added 'and other humors' *(lotium est sanquinis aliorumque umorum colatura)*: esteem for the ancient masters induces caution regarding the new theory! Theophilus' statement, on the contrary, is definite and undoubted (*De Urinis* 68–70):

'Such is the urine ... The urine is the blood's *percolation.*'

The interesting word 'percolation' had already been used by Dioscorides (*Materia Medica* 1, 73) to refer to the preparation of infusions and by Galen (in *Hippocratis Epidemiarum Librum Sextum Commentarius*, K XVII, 983). For Theophilus, this term assumed a very peculiar meaning, because it exactly represented the process of the

formation of urine directly in the kidney, going beyond the meaning of Aretheus (the loins divide the blood from the urine formed before). Theophilus' concept also exceeds the inclusive and vague reference to the humors, identifying just one humor alone, the blood, as the origin of the percolation forming urine. In fact, he says, the different humors have their own places of collection: the gallbladder gathers the yellow bile; the spleen gathers what is heavy; the watery or hematic secretion, through the median vena cava, reaches the loins, where it is transformed into urine. The blood, which originally is dense, is diluted in the liver by the watery solution to easily pass through the veins (*De Urinis* 70, 14).

Theophilus then describes the urine 'according to nature' and its physiologic composition. Urine 'according to nature' has a white, regular and smooth sediment; therefore, it is well balanced, owing to the well-balanced composition of the blood. Its property is moisture. It is possible to measure the moisture's density, which is described by the terms: lightness, thickness and 'middle course', i.e. equilibrium. This last, because it is 'according to nature', is inseparable. If the urine turns muddy with time, there is a coction principle (internal *cooking* or *burning*); if there is a sediment, the urine turns from heavy into light because of coction. Different colors are related to cold and warm, whereas consistency is related to dry and moist (*De Urinis* 86–88). Urine could thus have a light consistency with white color (De Urinis 78, 265); this finding was observed when people drank a lot, and also if there was diabetes, 'chamber-pot illness' 'thirst diabetes', or after a burning fever. It should be noted that Theophilus outlines very well the problems of total recovery of renal function after a febrile poisoning.

The different colors of urine are next described, divided according to a conventional chromatic scale (table 1). These chromatic scales form the most important part of uroscopy and can be referred to light urine as well as to heavy urine if chyme is present, there is inflammation of the joints, a 'cleansing of the black bile humor', a 'black bile suspension' occurred, or quartan fever (malaria) results in massive hemolysis (table 2). Theophilus (*De Urinis* 92) fixed the chromatic scale in 10 tonalities referred to the quantitative evaluation 'light'. The same couplings can be applied to 'thick' urines (*De Urinis* 100). Thus, thick and white urine derives from an abundance of chyme. Thick and milk-white urine shows renal and bladder lithiasis. Thick and light grey urine shows a bad condition of the humors. When heated, clot formation indicates fever; if bubbles appear on the surface, the fever is coming to an end. Thick and reddish urine shows the end of a chronic disease. Thick and red urine shows the expulsion of the hematic humor in the urine; the hematic humor, if expelled in a small quantity, could be dangerous; if fever, headache and pain are present in the hypochondrial region, icterus is about to occur. Thick and livid green urine shows a crisis when burning fevers are present with very painful headaches. Thick and winey urine in old people shows bladder staunching. Thick and dark blue urine results from strangury. Thick and black urine is connected with black bile coming from dried blood, as happens after quartan fever. The word quartan fever is very ancient (*Orphica, Lithica*, 635). It was remarked on by the ancient physicians, e.g. Galen (K XIII, 66; K XIV, 277) and was taken up by the epitomists (Alexander Trallianus, *De Febribus* 6, edited by Puschmann).

The statements on the different kinds of urine offer some interesting starting points. Theophilus, quoting Hippocrates, states that white pus, being like a good sediment, could deceive, because on the contrary it means a lesion of the loins or bladder (*De Urinis* 118, 17). Specific diseases and related types of urine are indicated, as is the case with phrenitis (*De Urinis* 81–82), which is an inflammation of the brain in Hippocrates (*Aphorisms* III, 30), but also a delirium in Galen (K XVI, 493); in Theophilus it seems to be either an inflammation of the brain or a delirium with ardent fever or an inflammation of the diaphragm, all related to an accumulation of yellow bile, as indicated by the excreted urine, which is white and light. It is worth noting that Theophilus' explanation is referred to as hepatic head disease (encephalopathy?). Diagrams are proposed in order to help the physician in the distinction of color-lightness and sediment (white, smooth or not smooth, regular or irregular in time, fig. 3).

Theophilus then dedicates individual chapters to the corpuscular sediments ('vetch-like', 'petal-like', 'bran-like', 'minced barley-like'), with prognostic considerations related to the authority of Hippocrates (*De Urinis* 126, 31; 128, 15; 130, 5; 13, 19). The treatise draws to an end with a new invocation to Christ, 'our True God' (*De Urinis* 138, 4–9) and finishes by stressing its own purposes – the improvement of those who want to learn.

The Legacy of Theophilus

Following Theophilus, the Arabs examined urine, under an indirect influence of the master of Byzantium, who was quoted by the most outstanding figures, Rhazes and Avicenna (*Canon* 1st book, II fen). The topic was treated by Isaac Judaeus (about 880–940 AD), whose *De Urinis*

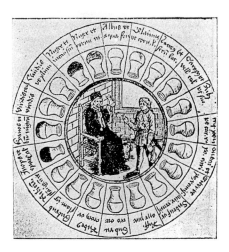

Fig. 3. A circular chart helpful for uroscopy (from the *Fasciculus Medicinae*, Venice, 1497). In the chart are shown 20 light and thick tonalities according to the *De Urinis* of Theophilus. It is worth noting that in the central part of the diagram the physician is examining urine in front of a relative of the patient and not in the presence of the patient. This indicates a role for uroscopy that anticipates laboratory medicine, which is related to but differentiated from clinical medicine.

was very popular in the Arabic world, thus explaining why no Syriac or Arabic translations of Theophilus have been found. The work of Isaac Judaeus was translated into Latin by Constantinus Africanus. It is divided into 10 *particulae:* (1) the science of urine, which derives from the 4 humors and, in particular, from the blood; (2) the importance of night urine; (3) different kinds of urine and the related pathology; (4) urine as the drainage of the humors; (5) different kinds of urine according to the color; (6) colors showing the organism's degradation; (7) limpid/clear, muddy/thick, honey-like etc … urine; (8) urinary sediment in relation to pathology; (9) kinds of urine in conjunction with sediments; and (10) other kinds of urine and sediments and their meaning. A copy of the treatise is carried in a Latin parchment codex of the 13th century (*Isaac Judaeus Filium Salomonis Liber Urinarum*) preserved in the university library in Pavia.

Works about urine and the pulse were included in many manuscripts of the Salerno-Cassino period (see in the *Codicum Casinensium Manuscriptorum Catalogus, Montis Casini*) 1915 ss.: ms 69v *Anonymi Varia Excerpta Medica* 551–562; *Incipiunt Signa Effemerorum Febrium De Urinis et Pulsis Secundum Precepta Dionisii*; ms 97v, *Galeni Hippocratis ps-Hipp. ac Aliorum Opera Medica* 26–33; and Galeni *De Urinis et Pulsibus* (Diels I, 128, 132).

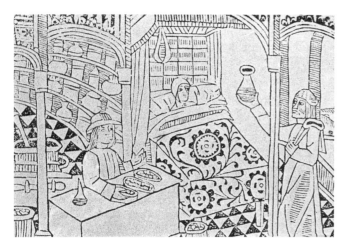

Fig. 4. A scene depicting uroscopy by the examination of *matula*, the special vessels for urine (right), and prescription of drugs (left) in the presence of the patient (from a 1494 edition of the 13th century work of Bartholomaeus Anglicus de Glanvilla, *De Proprietatibus Rerum – De las propriedades de las cosas,* Toulouse).

Commentaries on classical texts of medicine were recorded in the Salerno School of Medicine at the end of the 12th century by Magister Maurus: the works included *Aphorismi* and *Prognosticon* by Hippocrates, *Ars Parva* by Galen, *De Urinis* by Theophilus, *De Pulsibus* by Philaretes and *Isagoge* by Hunain ibn Ishâq (Johannitius). This corpus was the canon of teaching medicine, first in Salerno and then in the other European medical schools, and was printed as a short manual to teach the art and called *articella;* this canon was adopted until the 18th century [20–23].

The work of Theophilus *De Urinis* was largely used for Latin translations during the 12th and 13th centuries [24, 25]. The work is conserved in two Hebrew manuscripts translated from Latin (*Monacensis* III, 14th century; *Parisinus* 1165, 14th century) [26]. The area has been discussed in a number of reviews [27–30].

Thus, thanks to Constantinus, the study of urine became very important in the Salerno School of Medicine; it is not surprising, therefore, that Magister Maurus *(Regulae Urinarum)*, Magister Ursus *(Compendium de Urinis)* and Aegidius Corboliensis (Gilles de Corbeil) wrote on this subject. The last of these wrote the *Carmina de Urinarum Judiciis*, a book in verse in which are collected the works of classical medicine, i.e. those of Theophilus, Isaac Judaeus and the masters of the Salerno School of Medicine. In this way, Theophilus became one of the most important mediators between classical and medieval medicine. He developed the Byzantine medical tradition,

based on strict observation of signs; uroscopy is also based on this tradition, and in the 14th century was highly commended by Joannis Actuarius, an eminent physician working in the Xenodocheion of Constantinople, who wrote a ponderous treatise on uroscopy, divided into 7 volumes [31].

In the 16th century medical school of the Padua Studium, which mainly followed the doctrine of Aristotle and of Arabic medicine, the canon of official teaching of medicine was revised. There, great importance was awarded to the theoretic and practical course of uroscopy and the pulse; a Chair in these 2 fields was established on 20 October 1601 by a decree of the Venetian Senate. The Chair was given to Antonio Negro, was recorded as holding an annual theory course during the 2nd hour of the morning in Bo. The course was based on Arabic medicine: *Ad Lecturam Secundae seu Prima Canonis Avicennae.* Magister Antonio Negro was said to be obliged: 'andar all 'Ospital di s. Francesco dopo la lettura a far l'ostensione delle orine e la cognitione dè polsi ...' [32, 33]. If some specific treatises are taken into consideration, e.g. Philaretos *Peri Sphugmon – De Pulsibus*, the coupling *De Pulsibus et Urinis* is not uncommon in the earliest Byzantine treatises and in the following Latin vulgarizations. It is worth mentioning two versions of the *De Pulsibus et Urinis* written by an unknown Alexander, who lived during the early Middle Ages; this author refers to the fevers and to individual diseases [14, 34]. For diagnostic purposes, diagrams were very popular [35].

The teaching at Padua can thus be traced back to the Arabic tradition, which in turn developed from the legacy of Greek, Hellenistic and Byzantine medicine, including the work of Theophilus, who was appreciated as an eminent physician and the most important author on urology [36].

Summary

Neither Hippocrates nor Galen ascribed to urine a prominent semiologic value or linked its characteristics to a definite disease, except in the obvious cases of disease of the urinary tract. Urine was rather used, together with other physical signs (stools, vomit, sweat, facies, respiration etc.), in order to determine the prognosis in terms of the length and outcome of the illness. In the work of Theophilus, uroscopy attained a very important role and the urine became pathognomonic of specific diseases (fig. 4). The *De Urinis* owed its widespread popularity to this innovation as well as to its didactic character. After the

12th century, *De Urinis* occupied an assured position among the few texts making up the *Articella*, the Latin collection of ancient medical treatises used as a worldwide teaching canon in the medical schools of the Middle Ages and Renaissance.

Acknowledgements

This work was supported by grants from the Italian Ministry of Universities and Research and the National Research Council.

References

1 Thompson H: Assyrian prescriptions for diseases of the urine. Babyloniaca 1934;14:108–109.
2 Ebers: Papyrus of 24, 27, 37, 261, 265, 269, 270, 274, 276, 278, 282, 283
3 Edwin Smith: Papyrus 7.
4 Jouanna J: Hippocrate. Pour une Archéologie de l'Ecole de Cnide. Paris, Les Belles Lettres, 1974.
5 Jones WHS (ed): Anonymus Londinensis: The Medical Writings of *Anonymus Londinensis*. Cambridge, Cambridge University Press, 1947.
6 *Corpus Hippocraticum: Prognosticon* II, 12, 110–191; *Aphorismi*, IV, 458–609; *De Humoribus* V, 476–503; *Coacae Praenotiones* V, 588–733.
7 Giannopulos T, Kostakopoulos A, Sofras F Dimopoulos C: The operation of lithotomy in ancient Greece. Urol Int 1987;42:210–212.
8 *Corpus Hippocraticum: Jusjurandum* IV, 628–633.
9 Baader G, Keil G: Mittelalterliche Diagnostik: Ein Bericht, in Habrich C, Marguth F, Wolfs JH (eds): Medizinische Diagnostik in Geschichte und Gegenwart. Festschrift für Heinz Goerke zum 60. Geburtstag (Neue Münchner Beiträge zur Geschichte der Medizin und Naturwissenschaften, Medizinhistorische Reihe 7/8) 1978, pp 124–129.
10 Eknoyan G: The origins of nephrology. Galen, the founding father of experimental renal physiology. Am J Nephrol 1989;9:66–82.
11 Meyerhof M: Von Alexandrien nach Bagdad. Berlin, Sitzungsberichte der Preussischen Akademie der Wissenschaften. Philosophisch-Historische Klasse, 1930, pp 389–429.
12 Temkin O: Byzantine medicine: tradition and empiricism. Dumbarton Oaks Papers 1962;16:94–115.

13 Westernick LG: Philosophy and medicine in late antiquity. Janus 1964;51:169–177.
14 Baader G: Early medieval Latin adaptations of Byzantine medicine in Western Europe. Dumbarton Oaks Papers 1984;38:251–259.
15 Penella RJ: Greek Philosophers and Sophists in the Fourth Century AD. Studies in Eunapius of Sardis. Leiden, Brill, 1990, pp 1–9.
16 Hunger H: Die hochsprachliche profane Literatur der Byzantiner. München, Becksche Verlagsbuchhandlung, 1978.
17 Ideler IL (ed): *Theophili De Urinis*, in *Physici et Medici Graeci Minores*. Amsterdam, Adolf M Hakkert, 1963, pp 261–283.
18 Nutton V: From Galen to Alexander. Aspects of medicine and medical practice in late antiquity, Dumbarton Oaks Papers 1984;38:3–14.
19 *Magnus of Nisibus: De Urinis*, in Ideler IL (ed): *Physici et Medici Graeci*. Amsterdam, Adolf M Hakkert, 1963.
20 Angeletti LR: Transmission of classical medical texts through languages of the Middle-East. Medicina nei Secoli 1990;2:293–329.
21 Mujais SK: Nephrologic beginnings: the kidney in the age of Ibn Sina (980–1037 AD). Am J Nephrol 1987;7:133–136.
22 Riha O, Fisher W: Harndiagnotik bei Isaak Judaeus, Gilles de Corbeil und Ortolf von Baierland. Beobachtungen zur Bearbeitungstechnik. Sudhoffs Arch 1988;72:212–224.
23 Dal Canton A, Castellano M: Theory of urine formation and uroscopic diagnosis in the Medical School of Salerno. Kidney Int 1988;34:273–277.
24 Kristeller PO: Studi Sulla Scuola Medica Salernitana. Naples, 1st Ital Studi Filos 1986, pp 33, 55, 112.
25 Thorndike L: Relation between Byzantine and Western science and pseudo-science before 1350. Janus 1964;51:1–48.

26 Diels HA: Die Handschriften der antiken Ärzte. Leipzig, 1970.
27 Bussemaker C: Traité d'Etienne sur les urines, publié pour la première fois d'après un manuscrit de la Bibliothèque Royale. Revue de Philologie, de Littérature et d'Histoire Anciennes 1845;1:415–438, 543–560.
28 Dimitriadis K: Byzantinische Uroskopie. Dissertation, Bonn, 1971, pp 46–55.
29 Gottshalk L: Die Rezeption der antiken Wissenschaft durch den Islam. Anz Öst Ak Wiss Phil-Hist Kl 1965;102:111–134.
30 Kuzes AP: The apotheraputic of Theophilos according the Laurentian Codex plut. 75, 19. Prakt Akad Athen 1944–48;19:35–54.
31 *Ioannis Actuarii De Urinis*, in Ideler IL (ed): *Physici et Medici Graeci Minores*. Amsterdam, Adolf M Hakkert, 1963.
32 Bertolaso B: La Cattedra *De pulsibus et urinis* (1601–1748). Castalia 1960;3:109–117.
33 Bylebyl JJ: The school of Padua: humanistic medicine in the sixteenth century, in Webster C (ed): Health, Medicine and Mortality in the Sixteenth Century. Cambridge, Cambridge University Press, 1979, p 350.
34 Stoffregen M: Eine frühmittelalterliche Übersetzung des byzantinischen Puls- und Urintraktats des Alexandros: Text-Übersetzung, Kommentar. Dissertation, Berlin, 1977.
35 Jenkins GP: Diagnosis by diagram. The *matulae* disc from Johannes de Ketham's *Fasciculus Medicinae*, 1495. J Lab Clin Med 1989;114:439–440.
36 Stohmaier G: La ricezione e la tradizione: la medicina nel mondo bizantino e arabo, in Grmek MD (ed): Storia del Pensiero Medico Occidentale, l. Antichità e Medioevo. Laterza, Roma-Bari, 1993, pp 167–215.

Am J Nephrol 1994;14:290–294

Juan Riera Palmero

University of Valladolid, Valladolid, Spain

Nephrology from the Middle Ages to Humanism: The Italian Influence in Spain (12th–16th Centuries)

Key Words
Nephrology
Lithiasis
Renaissance
Spain
Anatomopathology

Abstract

The influence of medieval Italian medicine first reached Catalonia via Montpellier. Physicians from Salerno are known to have worked in Aragon, and many Italian medical and surgical texts circulated in Catalonia. By the end of the 15th century it was Valencia that maintained close ties with Italy, and in the 1st third of the 16th century, at the height of Renaissance humanism, the Castilian universities became the greatest Spanish patrons of medicine. Post-Vesalian anatomists were active and many Castilian doctors were educated in Italy. In both medieval and Renaissance Spain the most commonly described renal pathology was lithiasis. The works of Joanes Jacobi (14th century) and Julian Guttierez (15th century) are outstanding, and foreshadow the monograph on lithiasis by Sanchez de Oropesa (16th century) and the work of Francisco Diaz, probably the greatest Spanish contributor to modern nephrology. He devoted 3 books of his collected professional experience to lithiasis, renal ulcers and sores, kidney inflammation and other processes including haematuria. His view of renal anatomy was totally modern, and he strongly advocated autopsy as a means of determining the cause of death. This underlines the new anatomopathological approach to investigation that was adopted in Renaissance Spain.

Introduction

Nephrology throughout the Middle Ages [1–3] and the Renaissance constituted an integrated chapter of medical knowledge, renal lithiasis being the most common process described. Documents on the examination of urine were particularly well known, as uroscopy was the preferred diagnostic approach in internal diseases. Medieval nephrology, deriving from the Arabic influence, began in the Salerno School of Medicine *civitas hippocratica* – the first lay school of medieval medicine whose origins date back to the 10th century. The first translations from Arabic to Latin were made in Salerno by Constantinus Africanus (1015–1087), who is responsible for the translation of the book *De Urinis* by Isaac Judaeus, dedicated entirely to uroscopy. Numerous references to renal pathology are found in *Passionarius Galeni* by the Salerno master Gariopontus, describing the symptoms of renal and vesical calculi, with references to lithotomy. Gariopontus pointed out that stones originate in the kidney, descending towards the inferior urinary paths. Magister Maurus, in his *Regulae Urinarum*, elaborated additional valuable concepts later adopted up by Gilles de Corbeil. Clinical contributions on renal processes can be found in other

Juan R. Palmero
Sanz y Forés, 1,1° Dcha.
E–47003 Valladolid (Spain)

writers from Salerno, e.g. Urso, Mundisanus and Mattaeus Platearius. The most valuable contribution without doubt, can be attributed to Gilles de Corbeil (1165–1213), who although of French origin was trained in Salerno; his poem about urine, *Carmina de Urinarum*, was a milestone in the interpretation of urine examination in medical diagnosis.

Italian Influence in Catalonia

In Spain, the influence of Salerno was evident very early [4, 5], reaching the medieval Catalan doctors through Montpellier. Until the middle of the 13th century, Montpellier maintained a close political relationship with Catalonia, which has persisted in medicine until modern times. It is known that Barcelona had close commercial ties with Genoa and Pisa, which favored the presence in the Kingdom of Aragon of physicians from Salerno, e.g. William of Congenis and John of Procida. The latter was born on an island near Naples early in the 13th century, received his training in Salerno and was doctor to Emperor Frederick II and to King Manfred. Because of the French invasion, he took refuge in the Catalan court of Peter II (the Great) of Aragon. This communication was enriched by the diffusion in Catalonia of texts from Salerno, e.g. *Practica* by Bartholomy of Salerno and the treatise *De Egretudinem Curatione* by John Platearius.

The early conquest of Sicily by Peter II of Aragon intensified cultural relations with Italy, above all between Catalonia and Naples from the 13th century onwards. The Catalan presence in Sardinia dates from the beginning of the 14th century, which explains the abundant documental testimonies of Italian doctors in the court of James II of Aragon, e.g. those of Mascall of Cagliari and Dominic Crix of Naples. The Italian influence reached its climax in the rein of Alfonso V of Aragon, who spent almost his whole life on Italian soil, despite the cost of abandoning his interests in Catalonia and Aragon. Italian influence is evidenced by the circulation in Catalonia of surgical and medical texts, including the *De Mictu Sanguinis* by John of Tornamira and the works of Teodorico de Cervia, Saliceto, Peter of Argelata and Lanfranco, among others.

Towards the end of the 15th century, it was Valencia, the federated kingdom of the Catalan-Aragon crown, that maintained a stronger relationship with Italian medicine, to such a degree that the city itself was the entry point for Italian culture at the end of the 15th century. The Valencian doctor Gaspar Torella (born 1452), educated in

Siena, served Pope Alexander VI in the Roman court; other Valencian doctors, e.g. Pedro Pintot, Pedro Pamar and Geronimo Torella, also worked in Rome.

Italian Influence in Castile

From the 1st third of the 16th century, at the height of Renaissance humanism, the Castilian universities of Salamanca and Alcala de Henares were the most prestigious patrons of medicine, with an obvious influence of Italian humanistic medicine. The progress of anatomy at the University of Padua, based on the work of Andreas Vesalius, promptly produced echoes in Spain, through the post-Vesalian anatomists Pedro Jimeno, Luis Collado and Juan Valverde de Amusco. Their more detailed view of the human body facilitated advances in knowledge of the structure of the urinary apparatus, particularly of renal morphology.

The presence of Castilian doctors in Renaissance Italy was notable: Rodrigo de Reinoso, educated in Italy, taught in Alcala de Henares; Lorenzo Alderete, trained in Bologna, was Full Professor of Medicine in Salamanca. An extensive Castilian colony existed in Rome in the middle of the 16th century, with doctors as prestigious as Valverde de Amusco, Juan Aguilera (papal doctor) and above all Andres Laguna, a converted Jewish Segovian who had studied in Salamanca and Paris and obtained his doctorate in Bologna. Laguna lived in Rome from 1545 to 1554, serving as physician to Popes Paul III and Julius II. Evidently influenced by the Italian Alfonso Ferri, Laguna was the author of an excellent text on urinary tract diseases.

This historical framework explains the beneficial influence that Spain received from Italian medicine, from the early Middle Ages up to the decades of Renaissance humanism, a fruitful scientific influence confirmed by documents on renal pathology and diseases.

Nephrology in Medieval Spain

The most common renal pathology described in medieval Spain was undoubtedly lithiasis, on which a substantial number of scholastic and humanistic medical works focused, as demonstrated by two medieval *consilia*. The 'consiliar' genre, which arose in Italy, reached its maximum expression in the *Consilia Medica* of the Full Professor of Padua, Bartholomy Montagnana. In the Kingdom of Aragon in the 13th century, renal lithiasis was the subject of a valuable contribution by the Catalan doctor Arnau de Vilanova [6] (about 1311), who was born in Valencia, studied in Montpellier and later resided in either Naples or Salerno. Physician to King Peter II of Aragon and to James II, he was a personal friend of the Sicilian King Frederick. Arnau eased the sufferings of Popes Clement V and Boniface VIII. The Renaissance edition of *Opera Omnia* (Lyon, 1509) includes a nephrologic text titled *Tractatus contra Calculum*, 7 chapters long, which is dedicated to Pope Boniface VIII. The first 3 sections deal with general topics, while the last 4 focus on nephrologic areas. Arnau had acquired experience in Montpellier and treated Boniface's renal problems in August of 1301; he had earlier treated Cardinal Benedetto Gaetani when he was in Montpellier in the winter of 1290–91. In other works of Arnau, e.g. *Medicinalium Introductorium Speculum*, he addressed these same renal problems and considered bladder stones: 'as a preternatural disposition of the kidneys which quickly and notably damages their function, producing paroxystic pain'. The descriptions follow the traditional doctrines, which agree with the great treatises of the Bologna and Montpellier schools.

The best document on calculi in 14th century Spain is that of the Catalan doctor Joanes Jacobi [7], who was born in Lerida and later became Chancellor of Montpellier University from 1364 to 1384. He served as physician to kings and popes: he was doctor to Pope Urban V (1362–1370); in Avignon he visited Pope Gregory XI (1370–1378); and he was named doctor to Charles V, King of France, in 1378. Among his works are found *Tractatus de Calculis in Vesica* and a great medical text, *Secretarium Practicae Medicinae*, in which specific chapters deal with renal afflictions.

Medical texts addressing urinary tract diseases circulated throughout the territory of the Castilian crown during the 15th century [8, 9]. Alonso Chirino, doctor to Juan II of Castile, focused on the affliction called 'loin pain', a syndrome that encompassed both renal pain and nephritic colic. Before the end of the 15th century, the Castilian-converted Jewish doctor, Francisco Lopez de Villalobos published the *Sumario de la Medicina* (Salamanca, 1498), dedicating several chapters to the genitourinary system. The greatest contribution to nephrology in Castile in that century however, was *Cura de la Piedra y Dolor de Yjada y Colica Renal* (Toledo, 1498), prepared by Julian Gutierez de Toledo, doctor to the Catholic King and Queen [10]. This clearly written text concerning the urinary tract commences with a book written in Latin, *De Potu in Lapidis Preservatione*. Throughout the text, the *Cura de la Piedra* addresses the genesis of renal and vesical stones, clinical symptoms and diagnosis, and enumerates remedies.

Nephrology in Renaissance Spain

Renaissance humanism [11], the appearance of the printing press and the expansion of the Castilian universities encouraged better understanding of renal diseases. Apart from the works written in the 16th century specifically devoted to genitourinary pathology, treatises on general medicine can also be cited in which particular chapters on renal pathology are found. During the 1st half of the 16th century, renal pathology was addressed in *Remedio de Cuerpos Humanos* (Alcala, 1542) and in *Libro de las Cuatro Enfermedades Cortesanas* (Toledo, 1544), both by Luis Lobera of Avila, physician to Emperor Charles V. Nephrologic subjects are also presented in *Enchiridion Medicinae* (Zaragoza, 1549) by Alfonso Lopez de Corella.

During the 2nd half of the 16th century, medical humanism in Spain reached its apex, a fact which together with the popularity of Vesalian anatomy, favored increased knowledge of renal pathology. The number of medical texts increased, shedding new light on the nephrologic literature of the Renaissance. Among the medical treatises, specific chapters on renal disease were written by the Valencian Full Professor Juan Pascual and his compatriot Pedro Pablo Pereda. The great Castilian doctors of the century, Francisco Valles and Cristobal de Vega, reflected on these themes in their work at the University of Alcala. In Salamanca and Valladolid, the two Full Professors Agustin Vazquez and Luis Mercado are also worth citing.

What was known about renal illnesses in Renaissance Spain? Anatomy was beginning to be known from diffusion of the work of Vesalius. With respect to renal function, although medieval traditionalism was still in force, novel concepts, e.g. contributions to clinical symptomatology and the study of stenosis of the urinary tract, were also embraced. Nephrology formed a concise chapter treated in general medical texts, a topic about which the first monographs were written. Urinary tract surgery also progressed, particularly lithotomy, a technique revived in Italy by Mariano Sancto and disseminated in Spain by the Castilian surgeon Francisco Diaz. Renal pathology included inflammation and *apostemas* or renal tumors, 2 topics addressed by Diego Merino de Uruñuela and Luis Mercado [12]. Of greater importance in nephrology of the Spanish Renaissance were renal spasms and colic, processes which were considered to be different diseases.

Among clinical contributions, Luis Lobera de Avila, in his *Libro de las Cuatro Enfermedades Cortesanas*, established 2 differentiated clinical syndromes: renal colic and intestinal colic.

As in earlier centuries, the most common and thus the most carefully studied renal process in the Renaissance century was lithiasis or renal calculosis. The concept of stone formation followed the traditional doctrine of humors and elements. Incorporating medieval tradition, Luis Lobera de Avila states: 'The material from which the stone is engendered is dry earth mixed with viscous, sticky humidity because the viscous humidity is the cause of the mixing and strong amassing of the parts: and the dry earth part is the cause of the hardening of it all'. He similarly follows Aristotelian criteria in referring to the causes: 'Of these two causes, a material which is the viscous humidity with dry earth, and another efficient which is heat, the stone is engendered in miners as I said: and from the same cause it is formed in the kidneys and bladder.' Lobera describes the clinical symptoms, distinguishing between renal and vesical calculosis, processes for which he offers therapeutic recommendations. He states himself to be against the surgical method of nephrotomy: 'There are some that try to take out the kidney stone opening the patient at the loin or the back: but it is a fearful thing to do so and an operation of men lacking judgement.'

The greatest Spanish contribution to renal lithiasis comes from Francisco Sanchez de Oropesa, author of a valuable monograph on the subject. This monograph stands as an extensive, detailed study of the etiology, diagnosis, prognosis and cure of the morbid process. Sanchez de Oropesa, born in Valladolid and trained in Salamanca, was a disciple of Lorenzo Alderete. His work is of great interest as it compiles numerous clinical histories, including cases that caused the patients' deaths. Among his most valuable new ideas was the recommendation of cadaver dissection in order to ascertain the nature of the fatal disease. It is worth noting that hospitals had to provide facilities for necropsies to discover any internal illnesses. This is one of the first testimonies to the importance placed in the European Renaissance on the search for anatomopathologic lesions in urinary tract diseases. It seems that Sanchez de Oropesa assisted at some necropsies, including those performed by Mena and a medical graduate Salamanca (from Burgos), in which huge vesical stones were found. He cites one clinical case of acute renal failure which resulted in the death of the Bishop of Salamanca, Francisco de Soto, in 1577; after having been administered antimony powder by a doctor, the Bishop suffered acute anuria from which he died. Sanchez also relates the acute intoxication of the Archdeacon of Niebla, Francisco de Montoya, who died on 14 April 1587, from having eaten wild watercress which caused acute anuria.

Work of Francisco Diaz

The culmination of this growing interest in renal pathology in 16th century Spain was undoubtedly achieved in the work of Francisco Diaz, the greatest Spanish contributor to modern nephrology [13, 14]. Born in Burgos, he received his doctorate at the University of Alcala in 1559, though he graduated as a medical student in 1554. He trained at the University of Valencia together with two post-Vesalian anatomists, Luis Collado and Pedro Jimeno, dying in Madrid on 18 April 1590.

The professional experience of Diaz is collected in his *Tratado Nuevamente Impresso de Todas las Enfermedades de los Riñones, Vexiga y Carnosidades de la Verga* (Madrid, 1588). Renal pathology occupies the 1st of the 3 books which make up the *Tratado*. In these 15 chapters Diaz discussed lithiasis, renal ulcers and sores, kidney inflammation and other processes, e.g. hematuria. He began by detailing renal anatomy, in which he gave an excellent, totally modern, description of the kidney. In Diaz's opinion spasms, burning urination, vomiting and urinary tract pain characterized renal lithiasis. He judged the prognosis to be grave, possibly leading to anuria and death, and recommended therapeutic measures and dietetic remedies, completing the treatment with the use of hydrologic resources, e.g. medicinal water from fountains such as Alhama de Aragon, Caldas de Montbuy and Arnedillo, among others.

Diaz described the disease called 'kidney sore', a clinical syndrome of pain in the region affected and urine mixed with 'blood clots', i.e. hematuria. The disease was due to various causes: external factors, e.g. knife or sword wounds; and internal ones, e.g. renal tumors *(apostemas)* or vascular lesions, particularly those of some veins. Diaz reported a case history of this affliction, accompanied by the anatomopathologic necropsy of a patient who must have suffered renal and pulmonary metastatic tumors:

'Juan Velazques, Knight of the Order of Santiago and of the Order Council, very fair male, who having suffered a very severe burning on urination, with grave medical suspect that he had stones, only the medical graduate Ruy Garcia said he did not have stones in the kidney, nor in bladder, and seeing the distention, wished to assist on opening him; and we found in the bladder a sordid and black and malicious sore, [the diagnosis] which the medical student Ruy Garcia and I confessed to having, and not stones, and passing to the very healthy right kidney, but the left had a very hard cancre [cancer] the size of an egg yolk, a thing well forgotten by all. He had the lung damaged, almost totally cavitated and ruined ...'

This succinct quotation (for reasons of space the entire case history cannot be included) gives testimony to the anatomopathologic investigations that were undertaken in Spain throughout the 16th century, and which were the fruit of the influence of Vesalius' new anatomy. In this context, the autopsy references in which Diaz could show lesions of the genitourinary organs after anatomopathologic examination are numerous. One such is the case history and the autopsy performed on Prince Ruigomez of Portugal, in the service of Philip II of Spain. The Prince had suffered urinary problems for over 10 years, which eventually led to anuria and death. After opening the cadaver, Diaz relates, among other comments:

'Continuing with the dissection, we found the kidneys in very bad shape, which seem to have burned him with much inflammation and which fell to pieces upon only touching them with the tweezer.'

This paper has been restricted to the study of renal processes, omitting the important contribution of Spanish surgeons to urology in the Renaissance and the topic of ureteral stenosis (the so-called *carnosidades*), an area in which numerous Spanish doctors and surgeons worked in the Renaissance. Both of these fields are large and require discussions dedicated exclusively to them, and hence lie outside the scope of the present paper.

References

1 Balleger E (ed): History of Urology. Baltimore, 1933.
2 Kuss R, Gregoire W: Histoire Illustrée de l'Urologie de l'Antiquité à Nos Jours. Paris, Roger Dacosta, 1988.
3 Murphy LTJ: The History of Urology. Springfield, Illinois, C Thomas, 1972.
4 Planas AC: Historia de la Medicina a la Corona d'Aragó (1162–1479). Barcelona, Edit. Scientia, 1973.
5 Granjel LS: La Medicina Española Antigua y Medieval. Salamanca, Universidad, 1981.
6 Granjel LS: Retablo Histórico de la Urología Española. Salamanca, Instituto de Historia de la Medicina, 1986.

7 Ballester LG: El tratado del 'mal de la piedra'de Joan Jacme (siglo XIV), in Actas del Segundo Congreso Español de Historia de la Medicina. Salamanca, 1966, vol 1, pp 93–102.
8 Palmero JR: La urologia española en los textos medicos del Renacimiento, in Actas del Segundo Congreso Español de Historia de la Medicina. Salamanca, 1966, vol 1, pp 113–128.
9 Palmero JR: Historia de la urologia española, in Actas del Segundo Congreso Español de Historia de la Medicina. Salamanca, 1966, vol 1, pp 47–61.

10 Sancho de San Roman R: La Obra Urologica de Julian Gutierrez de Toledo. Lisbon, Imprensa Medica, 1958, vol 12, 236–246.
11 Granjel LS, Palmero JR: Medicina y sociedad en la España Renacentista, in Lain Entralgo P (ed): Historia Universal de la Medicina. Madrid, Salvat, 1973, vol 4: 181–189.
12 Juan Riera Palmero: Vida y obra de Luis Mercado. Salamanca, Universidad, 1968.
13 Palmero JR: La obra urologica de Francisco Diaz, in Cuadernos de Historia de la Medicina Española. Salamanca, 1967, vol 4, 77–128.14
14 Palmero JR: Cirujanos, Urólogos y Algebristas del Renacimiento y Barroco. Valladolid, Universidad, 1990.

Am J Nephrol 1994;14:295–301

Ellen L.P. Chan[a]
Tahir Masood Ahmed[b]
Marian Wang[c]
James C.M. Chan[d]

[a] Summer Fellow, Bowdoin College, Brunswick, Me., USA;
[b] MCV/VCU Visiting Professor, Postgraduate Medical Institute, Lahore, Pakistan;
[c] MCV/VCU Visiting Professor, University of Georgia, Athens, Ga.,
[d] Nephrology Division, Children's Medical Center, Virginia Commonwealth University's Medical College of Virginia, Richmond, Va., USA

History of Medicine and Nephrology in Asia

Key Words
Asia
China
Daoism
Alchemy
Ancient medicine
Nephrology

Abstract

The beginning of Chinese medicine has been attributed to 3 mythical emperors who gathered herbs for medicines. During the 2nd century BC, Han dynasty physicians developed cranial trephining and sedation with wine and herbs for anesthesia. Chiang Chung-Ching (142–212 AD) used the appearance of rashes in diagnosis, treated infections with anthelmintics and asthma with ephedra, described the symptoms of diabetes mellitus and expanded medical ethics. The specialties of obstetrics, pediatrics, ophthalmology and dentistry were described in the records of the Han and Tang dynasties, and methods of setting fractures and treating trauma were comparable with those of Roman military doctors. Shen Tua (1031–1095 AD) compiled a pharmacopeia and studied acupuncture and the pulses. Forensic medicine was developed during the 10th century by Sung Tse, who also advocated hand washing with sulfur and vinegar to avoid infection during autopsies. The Daoist physicians used androgens and estrogens to treat hypogonadism with therapeutic preparations of placentas. They also had an advanced knowledge of alchemy, claiming to achieve 'immortality' by their preservation techniques. Qualifying examinations for physicians were conducted by the Chinese state as early as the 1st century AD, and later incorporated philosophy and art to conform with the Confucian ideal. Throughout these eras, Chinese medicine profited from contact with western Asia. In ancient Chinese medicine, the excretory function of the kidney was attributed to the bladder. 'Kidney weakness', which refers to somatized depression, was treated by acupuncture along the 'kidney channel'. Pulse examination was also used to give a measure of the imbalance of renal Yin and Yang. The association of hardening of the arteries with high salt intake described in the 3rd century BC may be the earliest reference to nephrology; other references include acupuncture points related to the kidney and the castration procedure used in the Imperial Court. After the great voyages of Admiral Cheng Ho, which encompassed searches for new medicinal herbs and minerals, both industry and scientific pursuit declined and were eclipsed by the West.

James C.M. Chan, MD
Nephrology Division, Children's Medical Center
Virginia Commonwealth University's Medical College
1101 E Marshall Street, Box 498
Richmond, VA 23298-0498 (USA)

© 1994 S. Karger AG, Basel
0250-8095/94/0146-0295
$8.00/0

Introduction

With increasing interest in Asian culture, including 'alternative medicine' and with the rising importance of world commerce centered around the Pacific rim, it seems important and timely that we should begin to acquire a better knowledge of the history that molded medicine in this part of the world. For those who have lived in the region sometimes referred to as the Far East, it is home and it is neither 'far' nor 'remote', terms commonly used in the past to describe this part of the world. In fact, according to Asian experts, 'Far East' is an antiquated description and should be updated to 'East Asia'.

To the ancient Greeks, the land mass east of the Mediterranean had always been known as Asia Minor or simply the Orient. Today, it is probably a better geographic concept to refer to Asia Minor and the Middle East as 'West Asia' with the Himalaya and Tien Shan mountains as the divide between East and West Asia. To cover the history of medicine and nephrology in East and West Asia is an impossible task in a single article of this length. In terms of population, social organization and importance, ancient China is like the histories and influences of ancient Mesopotamia, Egypt, Persia, Greece, and Rome all rolled into one. Thus, this article will briefly comment on Chinese medical history with anecdotes and descriptions of medical exchanges that occurred between East and West Asia throughout history, particularly during the exciting age of the great ocean explorations of the 15th century, and the lessons that can be learned from such history.

Mythical Gods of Medicine

Verifiable Chinese history began with the Shang dynasty, but a previous dynasty named Hsia dating back to the 30th century BC (table 1) can be deduced from the records in the oracle bones and the royal tombs. The beginning of Chinese medicine has been attributed to 3 mythical emperors in the prehistoric period before the Hsia dynasty. These emperors, possibly a composite of several prehistoric characters, were reported to have gathered herbs for medicinal use.

The last of these prehistoric emperors, Huang Ti of the Hsia dynasty (table 1) was supposed to be the author of the medical classic Ney-Ching, which consisted of an exchange of questions and answers on health and diseases between Huang Ti and his ministers. Because there was a Confucian ideal of not taking credit for oneself but to attribute one's achievements to some other person, particularly ancient sages, it is not surprising that modern investigative scholars have since established that the Ney-Ching was actually written during the Han dynasty and was attributed retrospectively to the mythical Yellow Emperor, Huang Ti [1–5].

Medicine in Ancient China

According to Ssuma Chhien (145–?87 BC), possibly China's greatest historian, Han dynasty physicians of the 2nd century BC no longer practised magicoreligious medicine [6]. They relied on the medical history, physical examination of the patient and integration of the results of previous examinations with more current examinations for the formulation of a therapeutic strategy [6]. The theoretic premise of health founded on the equilibrium in the '5 elements' [5] and the balance between the Yin and Yang may not be based on quantifiable science, but the empiric observations, the categorization and correlations with past clinical experiences, and the deductive intellect employed for diagnosis and treatment were surprisingly contemporary.

The Han dynasty was one of the golden periods of Chinese civilization. During the Han dynasty of the 1st century AD (table 1), the invention of trephining of the cranium for release of intracranial pressure was attributed to Hua To (about 141–207 AD). Sedation with wine and herbs was used as anesthesia at this time. In later years, a cluster of legends grew around Hua To, who was worshipped as the Sage of Surgery [2]. According to the popular historical novel, the Romance of the Three Kingdoms, the paramount war lord of that period consulted him about a recurrent headache. Hua To's recommendation for trephining was wrongly taken as an assassination attempt and he was imprisoned for treason. Hua To's wife was so agitated by his imprisonment that she burned his surgical treatise, thus destroying his teachings. Surgery, which had had an early start, went into decline and was lost as an art of traditional Chinese medicine. In recent times, when missionary surgeons began operative removal of tumors in modern China, traditional medical doctors were filled with admiration, yet they also felt a sense of loss of their surgical heritage.

The legend recounted in the Romance of the Three Kingdoms and the accomplishments of Hua To were propagated in Japan, Vietnam, Korea and other Asian countries. This novel was based on historical events of the 2nd century, though it first appeared in the time of the

Table 1. Chronology of Chinese dynasties and medical personnel from ancient to modern times in comparison with events in Europe

	China		Europe, Asia Minor and Africa
30th–11th centuries BC	Hsia 夏 and Shang 商 dynasties	Oracle bones Fu Hsi 伏羲 She Nuy 神農 Huang Ti 黄帝 (about 2600 BC)	Phrygians migrated to Asia Minor Amenhotep IV of Egypt built Amarna Tutankhamun reinstated earlier deities Seti I, Ramses II and III built Memphis Israelites led by Moses left Egypt about 1240 BC
11th century BC to 249 BC	Chou 周 dynasty	*Ney-Ching* 易經 *(Book of Medicine)* Tsang Kung 倉公	The *Iliad* and *Odyssey* ascribed to Homer Hippocrates (460–370 BC)
221–206 BC	Chin 秦 dynasty	The 1st emperor, built the Great Wall	2nd Punic War
206 BC to 220 AD	Han 漢 dynasty	Chang Chung-Ching 張仲景 (Sage of Medicine) used ephedra to treat asthma Chun Yu Yen 淳于意 1st female obstetrician	3rd Punic War Asia Minor became 8th Roman province Venus de Milo carved Julius Caesar Augustus Caesar (27 BC to 14 AD)
220–280 AD	The Three 三國 Kingdoms	Hua To 華陀 (Sage of Surgery) Huang-Fu Mi 皇甫謐 pioneer in acupuncture	Goths invaded Asia Minor and Balkan peninsula
618–907 AD	Tang 唐 dynasty	Sun Szu-Miao 孫思邈 used seaweed for goiter, liver for blindness, beans for beriberi 'Silver paste'	The Hegira (Muhammed's flight from Mecca to Medina) Building of the Dome of the Rock, Jerusalem Charlemagne (768–814 AD) crowned 1st Holy Roman Emperor
960–1279 AD	Sung 宋 dynasty	Shen Kua 沈括 Tsien I 錢乙 1st pediatrician Sung Tse 宋慈 medical jurisprudence	Hospice of St Bernard, Switzerland Epidemic of St Vitus' dance El Cid of Spain St Mark's, Venice, completed
1206–1368 AD	Yuan 元 dynasty		Florence became leading city in commerce 'Pied Piper of Hamelin' Marco Polo's travels
1368–1644 AD	Ming 明 dynasty	Admiral Cheng Ho 鄭和 Li Shih Cheu 李時珍 encyclopedia of herbal medicine	Leonardo da Vinci Copernicus Gutenberg (1440 AD) Columbus' voyage (1492 AD) Ambroise Paré, French surgeon Vesalius, Dutch physician Brunfels, German botanist William Harvey
1644–1911 AD	Ching 清 dynasty	Wang Tsing-jen 王清任 reinterpretation of the medical classics	The plague 'Silver paste' Regnart (1818) Tavean (1837)

Yuan dynasty in the 13th century AD and underwent unknown numbers of revisions until its final form in the 16th century [7]. Reading it continues to be de rigueur for contemporary young people in China, Japan and other Asian countries, an uncommon phenomena for an old historical novel.

Chiang Chung-Ching (about 142–212 AD) of the Han dynasty, regarded throughout Chinese history as one of the country's great physicians, used the appearance and distribution of rashes to diagnose infectious diseases. He experimented with the treatment of parasitic infections using anthelmintics, treated asthma with ephedra (a green shrub containing ephedrine), categorized the symptoms of diabetes mellitus [2] and expanded on medical ethics.

Specialties of medicine, e.g. obstetrics, pediatrics, ophthalmology and dentistry, were described in the medical records of the Han and Tang dynasties [2, 6]. Military medicine of the Han dynasty prescribed methods of setting fractures and treating trauma which were as detailed as those found in the military manuals of Roman legions [6].

After the Han dynasty, however, China went into a period of chaos lasting 3 centuries, until it was reunited under the Tang dynasty, which ushered in another golden period of peace, prosperity and innovation. During the Tang dynasty lived one of the great doctors of China, Sun Szu-Miao (581–682 AD). He considered pulmonary tuberculosis a contagious disease brought about by microorganisms which invaded the lung, and he also described tumors of bone, adipose and vascular origins. He rejected appointment to the Imperial Court, and during his later years chose to live the life of a Daoist hermit in the high mountains. He was reputed to become 'immortal' because his body did not undergo decay after his death [1]. For a long time, this art of 'preserving the body frame after the spirit has left' was regarded by Western-trained scientists as a Daoist myth [1, 3]. Recent excavations and studies, however, provide a scientific basis for this Daoist alchemy [1], which will be discussed later in this presentation.

The Tang dynasty ended after 300 years and was succeeded by the Sung dynasty (table 1). Shen Kua (about 1031–1095 AD) of the Sung dynasty was commemorated throughout Chinese history as the compiler of a pharmacopeia and an advocate of studies on acupuncture and pulse [2]. According to the historian Ssuma Chhien [6], acupuncture was already practised at the time of Confucius. Modern scholars speculate that acupuncture originated through empiric observations during ancient warfare, when certain arrow punctures presumably resulted in anesthesia to specific parts of the body. (Physicians applying Western methods in modern times seem to believe that acupuncture anesthesia may be attributed to central nervous system endorphin released by the twirling acupuncture needle). Through further studies, acupuncture points presumably linked to specific internal organs were developed. Acupuncture needles were inserted into these points to regain balance of the Yin and Yang in the treatment of liver cirrhosis, gout, hearing loss, arthralgia and other diseases. Based on the conviction that each internal organ gave rise to its characteristic pulse, detectable by pulse reading (sphygmology) at specific points of the body, Shen Kua and other ancient Chinese physicians diagnosed multiple systemic diseases from studies of the pulses. Later, the study of the pulses developed into a major part of Tibetan medicine [4, 5]. Treatments with moxibustion and massage points [2] have also been used since the end of the Han dynasty (table 1) and continue to be practised in the rural areas of China as well as other parts of Asia.

Forensic medicine was developed during the Sung dynasty of the 10th century by Sung Tse (about 1186–1249 AD). He used the degree of rigor mortis to determine the time of death [8] and also advocated hand washing with sulfur and vinegar during and after the post-mortem examination to prevent the risk of infection to the examining physician [8]. He examined stomach contents in cases of poisoning and supposedly used a method of blood analysis to settle paternity disputes [8].

China had extensive libraries after typeset printing became available in the 11th century [1]. Books such as pharmacologic encyclopedias and medical treatises were widely available through these libraries, permitting physicians in China to be well versed in the literature. This printing innovation was not developed in Europe until 1440, when Gutenberg's movable press came into existence. The wide dissemination of knowledge generated by this printing technology gave momentum to the Renaissance in Europe. The equivalent of a Renaissance did not occur in China, however, and the reasons for such a difference in development between East and West remain the subject of keen interest and debate among modern historians [1].

Administration and Organization of Ancient Chinese Medicine

It may come as a surprise to many that there are records of qualifying examinations for medical practitioners [6] conducted by the state as early as the Han dynasty in the 1st century AD. By the Tang dynasty of the 7th century AD, the qualifying examinations for physicians consisted not only of diagnosis and knowledge of the pharmacopeia, but also of philosophy and art in order to conform with Confucian ideals of the physician as a scholar and to maintain the high regard in which physicians were held in Chinese society [6]. An Imperial Medical College was founded in the decade of 620–630 AD to award medical degrees to qualified medical students [6]. In the 9th century, Arabic visitors to Tang dynasty China recorded that there was an imperial edict for establishing a ratio of 20 medical students per 100, 000 families in every provincial city [6]. With the ascent of Buddhism in China during the Tang dynasty, hospital organization became a fusion of Confucian, Daoist and Buddhist philosophies. By the 10th century, Arab–Chinese contacts of the preceding 2 centuries had given rise to similar medical qualifying examinations in Baghdad [6].

Nephrology in Ancient China

The excretory function of the kidney was attributed to the bladder in ancient Chinese medicine. The kidneys were thought to be the site of *qi* (the force of life) [9]. Semen was thought to be stored in the kidney and the excessive loss of this 'life force' was thought to lead to an imbalance of the Yin and Yang, resulting in the development of neurasthenic symptoms, including lack of energy and depression.

It was also the theoretic premise of ancient Chinese medicine that 'kidney weakness' could be treated by acupuncture of the specific points along the 'kidney channel' [5] to re-establish the balance of renal Yin and Yang. Because it was thought that each internal organ gave rise to different pulses at specific points of the cardiovascular system, pulse examination provided a diagnosis of an imbalance of the kidney Yin and Yang. It should be recognized, however, that the points of reference are very different between modern Western medicine and medical terms based on ancient Chinese medicine. 'Kidney weakness' describes somatized depression [10], not the Western concept of chronic renal insufficiency. Western-trained physicians in their interactions with Asian patients need to become aware of such nuances of cultural difference.

The association of hardening of the arterial pulses and high salt intake [11] described in the 3rd century BC may have been the first references to nephrology in medical history. Other early references to nephrology include acupuncture points in relation to the kidney [2, 5] and the castration procedure used in the imperial court [1, 2]. After castration, a silver catheter was inserted into the urethra to prevent closure. The postoperative mortality rate resulting from infection was high [12].

Search for the Elixir of Youth and the Great Naval Expeditions of the Ming Dynasty

One of the most famous eunuchs in Chinese history was Admiral Cheng Ho, who led China's great naval expeditions in the 15th century. These 7 ocean voyages over 28 years, from 1405 to 1433 AD, rivaled the European global explorations several decades later [1, 13]. The saga of Admiral Cheng Ho and the organization of his grand armada, a force of over 37,000 men and 62 great ships, several of which were 400 feet long and displaced over 1,500 tons [1, 13], was a compelling story. In comparison, the contemporary European ships were much smaller. For example, in 1497 AD, none of Vasco da Gama's Portuguese ships, which sailed around Africa's Cape of Good Hope to India, displaced even 300 tons [1]. It was customary in the 15th century that youthful prisoners of war were castrated and those who did not die from the postoperative infections may be sent to the capital [14] to join the imperial corps of eunuchs, and sometimes, if they were fortunate, be appointed to positions of influence that could benefit the other family members. It was in this way that Cheng Ho served as a eunuch in the Ming court (table 1) and rose to a position of importance.

Admiral Cheng Ho [1] was able to win the approval of the Ming emperor for 7 long expeditions into the Indian Ocean. These expeditions were very different from those of the European voyages of discovery later in the century. These Chinese naval voyages were not expeditions of colonization, but were carried out under the aegis of gathering tribute from adjacent countries to glorify the Imperial Court. Recent scholars have established that these 'tribute-bearing' expeditions were actually state missions of trade. Whatever the Imperial Court received as 'tribute', Chinese products of equal value were returned. Cheng Ho, most of his officers and many of the sailors of the Grand Fleet were Moslems; thus, they made an expedition to Mecca in present day Saudi Arabia. They sailed also in the quest for medical herbs for the elixir of youth to ensure the Emperor's longevity. The Grand Fleet of the Ming dynasty probably had an additional purpose similar to that of the Great White Fleet sent around the world by President Roosevelt: a pronouncement of how a great nation saw itself and how it wanted to be seen by the rest of the world.

Of medical interest is the record that a complement of 180 medical officers sailed with Cheng Ho's fleet [1]. The ratio of 1 physician to 200 sailors was sufficiently high to suggest that a number of these physicians must have been scientific investigators searching for new medications. The 14th century was a time of serious epidemics, both in Europe (the Black Death) and China (bubonic and pneumonic plague). The search for new medicinal plants and minerals may have been another compelling reason for these voyages and the presence of so many physicians. Presumably, they must also have known how to prevent scurvy [1] on these long ocean voyages.

Conflicts continually recurred with the Confucian bureaucrats who objected to the large naval expenditures. After the death of the Emperor who supported these navigational exploits, the dockyards of Nanking, which had built these ships, were allowed to fall into decay [1]. This is a reflection of the attitude of the ruling class in China throughout history [1], which was directed towards development within the country, seeking inspiration from the Confucian classics and eschewing new knowledge and trade that could be gained by further exploration of the world.

China had a level of scientific and navigational skills during the Ming dynasty well ahead of western Europe in the early 15th century. It became eclipsed over the next 400 years by the European countries in their vigorous and persistent explorations. Was this the result of an inward turning of a nation [1] or the result of imperial over-reach [13]? Another example of this tremendous decline in productivity can be found in the iron ore industry of China. In the 11th century, China was manufacturing 125,000 tons of iron/year [13]. This level of iron production was not reached in western Europe until the later stages of the Industrial Revolution 7 centuries later, when England produced an equal tonnage [13]. By the 1700s, the iron works of Honan and Hopei in China were derelict [13]. The development of new medications also declined in East Asia despite the tremendous achievement of earlier times. Was this decline the culmination of imperial over-reach, or due to a lack of vision of the potential of international commerce or the natural rise and fall of great empires? These questions continue to perplex historians.

Finally, the lesson that can be learned from the inward turning of the Ming dynasty has a parallel in today's world. If we are to turn away from scientific investigations, and if we increasingly cut back on biomedical research efforts, this may be akin to the Ming dynasty's closing of ocean explorations. The entire state funding of the 7 ocean-going voyages of the Ming dynasty parallels the National Institutes of Health funding of medical research in the USA. If the linchpin is significantly reduced or removed, the whole enterprise may collapse. In the resetting of national priorities, particularly in such a fast-moving world, the long-term interests of a nation in maintaining its leading position in biologic research are compelling.

Early Contacts between East and West Asia

The astonishing surgical procedures of Hua To (141–207 AD) during the Han dynasty, including the cranial trephining described earlier, may have been influenced by Indian techniques [2]. The surgical skills in ancient India were extraordinary. Under deep anesthesia with *Cannabis sativa,* thoracotomy, cranial trephining, laparotomy and cataract operations were performed by Susrata (about 500 BC) and other Indian surgeons of antiquity [2].

In the early part of the 5th century AD, leprosariums were described as part of renowned hospitals in India, Persia and Baghdad [6]. In the 6th century AD, China learned from these experiences by contacts established through the Silk Road [2], and at this time, leprosariums began to appear in official Chinese history.

Quarantine for epidemic diseases, including imperial edicts barring officials from families with presumed infectious diseases from attending the Chinese Imperial Court for 100 days, was recorded [6] as early as the 6th century AD.

The hospitals in Iran in the 14th century under Rashid al-Din of Hamadan, Shiraz and Tabrig employed physicians from China, Syria and Arabia [1]. Considerable interchange between Iranian, Arabic and Turkish medical personnel took place during the Pax Mongolica of Genghis Khan and Kublai Khan [2].

In Vietnam, traditional medicine followed that of the Chinese pattern [2], and there was considerable resistance when Western medicine was introduced in the 19th century.

Daoist Alchemy and Its Modern Assessment

It was remarkable that Daoist physicians in the Sung dynasty (11th century AD) described the use of preparations of androgens and estrogens in purified and crystal-

Chan/Ahmed/Wang/Chan

line form in the treatment of hypogonadism [6]. The striking therapeutic use of human and animal placentas was recorded as early as the 8th century AD under the Tang dynasty and came into more common practice after the 14th century Ming dynasty. The extraction and use of sex hormones from urine [6] reported during the Ming dynasty is another extraordinarily early example of awareness of the influence of a subject's age and the need for separation of urine collection by sex.

As mentioned earlier, the Daoists had an advanced knowledge of alchemy [3]: in a recent discovery of the Lady of Tai who died 2000 years ago, laboratory examinations in China showed that there was still elasticity in her epidermal tissues [1]. There was no evidence of freezing, mummification, embalming, or tanning, but the tissue content of arsenic was high. In addition, she was entombed in an airtight and watertight coffin, her body encased with mercuric sulfide, and the coffin was surrounded by lime and charcoal [1]. These findings suggest that the level of understanding of tissue preservation by the Daoist alchemists were more advanced than previously assumed [1]. Sun Szu-Miao of the Tang dynasty (table 1), who gave up an Imperial Court appointment to practise Daoism [3], was known to have spent the remaining years of his long life in the high mountains where he experimented with arsenic elixirs because of the belief that this provided energy and led to preservation of the body [1]. He also aspired to the Daoist practice of a very restricted diet of pine resin and cypress cone. It is therefore possible that the tissues of his dead body contained arsenic levels high enough to poison bacteria, and it did not decompose because of the cold and dryness found in the high altitudes of the mountains [1]. These factors, coupled with the special diet [1] previously mentioned, resulted in 'immortality'.

Acknowledgements

The authors wish to thank C.Y. Lin, and Jin-Yao Lin (Taipei, Taiwan, Republic of China), S.K. Lam and John T.M. Chan (Hong Kong), Jonathan Spence (New Haven, Conn., USA), Joe Sung, H.S. Hsu and Kay Latta (Richmond, Va., USA) for helpful criticism of the manuscript and Betty Timozek and Linda L. Benson for secretarial and manuscript assistance.

References

1 Needham J: Science and Civilization in China. Cambridge, Cambridge University Press, 1961, vol 1; 1971, vol 4; 1974, vol 5.

2 Huard P, Wong M: Chinese Medicine. New York, World University Library, McGraw-Hill, 1968.

3 Yoon EJ: Daoism and the quest for immortality. Pharos 1991;54:30–33.

4 Matsumoto K, Birch S: Five elements and 10 stems. Brookline, Massachusetts, Paradigm Publishing, 1983, pp 236.

5 Maciocia G: The Foundations of Chinese Medicine: a Comprehensive Text for Acupuncture and Herbalists. Edinburgh, Churchill Livingstone, 1989.

6 Needham J, Lu GD: Chinese medicine, in Poynter FNL (ed): Medicine and Culture. Crewe, UK, Wellcome Institute of the History of Medicine/Frank Cottrell, 1969.

7 Latourette HS: The Chinese. Their History and Culture, 4th ed. New York, MacMillan, 1964, pp 221.

8 Chen CY: History of Chinese Medical Science. Hong Kong, Shanghai Press, 1968, pp 131.

9 Porkett M: The Theoretical Foundations of Chinese Medicine: Systems of Correspondence. Cambridge, Massachusetts, MIT Press, 1974, pp 1–368.

10 Kleinman A: Social Origins of Distress and Disease. New Haven, Connecticut, Yale University Press, 1986, pp 1–264.

11 Feld LG, Springate JE, Izzo JC Jr: Special considerations in hypertension, in Chan JCM, Gill JR Jr (eds): Kidney Electrolyte Disorders. New York, Churchill Livingstone, 1990, pp 565–599.

12 Wong KC, Wu LT: History of Chinese Medicine. New York, AMS Press, 1973.

13 Kennedy PM: The Rise and Fall of the Great Powers. New York, Random House, 1987, pp 6–9.

14 Levathes L: When China ruled the sea: The treasure fleet of the dragon throne 1405–1433. New York, Simon & Schuster, 1994, pp 1–252. Note: Cheng Ho (conventional Wade Giles system) = Zheng He (official pinyin system of the PR of China).

Early Contributors to Nephrology

Am J Nephrol 1994;14:302–306

The Aristotelian Kidney

Paolo Marandola[a]
Sergio Musitelli[b]
Hussein Jallous[a]
Alberto Speroni[a]
Tomaso de Bastiani[a]

[a] Scuola di Specializzazione in Urologia,
  Università degli Studi di Pavia, Pavia,
[a] Storico della Scienza, Milan, Italy

Key Words
Aristotle
Renal function
Renal structure
Urine formation

Abstract
Aristotle incorrectly observed the absence of the kidney in fish and birds and deduced that it was not essential for the existence of a living organism. This underlies his observations on structure and function of the kidney. From examination of rhesus monkeys he generalized that the right kidney is higher than the left. Aristotle did not consider that the renal pelvis is divided by a filter membrane into 2 chambers, and wrote that no blood reaches the renal pelvis. The theory of the 'filter kidney' cannot thus be attributed to Aristotle. The function of the kidney was described as being to separate the surplus liquid from the blood inside the renal meat (not in the renal pelvis) and to transform this liquid into what Aristotle called *residuum,* i.e. the urine. Aristotle also considered that the kidneys acted to anchor the blood vessels to the body. He only briefly considered renal pathology.

Introduction

Before examining the Aristotelian kidney, two explanatory notes are necessary. The first concerns the chronologic aspect. Aristotle refers to the kidney in 2 of his works: *Historia Animalium* (*Historia* meaning research) and *De Partibus Animalium* (*partes* meaning tissues and organs). Although it is difficult to date the zoologic and biologic works of Aristotle through historical and phylologic studies, it has been possible to establish that the 1st work was written between 347 BC and 343 BC [1, 2] and the 2nd between 335 BC and 330 BC [3–6]. This explains why, in the 2nd work, Aristotle frequently refers to his 1st. This, however, does not happen when Aristotle deals with the kidney. In fact, instead of simply referring to his 1st work he provides a novel consideration of it. This lack of interest towards the kidney in the 1st work *(Historia Animalium)* is explained by Aristotle himself, who says:

'The kidneys are not present for necessity in animals but have the functions of perfecting the animal itself.'

De Partibus III, 7, 670b, 23, 24

Aristotle did not consider the kidney worthy of any particular attention.

The second explanation necessary concerns what Aristotle intends when he says: 'not present for necessity'. It must be remembered that Aristotle followed the vitalistic theory, which dominated until the 17th century. This theory is characterized by 2 components, the first being the finalistic approach – if a function must be performed nature will provide the appropriate organ – and the sec-

Paolo Marandola, MD
Scuola di Specializzazione in Urologia
Università degli Studi di Pavia
I–27100 Pavia (Italy)

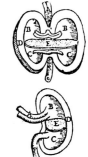

Fig. 1. The 'filter kidney' of Aristotle as represented by Andreas Vesalius.

ond component being that of 'necessity' – nature is forced to make the ultimate choice which is limited by the primary substance at her disposition. Aristotle incorrectly observed the absence of the kidney in certain animals (fish and birds, where the kidneys according to Aristotle are substituted by a mass of residual tissue) and therefore deduced that the kidneys are not essential for the existence of a living organism.

Aristotelian Renal Structure

Renal structure as described by Aristotle can now be analyzed. First, he says:

'The kidneys lie close beside the backbone, and resemble those of oxen. In all animals which have kidneys, the right one is placed higher than the left; it also contains less fat and is drier – this is so in all other animals too.' *Historia Animalium* I, 17, 496b–497a

The incorrect observation of the right kidney located higher in the abdomen than the left kidney is due to the fact that the studies were performed on rhesus monkeys, which do show this characteristic [7, 8].

Aristotle then examines the blood supply to the kidney:

'Passages lead to the kidneys both from the great blood vessel and from the aorta, though they do not lead into the cavity. I have not so far mentioned this cavity in the middle of the kidney. In some animals it is larger, in others smaller; but there is none in the seal's kidneys. These are similar to those of oxen and are more solid than those of all other animals. The passages which lead to the kidneys peter out in the mass of the kidneys themselves. That they do not continue

through the kidneys is shown by the fact that they contain no blood, nor does it congeal in them. (They contain, however, as has been said, a small cavity). From the cavity of the kidneys two sturdy passages lead into the bladder, and other strong continuous ones come from the aorta.' *Historia Animalium* I, 17, 496b–497a

The first two vessels to which Aristotle refers are the ureters, the last ones are the spermatic arteries. Aristotle then continues:

'To the middle of each kidney is attached a hollow and sinewy blood vessel, which extends alongside the back bone to the narrow regions; after that these blood vessels disappear into either loin, and then reappear extending to the loin. These branches from the small blood vessels go as far as the bladder.'

So far 2 important facts have emerged: first, the renal pelvis is not divided by a filter membrane into a lower and an upper chamber; secondly, no blood reaches the renal pelvis. The theory of the 'filter kidney' later to be ridiculed by Andreas Vesalius (fig. 1) cannot therefore be attributed to Aristotle.

The above facts are reconfirmed in Aristotle's second work:

'Kidneys are present in some animals, but not of necessity. They are present to serve a good purpose; that is to say, the particular nature enables them to cope with the *residuum* which collects in the bladder, in those cases where this deposit is somewhat abandoned, and to help the bladder to perform its function better.'
De Partibus Animalium III, 7, 670b

At this point an interesting observation on the relationship between the kidney and the bladder follows:

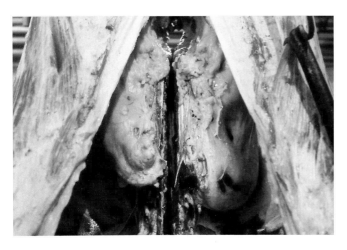

Fig. 2. The kidneys of an ox. Note that the right kidney is higher than the left and both kidneys are surrounded by a thick layer of perirenal fat.

'The bladder is not present in all animals. Nature seems to have intended only those animal which have blood in their lung to have a bladder. And this is quite reasonable, when we remember that such animals have an excess of the natural substance which constitutes the lung and are therefore more subject to thirst than any others, i.e. they need a larger amount of fluid food as well as of the ordinary solid food, and the necessary result of this is that a larger amount of residue also is produced, too large in fact for all of it to be concocted by the stomach and excreted with its own proper residue; hence it is necessary to have some parts that will receive this additional residue. This shows us why all animals which have blood in their lung possess a bladder too.' *De Partibus Animalium* III, 7, 670b–671a

It can be deduced from the above passage that the bladder has a passive function of collecting urine which will then be eliminated via the urethra. This deduction is reconfirmed:

'But, as I said before, all the other animals whose lung contains blood have kidneys, since nature makes use of them for two purposes (1) to subserve the blood vessel; and (2) to excrete the fluid residue (a channel leads into them from the great blood vessel.' *De Partibus Animalium* III, 7, 671a–671b

Aristotelian Renal Function

Aristotle attributes 2 functions to the kidney. The first is the anchoring of the blood vessels to the body:

'The viscera which are below the diaphragm are all of them present for the sake of the blood vessel, in order that the latter may have freedom of carriage and at the same time be attached to the body by means of the viscera, which act as a bond. Indeed, there are, as it were, anchor-lines thrown out to the body through the extended

parts: e.g. from the great blood vessel to the liver and to the spleen, for these viscera act, as it were, like rivets and fasten it to the body; that is to say, the liver and the spleen fasten the great blood vessel to the sides of the body, while the kidneys fasten it to the rear parts.' *De Partibus Animalium* III, 7, 670a, 10ss

The second and most important function is the secretion of residual fluid:

'... and to the kidneys – to each of them – there is a blood vessel passing not only from the great blood vessel, but also from the aorta. These advantages, then, accrue to the animal organisms from the lower viscera. Liver and spleen also assist in the concoction of the food, since they both have blood in them and so are hot. The kidneys assist in connection with the *residuum* which is excreted into the bladder.' (ibid.)

Aristotle then states that the kidney does not depend on the bladder, but that the contrary is true [9, 10]:

'There is always a hollow [lumen], varying in size, in the kidneys, except in the seal, whose kidneys are more solid than any others and in shape resemble those of oxen Human kidneys too resemble those of the ox: they are, as it were, made up of a number of small kidneys, and have not an even surface like those of the sheep and other quadrupeds.' (ibid.)

It is necessary to clarify that the anatomic studies by Aristotle were evidently performed on the kidneys of aborted fetuses, which are divided into several lobes (figs. 2–4), a view confirmed in *Historia Animalium* VII, 3, 583b. Aristotle continues:

'... thus when once an ailment attacks the human kidneys, the trouble is not easily removed, because it is as though the patient had many kidneys diseased and not only one; and so the cure is more difficult to effect. The channel which runs from the great blood vessel to the kidney does not debouch into the hollow part of the kidneys, but the whole of what it supplies is spent upon the body of the kidneys; thus no blood goes into the hollows, and at death none congeals there. From the hollow part of the kidneys two sturdy channels lead into the bladder, one from each; these contain no blood. Other channels come from the aorta to the kidneys; these are strong, continuous ones. This arrangement is on purpose to enable the residue from the moisture to pass out of the blood vessel into the kidney, and so that when the fluid percolates through the body of the kidneys the excretion that results may collect into the middle of the kidney, where the hollow is in most cases. (This explains, incidently, why the kidney is the most ill-scented of all the viscera). From the middle of the kidney the fluid is passed off through the aforesaid channel into the bladder, by which time it has practically taken on the character of the excremental residue. The bladder is actually moored to the kidneys as has been stated, they are strong channels extending from them to it.'

In the 2nd work, Aristotle repeats the error already noticed in *Historia Animalium* regarding the position of the 2 kidneys:

3   **4**

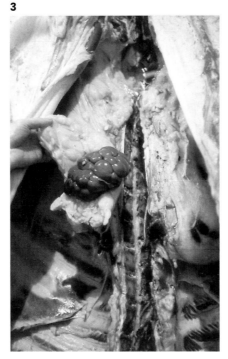
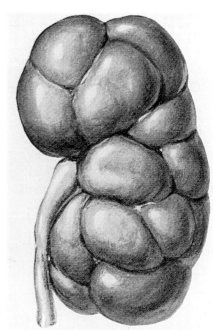

Fig. 3. The lobulated kidney of an ox
after removal of the perirenal fat.
Fig. 4. Persistent fetal lobulation of the
human kidney.

'The right kidney is always higher up than the left. The reason for
that is that as motion always begins on the right-hand side, the parts
that are on that side are stronger than those on the others; and owing
to this motion they are bound to make their way upwards before the
ones on the left.'   (ibid.)

The fact that Aristotle claims that the position of the
kidney is due to movement means that the kidney itself
possesses 'movement' which is due to its function. In fact,
Aristotle says:

'The kidneys contain more fat than any other of the viscera. This
is partly a necessary consequence upon the percolation of the residual
through the kidney, in other words, the blood which gets left behind
there is easy concoction and the final products are lard and suet. This
fat is not formed actually in the kidneys themselves, because they are
so dense it collects outside them. This formation of lard, then, about
the kidneys is the necessary consequence upon the conditions which
necessarily obtain in animals that possess kidneys. But there is another reason for this formation and that is on purpose to safeguard the
kidneys themselves and to preserve the natural heat. These are the
reasons why the kidney has fat. In all animals, however, the right
kidney has less fat than the left. This is because the right side is dry
and solid and more adapted for motion than the left; and motion is
an enemy to fat because it tends to melt it.'   (ibid.)

As can be seen, for Aristotle the kidney had 2 functions: to separate the surplus liquid from the blood and to
modify this liquid which will be eliminated via the ureters, bladder and urethra. These activities, representing

the 'movement' of the kidneys, gave origin to the formation of the perirenal fat observed in oxen and sheep and
therefore were thought to be present in humans as well
(fig. 2).

Aristotelian Renal Pathology

Renal pathology is also briefly examined by Aristotle:

'Thus, too, in the case of human beings who suffer from their
kidneys, although it is an advantage for them to have fat yet if they
become unduly fatty, pains result which prove fatal.'   (ibid.)

In this passage he refers to the renal fat as the cause of
renal cancer and gangrene, for the fat embottles the air
that is localized inside the kidney and therefore the air
would directly cause the gangrene. He then writes:

'Very often the kidneys are found to be full of stones, growths, and
small abscesses; so is the liver, and the lung, and especially the
spleen.'   *De Partibus Animalium* III, 4, 667b

Summary

Aristotle's view of the kidney can be summarized as follows:

(1) Blood does not reach the renal pelvis;

(2) There is no transverse membrane which divides the renal pelvis into two cavities, a superior and an inferior cavity;

(3) The surplus liquid is separated from the blood inside the renal meat and not inside the renal pelvis;

(4) The kidney not only filters the surplus liquid but also transforms it into what Aristotle called *residuum,* otherwise known as urine;

(5) Urine is transported via the ureter into the bladder and then eliminated during micturition.

As can be seen, there is no trace whatsoever of the famous 'filter kidney' in Aristotle's works, and this concept is also absent from the work of Galen. The question thus remains of how, where, when and why did the 'filter kidney' originate, for this theory lasted through the whole of the Middle Ages, only to be demolished first by Berengario de Carpi and then by Andreas Vesalius, Bartolomeo Eustachi, Lorenzo Bellini and above all by Marcello Malpighi. Only future studies on the history of urology will be able to solve this problem.

References

1 Louis P: Histoire des Animaux. Paris, 1964–1969.
2 Peck AL: History of Animals. Cambridge, Massachusetts, 1965–1970.
3 Ogle W: De Partibus Animalium. Oxford, 1912.
4 Düring I: Aristotle's *De Partibus Animalium.* Critical and Literary Comments. Goeteborg 1943.
5 Louis P: Les Parties des Animaux. Paris, 1956.
6 Peck AL: Parts of Animals. London, Cambridge, Massachusetts, 1961.
7 Hartmann N, Strauss J: The Anatomy of the Rhesus Monkey. Baltimore, 1933.
8 May M: Galen on the Usefulness of the Parts of the Body. Ithaca, New York, 1968.
9 Blass H: Studien über Aristoteles als vergleichenden Anatom. Archivio di Storia della Scienza 1924;5–11.
10 Lanza D, Vegetti M: Opere Biologiche di Aristotele. Torino, 1971.

Am J Nephrol 1994;14:307–312

Shaul G. Massry

Division of Nephrology, Department of
Medicine, The University of Southern
California School of Medicine,
Los Angeles, Calif., USA

Maimonides: Physician and Nephrologist

Key Words

Maimonides
Body homeostasis
Nephrology
Uroscopy

Abstract

Maimonides (Moses ben Maimon) was born in 1135 in Cordoba, the son of a Jewish rabbi. After a seminomadic upbringing in Spain and North Africa during the rule of the Almohades, Maimonides settled in Fostate (Old Cairo), where he became renowned as a physician, eventually being appointed as court physician to Saladin and his son. Maimonides wrote both religious and medical treatises, the latter including the *Medical Aphorisms of Moses* in which he deals with almost all aspects of health and disease. His aphorisms on urine and the kidney were influenced by Galen, to whose contributions he added new dimensions. His aphorisms dealt with a variety of renal diseases recognized today.

Introduction

In the 12th century, the Almohades (Al Muahhidin), i.e. Unitarians, ruled what is now known as North Africa from the Atlas Mountains to the borders of Egypt and Spain. The Almohades were Islamic zealots who persecuted believers of other faiths. They destroyed churches and synagogues and offered the Jews 3 options: they could convert to Islam (real convert), they could accept publicly that Muhammad was the Prophet but could then practise their Jewish laws in secret (pseudoconvert), or they could leave for other lands. Jews who defied the Almohades, refused to accept any of these options and continued to practise Judaism in public were imprisoned, tortured and executed.

The Life of Maimonides

In these oppressive and terrifying times for Jews, there lived in Cordoba, Spain, the family of Rabbi Maimon, a scholar and judge, who apparently was a descendent of King David. On 30 March 1135 (the Passover eve of the Hebrew year 4895), Rabbi Maimon had a son whom he called Moses. His mother died at birth. Later the Rabbi had another son, David, from a second wife.

Moses is now known as Maimonides, which is the Greek word for 'son of Maimon'. In the Hebrew language the word 'ben' stands for the English word 'son', and so Maimonides is known among the Jews as RMBM (pronounced Rambam), an acronym for Rabbi Moses ben Maimon. The Arabs called him Abu Amram Musa ibn Maimon (fig. 1).

The Almohades conquered Cordoba in 1148 when Maimonides was 13 years old. The Maimons remained in Cordoba under the rule of the Almohades for a short time and practised their Judaism secretly at their home. They thus lived a double life which was worrisome, irksome and dangerous. The Maimon family left Cordoba and wandered into southern Spain and North Africa to finally settle in 1160 in the city of Fez, Morocco. It is not clear why they chose Fez, as it was also ruled by the Almohades. It is possible that they believed that Fez would be a safer place to live because they were strangers and their religious disguise would not be detected. Another reason might have been the desire of Rabbi Maimon that his children study with and be tutored by the great scholar of the time, Rabbi Judah ibn Shoshan. When this teacher was

Shaul G. Massry, MD
Division of Nephrology
University of Southern California School of Medicine
2025 Zonal Avenue
Los Angeles, CA 90033 (USA)

© 1994 S. Karger AG, Basel
0250–8095/94/0146–0307
$8.00/0

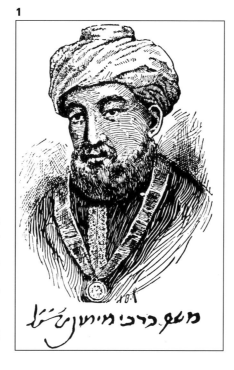

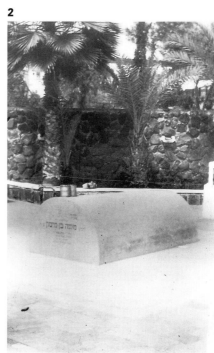

Fig. 1. A portrait of Maimonides, with his name in Hebrew. With permission from the New York Academy of Medicine.

Fig. 2. The tomb of Maimonides in Tiberias. The inscription in Hebrew says:
'From Moses unto Moses, there was none like Moses
Here rests the dust of the Great Eagle
The Giant of the Bible, understanding and medicine.'

arrested and executed in 1165 by the Almohades for practising Judaism, the Maimon family fled to Palestine and settled in Acre.

Their stay in Acre was brief, and at the end of 1165 they moved to Egypt. During this journey, or shortly after their arrival in Egypt, Rabbi Maimon died and his two sons, Moses and David, settled in the city of Fostate (Old Cairo). The desire of Rabbi Maimon was that David should engage in commerce and be the breadwinner, so that Moses could devote his time to scholarly endeavors related to the study of Judaism and the Bible. David did indeed become a merchant and dealt in precious stones, a business that provided him with the means to support his own family as well as his brother Moses. Not long after their arrival in Fostate, however, David died in a shipwreck in the Indian Ocean while on a business voyage.

Maimonides was then faced with the task of supporting his brother's family and earning his own living. He refused to receive payment for his religious services as a rabbi, and instead began to utilize his knowledge in medicine to practise the art of healing. His medical endeavors were very successful. They brought him recognition and fame and led to his appointment as court physician to the famous Muslim military leader Saladin, as well as to his son Al Afdal, thereafter. He was offered the post of physician to Richard Coeur de Lion of England, but he declined.

In 1187, at the age of 52 years, Maimonides had a son, Abraham from a late marriage. Abraham grew to be a Jewish scholar and a physician. Maimonides died on December 13, 1204 (Tebeth 20 of the Hebrew year 4965). He is buried in Tiberias, Israel, on the shores of the Sea of Galilee (fig. 2). It is not clear why his burial site is so distant from the place of his death. A legend claims that his family and friends could not decide where to bury him because he did not leave instructions. They therefore placed the coffin on the back of a camel and let it loose. The camel walked without stopping for 7 days and 7 nights across the Sinai desert and then northward toward Tiberias where it stopped. This was taken as a sign that Maimonides wished to be buried in Tiberias and his wish was fulfilled. It is also said that Maimonides wanted to spend the last years of his life in the Holy Land. He died before his wish could be realized, but his remains were brought from Egypt for burial in Tiberias.

The Writings of Maimonides

Maimonides wrote both religious and medical treatises. His religious writings were in Hebrew, while his medical treatises were in Arabic. He produced 7 religious contributions (table 1). The most important among them is *Mishneh Torah* (*Commentary on the Mishneh*). The *Mishneh* is

Table 1. Religious writings of Maimonides

Original name (Hebrew)	English translation
Mishneh Torah	Commentary on the *Mishneh*
Morahe Nibokhim	Guide for the Perplexed
Ma'amar Hahigayon	Book on Logic
Safer Ha-mitzvot	Book of Commandments
Iggereth Hashmad	Epistle to Yemen
Ma'amar Techiyath Ha-methim	Treatise on Resurrection

Table 2. Medical writings of Maimonides

Original name (Arabic)	English translation
Al Mukhtasart	The Extracts
Fusul Musa fi al Tibb	The Medical Aphorisms of Moses
Sharh Fusal Abuqrat	A Commentary on the Aphorisms of Hippocrates
Fi al Jima'a	On Coitus
Fi al Bawasir	On Hemorrhoids
Maqalah fi al Rabu	A Discourse on Asthma
Kitab al Sumum Wa al Metahhariz min al Adiwiya al Qittalah	A Book on Poisons and the Protection against Lethal Drugs
Sharh Asma al Uqqar	A Commentary on the Names of Drugs
Fi Tadbir al Sihhah	On the Regimen of Health
Maqalah fi Bayan Ba'd al A'rad Wa-al Jawab anha	A Treatise in Elucidation of Some Accidents and the Response

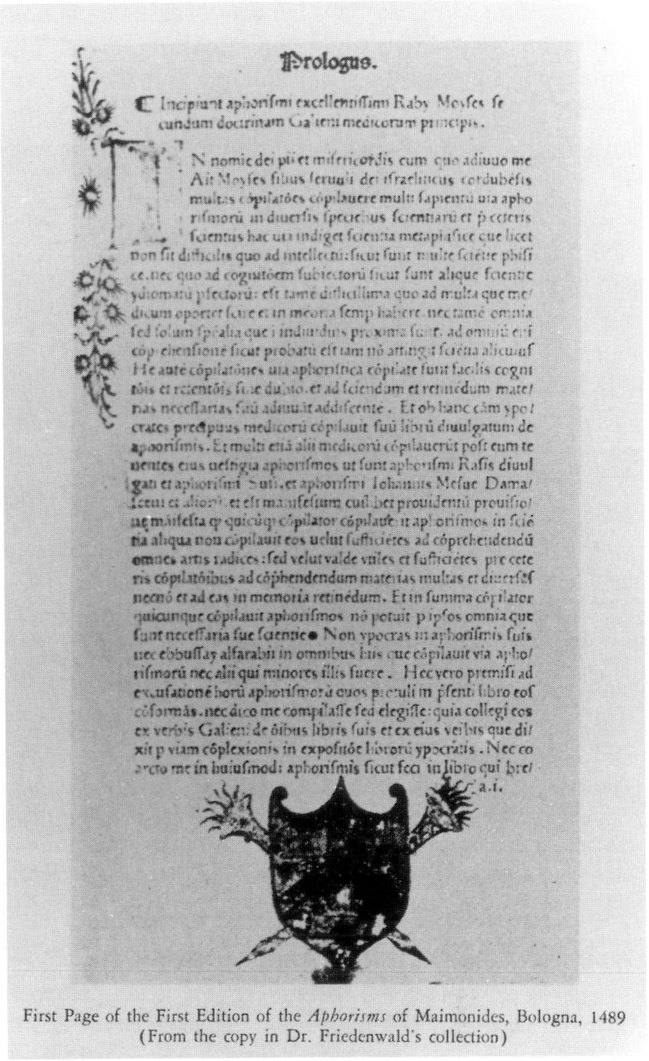
Prologus.

Incipiunt aphorismi excellentissimi Raby Moyses secundum doctrinam Galieni medicorum principis.

First Page of the First Edition of the *Aphorisms* of Maimonides, Bologna, 1489
(From the copy in Dr. Friedenwald's collection)

Fig. 3. The 1st page of the 1st edition of the Latin translation of the Medical Aphorisms of Maimonides, Bologna, 1498. With permission of Dr. Friedenwald.

an authoritative postbiblical collection of Jewish oral laws, compiled by many scholars over the first 2 centuries AD. Thus, the *Mishneh* represents *Torah Baal Peh,* the Hebrew oral law. A parallel to *Torah Baal Peh* is found in Islam and is called the *Hadith,* the 'conversation'. The *Mishneh* was codified in the 3rd century AD by Judah ha-Nasl; it was then subjected to intensive study both in Babylon and Jerusalem. These studies produced a wide range of critical notes called *Gemara,* which means 'completion'. The *Mishneh* and the *Gemara* make the *Talmud.* Thus, although there are 2 *Talmuds,* a Babylonian and a Jerusalem *Talmud,* they contain 1 *Mishneh* but 2 *Gemaras.* The *Mishneh Torah* of Maimonides includes important, critical commentary on the *Mishneh* and remains a classic even today.

Maimonides wrote 10 medical contributions (table 2). The most important of them is *Fusul Musa fi al Tibb*, or the *Medical Aphorisms of Moses* (fig. 3). This treatise dealt with almost all aspects of health and disease, and it is in the *Medical Aphorisms of Moses* that the contribution of Maimonides to the origins of nephrology can be found. *Fusul Musa fi al Tibb* was composed between 1187 and 1190, written in Arabic and translated into Hebrew and Latin. It contained 1,500 aphorisms, most of which are derived from Galen.

Maimonides the Physician-Scientist

It is not known where and how Maimonides gained his knowledge in medicine. It is accepted, however, that he acquired the foundation of the art of healing in the West, i.e. Spain and Morocco. This concept is based on certain statements made in the writings of Maimonides, e.g.: 'This is what we have received from the Elders of the Art' and 'This we have seen the outstanding Elders do in the land of Andalusia', though he did not mention the names of those Elders. It has been said that he might have learned medicine from 2 famous physicians of the time, Abu Marwan ibn Zuhar (Avenzoar, 1091–1162, fig. 4) and Ibn Rushd (Averroes, 1126–1198, fig. 5). It should be mentioned that there is nothing in the writings of Maimonides to attest to this claim.

Maimonides was very critical in his medical thinking and practice and demanded the same from others. He was a true scientist. His medical thinking and writings were governed by 3 principles that he detailed as follows:

'Man should believe nothing which is not attested (1) by rational proof as in mathematical science; (2) by evidence of the senses; or (3) by the authority of prophets and saints.'

He further declared:

'Do not allow your mind to be swayed by the novelties which he tells you, but look into his theory and his belief, just as you should do concerning the things which he declares that he has seen; look into the matter he declares that he has seen; look into the matter without letting yourself be persuaded. And this is true, whether the person in question is notable, or one of the people. For a strong will may lead a man to speak erringly, especially in disputation.'

He continues:

'In this aphorism, it is my purpose to bring before you something well deserving your examination and belief: if anyone declares to you that he has actual proof, from his own experience, of something which he requires for the confirmation of his theory, even though he be considered a man of great authority, truthfulness, earnest words and morality, yet, just because he is anxious for you to believe his theory, you should hesitate.'

Maimonides was a dedicated physician and worked extremely hard in the service of patients. He described his day as follows:

'I dismount from my animal, wash my hands, go forth to my patients, and entreat them to bear with me while I partake some light refreshment, the only meal I eat in 24 hours. Then I go to attend my patients and write prescriptions and direction for their ailments. Patients go in and out until nightfall, and sometimes until 2 hour and more in the night. I converse with them and prescribe for them even while lying down from sheer fatigue. When night falls, I am so exhausted that I can hardly speak.'

Maimonides the Nephrologist

The aphorisms of Maimonides on medicine and health and those related to urine and the kidney, and thus to nephrology, were influenced by Galen. He added new dimensions, however, to the contributions of Galen. He was praised by one of the authorities of his time in comparing him with Galen:

'I deem Galen's medicine fit for the body,
But Abu Imran's [Maimonides] for both body and mind.
Had the medicine of the time on him come to call,
Through knowledge he would have cured it of ignorance ills.'

Maimonides was also influenced by the medical aphorisms of the Old Testament and the Jewish prayers. Figure 6 provides the original Hebrew text of a Jewish morning blessing and its English translation. This blessing speaks of the life-threatening consequences of excessive and severe urinary losses or diarrhea and of urinary or intestinal obstruction. It ends by thanking God for acting 'wondrously'. This is interpreted to indicate the wondrous coordination of body function, and in medical lexicon, 'body homeostasis'. Two of the aphorisms of Maimonides deal with the same issues presented in the Jewish morning prayer. First:

'Bodies whose excretory passages are patent, their health status is more permanent. When they become ill, they heal very easily. The bodies whose passages are obstructed have opposite conditions prevailing.'

In this aphorism, Maimonides recognizes the importance of a patent urinary tract for health and emphasizes the danger of urinary obstruction. In the second aphorism he states:

'Elimination of excessive moist liquid occurs in one of three manners: either through diarrhea, through the sweat, or in the urine. Nature will push these fluids from whichever site we desire and will seal off the other two sites. Therefore, should a crisis be near while the patient is constipated or in urinary retention, then of necessity, shivering should be induced and profuse sweating will ensue through which the patient will lose his bad humor.'

This is an interesting description of how to maintain fluid balance of the body and certainly describes body homeostasis. It should be mentioned that even in modern times, sweating has been used to treat uremic patients.

In the aphorisms of Maimonides, the word 'cooking' or 'cooked' is often encountered. Cooking means that the organs of the body are doing their tasks adequately, and complete cooking indicates successful achievement of

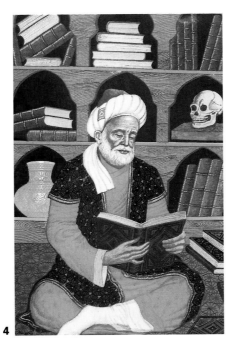

4

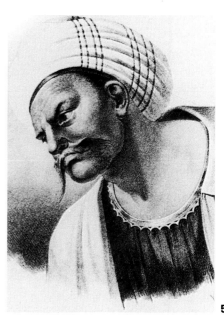

5

Fig. 4. Abu Marwan ibn Zuhar (Avenzoar).
Fig. 5. Ibn Rushd (Averroes). A lithograph by Vigneron, in the collection of the Wellcome Foundation, with permission.
Fig. 6. Jewish morning blessing. Both the Hebrew text and the English translation are provided.

'Blessed are you our God, King of the Universe, who fashioned man with wisdom and created within him many openings and many cavities. It is obvious and known before your Throne of Glory that if but one of them be opened excessively or but one of them were to be blocked, it would be impossible to survive and stand before you. You are our blessed God who heals all flesh and acts wondrously.'

בָּרוּךְ אַתָּה יְיָ, אֱלֹהֵינוּ מֶלֶךְ הָעוֹלָם, אֲשֶׁר יָצַר אֶת הָאָדָם בְּחָכְמָה, וּבָרָא בוֹ נְקָבִים נְקָבִים, חֲלוּלִים חֲלוּלִים. גָּלוּי וְיָדוּעַ לִפְנֵי כִסֵּא כְבוֹדֶךָ, שֶׁאִם יִפָּתֵחַ אֶחָד מֵהֶם, אוֹ יִסָּתֵם אֶחָד מֵהֶם, אִי אֶפְשַׁר לְהִתְקַיֵּם וְלַעֲמוֹד לְפָנֶיךָ (אֲפִילוּ שָׁעָה אֶחָת). בָּרוּךְ אַתָּה יְיָ, רוֹפֵא כָל בָּשָׂר וּמַפְלִיא לַעֲשׂוֹת.

6

these objectives. It also indicates that nature has already triumphed over the illness and has begun to excrete the illness-producing liquids. Hence, the description that the excretions of various organs are 'maximally cooked' reflects healthy conditions.

Maimonides defined normal urine as follows:

'Maximally 'cooked' urine in the healthiest people is urine which is even in thickness and whose yellowness leans to a tinge of redness to deepen the yellow color. This urine may have white turbidity in it which is flat and even and should settle to the bottom of a vessel.'

This sediment described by Maimonides is most probably urate. He recommends that urinalysis be done in all patients with fever because the character of the urine may provide information on the illness. This ancient advice by Maimonides is commonly practised today.

He provides several aphorisms on the value of urine examination in diagnosing various illnesses. He states:

'If the urine is fatty and its appearance and consistency as that of oil, this is a bad [sign], causing death by dissolving the flesh because heat [disease] which melts the flesh is dangerous' ... 'urine in which foam [protein] accumulates reflects the chronicity of the illness.'

This description probably reflects the lipiduria and proteinuria seen in nephrotic syndrome.

In another aphorism he describes macroscopic hematuria and (probably) acute glomerulonephritis. He states:

'There is a type of kidney ailment in which the patient micturates rusty, thin urine similar to early excretions of a sick liver, and this one contains more blood than others.'

He also describes the character of the urine in blackwater fever or hemoglobinuric fever:

Table 3. The medical writings of Maimonides on nephrology. References to these functions and conditions are found in his writings

Body homeostasis
Kidney function
Obstruction of the urinary tract
Polyuria of diabetes mellitus and/or diabetes insipidus
Nephrotic syndrome
Hemoglobinuria and/or blackwater fever
Proteinuria as an indication of the chronicity of illness
Macroscopic hematuria as an indicator of glomerular diseases
Use of sweating as a therapeutic modality in conditions with urine retention*

* Sweating has been used in the treatment of uremia even in modern times.

'Black urine and black sediment are extremely malignant and indicate serious illness. They occur in association with what resembles the death of natural resources.' ... 'I have never seen anyone who urinated black urine who survived.'

He also warns about the dangers of polyuria:

'When urine resembling water is micturated repeatedly as occurs in people with the illness diabetes, this is the most unfavorable of all uncooked urine.'

The word diabetes in this aphorism may indicate either diabetes mellitus or diabetes insipidus.

It is apparent that the medical writings of Maimonides contain many statements related to nephrology and describe many of the nephrologic concepts and renal diseases known today (table 3). The name of Maimonides should be added to the list of scholars who contributed to the origins of nephrology.

Further Reading

Bar-Sela A, Hoff HE, Faris E: Moses Maimonides' two treatises on the regimen of health. Trans Am Philos Soc 1964;54:3–50.

Brodie A: The moral philosophy of Maimonides. J Med Ethics 1988;14:200–202.

Posner F, Muntner S: Studies in Judaica. The Medical Aphorisms of Maimonides. New York, Yeshiva University Press, vol 1, 1970.

Posner F, Muntner S: Studies in Judaica. The Medical Aphorisms of Maimonides. New York, Yeshiva University Press, vol 2, 1971.

Posner F, Muntner S: Moses Maimonides' aphorism regarding analysis of urine. Ann Intern Med 1971;71:217–220.

Posner F: The medical writings of Moses Maimonides. N Y State J Med 1987;87:656–661.

Early Contributors to Nephrology

Am J Nephrol 1994;14:313–316

Raffaele A. Bernabeo

Chair of History of Medicine,
University of Bologna, Bologna, Italy

The *Consilium ad Calcolum* of Alberto de' Zancari

Key Words
Bologna
Alberto de' Zancari
Nephrolithiasis

Abstract
Zancari was born in 1278 and practised medicine in Ravenna and Bologna. He is mentioned in the Decameron of Boccaccio and in court records of Bologna in connection with 4 of his students who were accused of exhuming a body for medical research. Zancari's writings are found in several manuscript versions and include commentaries on Galen and *Consilium ad Calcolum*, which deals with renal calculosis. His therapeutic rules are summarized in 74 lines and cover both acute and quiescent calculi and prevention. The treatments prescribed do not differ from those in general use at the time, nor are any new concepts introduced.

Introduction

In the Decameron (1348 AD), giornata 1, novella 10 [1], Giovanni Boccaccio mentions a certain Maestro Alberto da Bologna who is afflicted with a passion of love for a young girl, though he is 70 years old:

'Egli non sono ancora molti anni passati, che in Bologna fu un grandissimo medico e di chiara fama quasi a tutto il mondo, e forse ancora vive, il cui nome fu Maestro Alberto; il quale essendo già vecchio di presso a settanta anni, tanta fu la nobilità del suo spirito che, essendo già del corpo quasi ogni natural caldo partito, in sè non schifò di ricevere l'amorosa fiamma, per che avendo veduta ad una festa una bellissima donna vedova, chiamata, secondo che alcuni dicono, Madonna Malgherida de' Ghisolieri, e piaciutagli sommamente, non altramenti che un giovanetto quella nel maturo petto ricevette ...'

Salvatore de Renzi (1800–1872), general pathologist and medical historian in Naples, thought this figure could only be the Bolognese Alberto Ferri or Dal Ferro, called to hold *lettura di medicina* in 1310 and mentioned among the Anziani in 1313/1314 [2]. Local gossip, registration documents and chronologic data, however, agree on the identification of this man as Alberto de' Zancari, the son of Maestro Galvano and Beatrice di Jacopo de' Faffi, who in 1337 lived near the Chapel of Santa Tecla, Porta Nuova district, where the medical schools were situated at that time [3].

The Life of Alberto de' Zancari

According to the poor biographic records that are available, Alberto de' Zancari was born on an uncertain date in 1278 and was already a well-established *doctor physicae* when he signed the *contratto nuziale* with Egidia di Fabiano Malpigli [4] on 20 June 1310. On 24 February 1314, he was assigned to the post of municipal doctor for 1 year (from 1 April) by Guido, the Ruler of the Church of San Fabiano in Ravenna and Procurator of the Podesta Lamberto da Polenta. He thus became obliged to treat all the sick living in that town and in its suburbs, according to social status and disease, for a salary of 300 *bolognini* lire;

Raffaele A. Bernabeo, MD
Chair of History of Medicine
University of Bologna
I–40100 Bologna (Italy)

in addition, he used to receive a gratuity from each patient he visited, which, however, was not higher than 3 *ravegnani* lire [5].

From 1326 to 1347 Zancari undertook the *lettura di medicina pratica* in Bologna, succeeding Mondino de' Luzzi, to whose last wishes he acceded on account of their close friendship, on 17 February 1326 [6]. He made his will just before his death on 15 August 1348 and declared that he wanted to be buried at the Monastery of the Preaching Friars of San Domenico (where, however, no trace of his burial has been found) [7].

Maestro Alberto is also mentioned in the *Atti Giudiziari* of the ancient Criminal Court of Bologna in connection with a trial held from 21 November to 8 December 1319 of 4 of his students – Paxino, Laurenti, Albertino Milanesi and Jacopo of Piacenza, who were accused of exhuming a body: '... causa faciendi notomiam et ad hoc ut Magister Albertus predictus doceret eos videre ea quae vivenda sunt in corpore hominum'. Indeed, according to the evidence the 4 men, on 19 November: '... noctis tempore accesserunt ad ecclesiam S. Barnabe, et entraverunt in cimiterio, et de dicto cimiterio et sepulcro estraxerunt et exportaverunt queddam corpus cuiusdam Pixe ... qui fuit suspensus dicta die ad furcas positas ad pontem Reni'. The body was then brought: 'in domo scolarum in quibus legit Magister Albertus Bononiensis, posita in cappella Sancti Salvatoris ...', where according to a servant, a certain Carlino di Bonetto from Bergamo: '... et Magister Albertus et alios complurimos cum rasuriis et cultellis et aliis artificiis, et sparantes dictum ominem mortuum et alia facientes que spectant ad artem medicam' [8].

The Writings of Alberto de' Zancari

Bibliographic research reveals that the writings of Alberto de' Zancari are kept not only at the National Library of Paris and the Palatine Library in Vienna, but also at the Vatican Library in a number of codices. Some examples are given here: Codex 2000, 'Alberti Bononiensis in Galeni libros de accidente et morbo commentarius'; Codex 2418, folio 145, 'Consilium magistri Alberti super passione calculosa renum per solam medicinam constructum, quaestio disputata anno 1314', folio 164, 'Utrum principium motum pulsus arteriarum et cordis sit virtus aliqua animae ...', folio 165, 'Utrum corpus collericum, vel flegmaticum ex generatione sanguinem, vel melanconicum possit reduci ad temperamentum per res temporales', folio 168, 'Utrum corpus sanum et nunc habeat sanitatem acquisitam a rebus temporalibus ...', folio 169,

'Utrum membrum solum, vel simul actuatum cum spiritu sit subiectum sanitatis et aegritudinis', folio 187, 'Magistri Alberti Bononiensis quaestio utrum ex colera non putrescente sit possibile accendi febrim humoralem'; Codex 2391, folio 159 v, 'Breves quaedam glossae in Aphorismos Hippocratis'; Codices 2414 and 4456, 'Libellus de cautelis seu documentis medicorum habendis ...'; Codex 4452, folio 59, 'Alberti Bononiensis expositiones super libro de pharmacis Hippocratis'.

Zancari's writings can also be found in the *Donazione Vittorio Putti* of the Orthopedic Institute Rizzoli of Bologna (*Medical Miscellanies*, parchment manuscript of the 14th century of 30 folios, 177 × 250 mm, written by different hands in 2 columns with rubrics in red, where F. 29th line reads: 'explicit libellus de cautelis medicorum habendis, editus a magistro Alberto de Zancharys Bononiensi'), and at the Malatestiana Library of Cesena [9]. These last libraries in particular were ignored by medical historians interested in Zancari until Bernabeo and Busacchi began to study them [10, 11].

Apart from three commentaries on works by Galen *(De Accidentus et Morbus, De Diebus Criticis, De Simplicibus Pharmacis)*, a treatise called *Consilium ad Calcolum* (a copy of which can be found at the Vatican Library) is also kept at the Malatestiana Library. This treatise contains concepts concerning the medical therapy *de renum lapidis vitium* [12], which are certainly not original and which were common at that time.

Alberto de' Zancari and the *Consilium ad Calcolum*

The study and treatment of urinary afflictions, which originated with the Hippocratic observation of humoral dyscrasia affecting the quality and quantity of urine through its effects on the blood, were very successful in the Middle Ages, when a vast literature on the subject accumulated. The affliction *mal della pietra,* which was then considered as a nosologic entity pertaining to the genital tract, was discussed by various authors based on their classical knowledge.

The Salerno School of Medicine played an important role. Its masters collected and commented on the earlier work of Greek and Roman physicians, often transmitted via Arab physicians, e.g. the Latin translation, *De Urinis,* from the Arabic work of Isaac Judaeus, made by Constantinus Africanus. Thus, Abbott Hugo de Flavigny (Verdun, 1065–1115) wrote in *Cronachae Yverdunenses* that in 984 the Bishop of Verdun, Adlaberone, had gone to Salerno to be treated for calculosis affecting him for many years, after consulting the well-known Monk Gerberto in vain. The masters at Salerno codified the principles of uroscopy and gave it an essential diagnostic and prognostic role in support of the information gained by study of the pulse. Moreover, they spread the concept that urinary fluid varied in: 'color, substantia, quantitas et contentum' according to the affected region of the body or the altered circulating humors, so that therapy had to be adapted to the requirements of each individual case. Blood-letting through the saphenous or dorsalis pedis artery was still the main remedy, however, as it allowed diversion of morbid matter out of the body. According to tradition, the medical science of Salerno was introduced to Bologna by Guglielmo da Saliceto (1210–1276). He devoted a whole chapter of the 1st book of *Summa Conservationis et Curationis Corporis*, written in 1275, to renal afflictions 'according to Maestro Mauro Salernitano'.

The text in the Malatestiana Library that refers to Zancari is contained in miscellaneous parchment folios of 185 × 260 mm. They are handwritten in 2 columns with a space of 1 cm between, and some have miniature initial letters. The text starts at the bottom of the paper, 13th line in the lefthand column, with the attribution to *Magistre Alberti de Ravenna*, apparently referring to the period when he worked as a medical officer in that town (1314–1315). It continues at the beginning of the righthand column at the top of the page.

Zancari quoted from Giovanni Mesue the Elder (Juhannà ibn Massawaih, 777–857), who maintained in *De Compositione Medicamentorum* that the main task of a doctor is: 'to treat and effectively help his patients'. Zancari then observed that above all it is necessary to know how to respond to a recurrent and painful affliction, e.g. nephrolithiasis. He made no reference to pathophysiologic assumptions, excluding any attempt at differential diagnosis, and he did not dwell on urinalysis, on which (as he wrote in *Libellus de Cautelis Medicorum*) the physician does not have to rely, as it is merely subjective and susceptible to totally arbitrary deductions. He summarized a series of therapeutic rules with short but highly impressive concepts in 74 lines. According to him, these are the rules that an expert doctor must adopt in cases of renal calculosis in its fully developed form.

In the acute phase, to facilitate the calculus to be discharged and to soothe pain, he suggested that the patient abstained from eating and was administered abundant emetics for 2 days at least, plus 2 pounds of a syrup made of: '... 1 pound of celery and fennel seeds, 1½ pounds of sponge stone, 1 pound of breakstone, 2 pounds of stinging nettle seeds, the whole pulverized and mixed with ⅓ of

Table 1. Medicinal herbs mentioned in *Consilium ad Calcolum*

	Classical use	Actual use
Aloe (*Aloe* F.M.)	Purgative	+
Altea (*Althaea* off. L.)	Emollient	+
Appio (*Apium* G.L.)	Diuretic	+
	Lithotritic	–
Aristolochia (*Aristolochia* C.L.)	Depurative	+
	Sudorific	+
Camomilla (*Matricaria* C.L.)	Analgesic	+
	Antispasmodic	+
Cappero (*Capparis* S.L.)	Antispasmodic	+
	Diuretic	+
Cardamomo (*Eletteria* C.R.X.)	Carminative	+
Cariofillato (*Geum uranum* L.)	Diaphoretic	+
Ciliegio (*Prunus* C.L.)	Diuretic	+
Cipolla (*Allium* cepa L.)	Diuretic	+
	Emollient	+
	Lithotritic	–
Fieno greco (*Trigonella* F.G.L.)	Emollient	+
	Laxative	+
Finocchio (*Foeniculum* V.G.)	Diuretic	+
Genziana (*Gentiana lutea* L.)	Stomachic	+
Malva (*Malva* S.L.)	Emollient	+
Miglio (*Panicum* M.L.)	Diaphoretic	+
	Diuretic	+
	Emollient	+
Oregano (*Origanum* V.L.)	Antispasmodic	+
	Diaphoretic	+
Ortica (*Urtica* D.L.)	Diuretic	+
Parietaria (*Parietaria* off. L.)	Diuretic	+
	Emollient	+
Pepe (*Piper* L.)	Stomachic	+
Pesco (*Prunus* P.L.)	Antispasmodic	+
	Laxative	+
Polipodio (*Polypodium* V.L.)	Laxative	+
Rafano (*Nasturtium* A.F.)	Diuretic	+
Sassifraga (*Saxifraga* G.L.)	Diuretic	+
	Lithotritic	–
Serpillo (*Thymus* S.L.)	Antispasmodic	+
	Carminative	+
	Diuretic	+
Tarassaco (*Taraxacum* off. W.)	Depurative	+
	Diuretic	+
Viola (*Viola* O.L.)	Diuretic	+
	Emollient	+

oxymel' and a sedative enema made of '... herb bennet and fenugreek, 1 pound ana, boiled in 2 pounds of water'. On the 3rd day, he recommended the repeated intake of a large glass of warm infusion of radish root in vinegar and abundant phlebotomy from the dorsalis pedis or internal tibial artery, with a long warm bath in a water solution of: '... malva, pellitory, althaea, cabbage, chamomile, and leek roots'. After the bath, a revulsive oil must be applied on the renal, abdominal and pubic regions. This oil must be made by filtering the crushing of: '... birthwort, gentian and caper roots, 1½ pounds', dissolved in sweet almond oil, exposed to the sun for a week in a closed pot and then enriched with 8 pounds of scorpion powder dried under the sun for 3 days.

To remove calculi in the quiescent phase or to prevent their formation and for prophylactic purposes, he suggested taking a large glass of aperient and diuretic infusion for 3 days at daybreak in Spring and Autumn. This infusion must be made of: '... violet flowers, stinging nettle and cankerwort seeds, leaves of oregano, pellitory, polypody, breakstone and wild thyme, gentian and radish roots'. A therapeutic cycle then followed in order to purify the body, thus eliminating the *superfluitates* responsible for the renal and vesical concretions. To achieve this, he suggested drinking a glass of hot white wine (or of course, boiling wine at the wine-making) before eating, early in the morning. This wine must include 1½ pounds of an electuary made of:

'... fennel, pellitory, celery, radish, Macedonian oregano, pennyroyal, wild thyme, millet, breakstone, herb bennet, polypody and red polypody, aloe, agaric, cardamom 5 pounds ana, 1 peach stone and 1 cherry stone, plus ash of scorpion ventricles, a root of rural colewort, hair of a hare, sponge stone, shell of eggs from which chicks have hatched, cauda tremula, Judaic gravestone, with pepper and human calculi or pulverized edible boletus, the whole dissolved in maple honey and sugar in the measure of a part and a half.'

Medicated enemas and blood-letting, however, must not be neglected.

As these extracts show, this short *libellus* by Zancari does not introduce any new concepts, nor does it contain any original treatments that differ from the other remedies of that time (table 1). It should be said, however, that owing to its various terminologic mistakes and incorrect usages (which make the text very difficult to transcribe and read and sometimes even impossible to interpret), it appears to be a page of one of the notebooks (petiae) used by students or obliging school porters to collect and summarize the lessons of the masters.

References

1 Boccaccio G: Il Decamerone, giornata 1, novella 10, in Petronio G (ed): Torino, Einaudi, 1950, vol 1, p 174.
2 De Renzi S: Storia della Medicina in Italia. Napoli, Filiatre Sebezio, vol 2, 1845/48, p 249.
3 Frati L: Alberto de' Zancari, Riv. di Storia Critica delle Scienze Mediche e Naturali. A.V, 1914;5:329–338.
4 Memoriale di Guido dalle Quercie. Archivio di Stato di Bologna, B 310, c. Lir.
5 Memoriale di Pietro di Alberto Mattesillani. Archivio di Stato di Bologna, B 1314, p 23.
6 Pasquali Alidosi N: Li Dottori Bolognesi di Teologia, Filosofia, Medicina e d'Arti Liberali dall'Anno 1000 per Tutto Marzo 1623. Bologna, Tebaldini, 1623.
7 Testamentum Magistri Alberti de Zanchariis de Bononia medicine doctori, rog. Franciscus de Castelfranco et Jacobus Angelelli. Archivio di Stato di Bologna, San Salvatore, B 136/2583, Cass. 127, number 4.
8 Mazzoni Toselli O: Op. cit., vol 3, 1870, pp 113–127.
9 Zazzeri R: Sui Codici e Libri a Stampa della Biblioteca Malatestiana di Cesena. Cesena, s.e., 1887.
10 Bernabeo RA: Lo sconosciuto *Consilium ad Calcolum* di Maestro Alberto de' Zancari della Malatestiana di Cesena. Atti II Conv. Marca per la Storia della Medicina. Fermo, 1957, pp 19–23.
11 Busacchi V: op. cit. 10, pp 15–18.
12 Magistri Alberti: Consilium ad Calcolum, cataloged in Pluteo 24, 3, 3D.

Am J Nephrol 1994;14:317–319

Sergio Musitelli[b]
Paolo Marandola[a]
Hussein Jallous[a]
Alberto Speroni[a]
Tomaso de Bastiani[a]

[a] Scuola di Specializzazione in Urologia,
  Università degli Studi di Pavia, Pavia,
[b] Storico della Scienza, Milan, Italy;

The Medical School at Ravenna

Key Words

Ravenna School of Medicine
Galenic medicine
Ambrosian codex
Early medieval medicine

Abstract

The existence of the Ravenna School of Medicine can be deduced from a codex in the Ambrosian Library of Milan, which contains Latin translations of 3 Hippocratic works and commentaries on 4 works by Galen. Although it was written in the 9th century, the codex appears to be a copy of an earlier work, probably 7th century. The Ambrosian commentaries follow other commentators on Aristotle, rather than the original Aristotelian works, and contain a number of misinterpretations. Nevertheless, the commentaries make it clear that the earliest literature in Salerno had its roots in the studies of classical medicine at the Ravenna School of Medicine, where the teaching was essentially Galenic in structure.

Clues to the Existence of a Medical School at Ravenna

In 1870 Daremberg wrote in his monumental *Histoire des Sciences Médicales* (1, page 257):

'Un manuscrit de Milan contient la preuve qu'il y avait à Ravenne, vers la fin du VIIIe siècle, des leçons publiques sur Hippocrates et sur Gallien.'

Evidently Daremberg must have consulted the codex G. 108 inf. conserved in the Ambrosian Library of Milan, which contains the Latin translation of 3 Hippocratic works and, most importantly, the commentaries on 4 works by Galen *(De Sectis, Ars Parva, De Pulsibus, Therapeutica ad Glauconem)*.

Henry Sigerist also consulted the codex G. 108 inf. in 1934 and published an article [1] in which he wrote (page 39):

'The manuscript was written at the end of the 9th or at the beginning of the 10th century, and contains in its first part Latin translations of Hippocratic writings. Whoever was interested in the Hippocratic texts studied this manuscript, and I found in it traces of Daremberg, Kuehlewein, Roscher and others. I was most anxious to see the manuscript ... this manuscript proved to be the most important of all the manuscripts I saw ... All the scholars who examined this manuscript were interested in Hippocrates. But the second part of the manuscript proved to be far more important than the beginning. It ... proves that in the early Middle Ages, Galenic treatises were already translated into Latin, and were interpreted; but more than this, we even know where and by whom these texts were discussed, for, in the manuscript, at the end of three of these treatises, we find mentioned: 'ex voce Agnello iatrosofista ego Simplicius deo iuvante legi et scripsi in Ravenna feliciter'. *Iatrosofista* at that time meant 'professor' of medicine, and so we know that in Ravenna there were teachers of medicine who had, and probably did, translations of Galenic works, and interpreted them. Our manuscript was written at the end of the 9th century, but in all probability it is not an original, but a copy of an older manuscript. The text of the Milan manuscript was never printed before and will therefore be published in the second volume of my work.'

Paolo Marandola, MD
Scuola di Specializzazione in Urologia
Università degli Studi di Pavia
I–27100 Pavia (Italy)

Sigerist never fulfilled this intention. Parts of the manuscript had, in fact, already been published by Kuehlewein in 1890 and 1905, by Ilberg in 1894, by Gundermann in 1911 and by Roscher in 1913, but all these authors concentrated on Hippocrates and paid no attention to Galen.

Finally, in 1956 Augusto Beccaria examined the codex G. 108 inf. completely in his work *I Codici di Medicina del Periodo Presalernitano* [2]. He then started a historical-philologic examination of the codex which he never completed because of his death. Only 3 of the 5 planned articles were published in *Italia Medioevale e Umanistica* [3–5]. In 1981 Westerink, helped by a group at the State University of New York at Buffalo [6], published a critical edition of the commentary to *De Sectis*. In the same year Palmieri published a mediocre edition of *Therapeutica ad Glauconem*. In 1982 Pritchet published a commentary on *De Sectis* using the printed editions (Venice, 1490; Venice, 1502; Pavia, 1515) [7]; this work contains many errors and misinterpretations. For example, it erroneously ascribes the comments to Giovanni Alessandrino and states that Burgundione of Pisa was the translator of the commentary, when in actual fact Burgundione was (this still has to be proved) probably only the translator of the text of Galen, whose *lemmata* have been inserted in the commentary. It would therefore be better not to consider Pritchet's work but to return to the Ambrosian codex.

The text of the Ambrosian codex can also be found in 2 fragments of the Karlsruhe codex (Codex Reichenau 120). Both of these codices were written halfway through the 9th century and both appear to derive from an original text of the 6th century, as the Latin used in the codex is that of the 6th century.

It can thus be deduced that a medical school existed in Ravenna between the 6th and 7th centuries AD. The school concentrated its attention on the thoughts of Galen, and in particular on the 4 works that were considered the basis of medical teaching by the School of Alexandria and in the Arab world.

The Ambrosian Codex

The Ravenna School of Medicine is referred to in the colophon of the first 3 commentaries:

'Explicit scolia peri hereseon Galeni actio trigesima tertia feliciter. Ex voce Agnello iatrosophista ego Simplicius deo iuvante legi et scripsi in Ravenna feliciter.'

'Ex vocem Agnello archiatro deo iuvante ego Simplicius medicus legi contuli et scripsi in Ravenna feliciter.'

'Ex voce Agnello iatrosophista ego Simplicius audiui legi contuli Deo iuuante et scripsi feliciter.'

Ex voce means that Simplicio wrote under direct dictation of Maestro Agnello or took notes from his lessons.

The structure of the first 3 commentaries is derived from the scheme initiated by Ammonius, which was followed by the School of Alexandria and perfected by Olympiodorus in the 6th century. The commentary is divided into 'lessons' *(actiones),* each of which begins with a general introduction *(theoria)*; it then quotes only *lemmata* from the works of Galen with some explanation. At the end of each *theoria* and each *actio* are fixed expressions: *finit theoria* or *finit actio.*

The 4th commentary does not have a detailed colophon as do the previous 3, nor does it have a similar structure. It is divided into chapters without a specific scheme.

Agnello and Simplicio based their commentaries on the line of thought followed by the commentators on Aristotle (Ammonius, Olympiodorus, David, Elias, etc.) rather than on the original Aristotelian works, and above all they were subjected to the influence of Boezio. Even so, a number of elements confirm that Agnello and Simplicio are not the true authors of the commentaries. For example, they confuse *kion* (column) with *khion* (snow) or *porus* written with omega (ω) (corn) with *porus* written with omicron (o) (hole). It is thus easy to understand how misinterpretation of Galen's work was possible for these authors. Moreover, many other points confirm that Agnello and Simplicio combined several sources of information, ranging from Greek texts, lexicons that were the sources for Esichio and Zonara, and their own experience, to organize the commentaries.

After reading these commentaries it can be deduced that the earliest literature in Salerno had its roots in studies of classical medicine mainly carried out by the Ravenna School of Medicine.

It should be noted that De Renzi in his *Collectio Salernitana* (cfr. vol I, page ff.; particularly page 143) affirms that Gariopontus of the Salerno School of Medicine was the first to Latinize certain Greek words, e.g. *gargarizare, cicatrizare, cauterizare,* when in actual fact these words were already present in the works by Agnello and Simplicio of the Ravenna School of Medicine. Moreover, the Latin translation and the commentary on Hippocrates' *Aphorisms* that are found in a great number of Beneventan manuscripts are the same as those produced in Ravenna in the 6th century. In this way a map can be drawn of a medieval Italy crossed (from Ravenna to Benevento, to Cassino, and to Salerno) by a line of Greek tradition, which has its roots in the works of Hippocrates and Galen.

The Galenic commentaries outline the essential structure of the Ravenna School of Medicine. They also give an introductory note on the medical studies performed at this school. Any further information concerning the medical studies would be found in the more advanced and detailed lessons of the Ravenna School of Medicine.

As the works by Galen are simply propedeutic in nature, it becomes clear why Agnello dedicates only two brief passages to the discipline of urology in his commentary to *Ars Parva*. The first passage reads:

'In fact the concave and porous parts are attacked by this pathology, known as obstruction, when fat and glutinous humor such as clotted blood and phlegm accumulate there, but this pathology can be caused by unnatural situations, for example a stone in the bladder, in the ureters, or in the urethra. In fact in these hollow organs, fat humor collects. In these cases we intervene with those preparations that

break, extract and thin ... If the obstruction is caused by blood we evacuate the blood by phlebotomy. If it is caused by feces we use an enema. If the cause is a stone we must use preparations that can break it down. If with these preparations we are unsuccessful we must then use those instruments that are able to move the stone from its position, for example a catheter. If the catheter is also unsuccessful we must then proceed with a surgical procedure that we call lithotomy.'

The second passage reads:

'In the pathology of the colon the urine may change its characteristics or difficulty may be encountered when urinating. This occurs because the colon swells producing the suffering of the urethra and the bladder.'

As can be seen, Agnello knew and probably practised what the doctors of the ancient Greco-Roman period knew and practised (from Eliodorus to Celsus, Galen, Aretaeus and Oribasius). The importance of the Ravenna School of Medicine in the history of medieval medicine can now be appreciated. Above all, it provides a fundamental new source in the interpretation of the great Salerno School of Medicine.

References

1 Sigerist H: Medical literature of the early Middle Ages. Bull Hist Med 1934;2:26ff.
2 Beccaria A: I Codici della Medicina del Periodo Presalernitano. Rome, 1956.
3 Beccaria A: Sulle tracce di un antico canone di Ippocrate e di Galeno, in Italia Medioevale e Umanistica', vol 1, part 2, 1959, pp 1ff.

4 Beccaria: Sulle tracce di un antico canone di Ippocrate e di Galeno, in Italia Medioevale e Umanistica'. vol 2, part 4, 1961, pp 1ff.
5 Beccaria A: Sulle tracce di un antico canone di Ippocrate e di Galeno, in Italia Medioevale e Umanistica. vol 3, part 14, 1971, pp 1ff.
6 Westerink LG: Agnellus of Ravenna: Lectures on Galen's De Sectis. Latin Text and Translation. New York, Seminar Classics 609, 1981.

7 Pritchet CD: Iohannis Alexandrini Commentaria in Librum De Sectis Galeni, Recognovit et Adnotatione Critica Instruxit. Leiden, 1982.
8 Temkin O: Studies in Alexandrian medicine. I. Alexandrian commentaries in Galen's De Sectis ad Introducendos. Bull Inst Hist Med 1935; 3:405ff.

Early Contributors to Nephrology

Am J Nephrol 1994;14:320–324

Carl W. Gottschalk

Department of Medicine and Physiology, University of North Carolina at Chapel Hill, Chapel Hill, N.C., USA

Alexander Schumlansky's *De structura renum*

Key Words
Schumlansky
Renal anatomy
Renal microstructure
Renal tubule

Abstract
The overall structural organization of the kidney, its vasculature and its excretory units, the nephrons, was the subject of intense study and disagreement for hundreds of years. In 1783, Schumlansky received a doctoral degree with the dissertation *De structura renum*, in which he presented a detailed and comprehensive description of the major blood vessels of the kidney, the blood vessels of the medulla and pyramids of Ferrein and the malpighian glandula. He concluded the dissertation with a description of 3 experiments on a pig kidney, deducing a connection between the glomerulus and the uriniferous tubule, though his illustration of it was far from convincing. It was only 59 years later that Bowman proved Schumlansky to be correct.

Introduction

The overall structural organization of the kidney, its vasculature and its excretory units, the nephrons, was the subject of intense study and disagreement for hundreds of years. It was not until 1862 that Henle [1] described the hairpin-shaped medullary loop of the tubule that now bears his name. It remained for Schweigger-Seidel in 1865 to establish the origin and termination of the loop of Henle [2], thereby completing the overall description of the major nephron segments.

The relationship of the malpighian corpuscle to the uriniferous tubule was particularly controversial, until William Bowman definitively settled the issue in 1842 [3]. Malpighi, in his famous work of 1666, had already described the 'glands', now called glomeruli, of the kidney and their arterial and venous connections [4]. He believed that they corresponded in number and probably were connected to the urinary vessels, of which, he stated, the outer part of the kidney is chiefly composed.

'I worked a long time in order that I might subject to the eye this evident connection which reason sufficiently attests ... In spite of many attempts (but in vain) I could not demonstrate the connection of the glands and the urinary vessels.'

Malpighi goes on:

'If, indeed, as is probably agreed by all, the material of the urine is derived from the arteries, and since it is clear from the evidence above that the ends of the arteries lie open in these very numerous glands, and since the urine is eliminated into the pelvis through the fibers of the kidney as though through its own peculiar excretory vessels, there must of necessity be granted a continuity and communication between them, for otherwise no secreted fluid would be strained out from the arteries into the pelvis' [5].

This paper reviews the contributions of Aleksandr Mikhailovich Shumlyansky to this subject, particularly as they relate to the glomerular-tubular relationship.

Carl W. Gottschalk, MD
University of North Carolina
Department of Medicine
3034 Old Clinic Building CB 7155
Chapel Hill, NC 27599-7155 (USA)

© 1994 S. Karger AG, Basel
0250–8095/94/0146–0320
$8.00/0

The Life of Shumlyansky

Shumlyansky, who lived from 1748 to 1795, is little known outside his native Russia, but Russian anatomists consider him the discoverer of the glomerulus. Only short entries about him appear in non-Russian biographic sources. According to Hirsch's *Biographical Lexicon* [6], Schumlansky (the Latinized version of his name), was born in Pultava, and studied and received a doctoral degree in 1783 in Strasbourg with the inaugural dissertation *De structura renum* (1782), which was republished in 1788 [7]. After his return to Russia he became professor of pathology and clinician at the Military Hospital in Moscow, a privy counselor and director of the maternity hospital. He published *Thoughts of a Friend on the Truth about the Improvement of the Science Most Useful for Mankind* (Petersburg, 1787) and translated Tissot's *Treatise on the Health of Scholars* into Russian (Petersburg, 1787).

Schumlansky was an obstetrician and trained in obstetrics before and during his 4 years in Strasbourg and for the 2 years following in various European cities. On his return to Russia in 1784 he was greeted warmly, but not allowed to continue his research. In fact, for a number of years he could not find work and lived in poverty. At that time almost all administrative and teaching positions in Russian medical schools were held by foreigners. In 1784 he was appointed a Professor at the Petersburg Medico-Surgical Institute and in 1788 moved to Moscow. Finally, in 1793 he received an appointment in the Moscow Obstetrics School with the title of 'Civil Obstetrician'. He died 2 years later, on 25 June 1795, at the age of 47 years [8, 9].

Schumlansky's *De structura renum*

Two short articles recently published in Russia to honor the 200th anniversary of Schumlansky's *De structura renum* review his career and his scientific contributions [8, 9]. They renew the contention that Schumlansky has not received due credit for his observations. While acknowledging that Bowman, with his achromatic microscope, could visualize structures that Schumlansky could not see with his lens, they contend that the structure in question should be termed 'Schumlansky's capsule' and not 'Bowman's capsule'.

De structura renum is apparently Schumlansky's only publication on the kidney. The material is presented in a very detailed, meticulous fashion. At times he wrote in a very flowery style, particularly when referring to some of his most famous predecessors. Malpighi, for example, is: 'that famed priest of nature's mysteries'. At other times he is reflective or philosophic, even self-deprecating. As an example of the latter:

'However, if mocked by my dull wit I have not put my finger on the answer, am I to blush at admitting my ignorance which is shared by such eminent men or at admitting my error which perhaps was induced by the bewitching appearance of truth?'

De structura renum is a small (20 cm × 12 cm) book of 138 pages with 2 copper plates, printed in Strasbourg in 1788. It is divided into 47 sections concerned with the macroscopic and microscopic structure of the kidney, followed by a description of 3 experiments also dealing with the gross and microscopic structure of a kidney from a pig.

Schumlansky presented a detailed and comprehensive review of the descriptions of the macroscopic anatomy of the kidney by previous workers, back to the time of Aristotle, and compared their findings with his observations. Humans and many other vertebrate species were considered. It is beyond the scope of this presentation to give an account of those findings with which he agreed and with which he disagreed. Most importantly, the final overall description including that of the major vasculature agrees well with current understanding, as illustrated in figure 1. The inset is a microscopic view of the kidney surface. It is very reminiscent of the micropuncturist's view of the surface of the kidney. It is doubtful, however, whether the reticulated network depicted is of such small structures as the peritubular capillaries.

Schumlansky also presented a lengthy section entitled *Notes on What Can Be Discovered in the Kidney when Observed with a Microscope and with the Aid of More Refined Techniques*. By the latter he was referring to vascular and tubular injections with dye-stained aqueous solutions, mercury, or air. To quote Schumlansky:

'These are the invisible parts which are, so to speak, the abyss where reason deprived of the senses wonders beyond the limits of understanding, often falls into error and lapses into curious fiction. These are the shadowy areas into which I now descend. I wish that the jealous skill of nature would come to the aid of my feeble senses so that after descending into the depths, I may come out, not as the saying goes, handsomer, but sounder in mind. True is the observation: 'There is a limit in things. There exist definite fixed boundaries within which and beyond which the truth is hard to establish.' Science has given to man the tools with which nature's rich store of guile is often unmasked by indefatigable labors.'

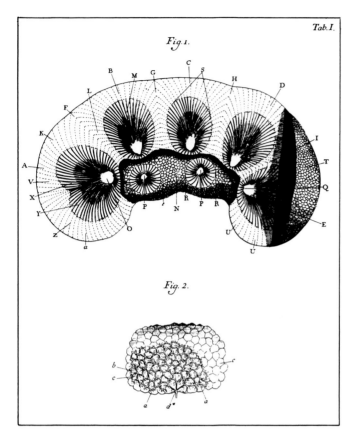

Fig. 1. Schumlansky's diagram of a vertically bisected human kidney (above) and the microscopic appearance of the kidney surface (below).

His general description of the major vessels, which he always carefully compared and contrasted with that of earlier workers, compares well with current knowledge. Of the bifurcating renal arteries and veins, interlobar and arcuate vessels, he wrote:

'From their entire convexity there extend perpendicularly arterioles and their companion veins ... they proceed on their course through the thickness of the cortex ... all the way up to the surface. All along this path they are surrounded by some pulpy, gelatinous substance which is white, semidiaphanous and impervious to wax [obviously the convoluted tubules] ... the branches of the arteries in turn send out small, short capillary branches, more or less numerous, to which granules are appended by stems, one granule per stem; when swollen with matter, the granules look like poppy seeds. The whole branch when viewed with its stems and little granular bodies, resembles a cluster of currants. These are the famous glandula of Malpighi.'

Schumlansky continued with a description of the blood vessels of the medulla and the pyramids of Ferrein. This is followed by a section on the glandula. He states: 'I will discuss what is meant by malpighian glandula'. (As an aside and in an effort to avoid confusion, glandula is the Latin word Malpighi [4] used and which Hayman [5] translated as 'gland'.) Like Malpighi, Schumlansky was able to fill the glandulae by arterial, but not by venous, injection of various solutions. He summed up a presentation of the conflicting results of numerous other workers on the glomerular-tubular connection with the question:

'How am I to extricate myself from this crowd? So many approximations of the truth flock together, producing a knotted and thorny problem. At any rate, let us see if the truth, that royal queen, has shed some light on these matters for us.'

Schumlansky concluded his treatise with the description of 3 experiments on the kidney of a pig which he perfused arterially with a yellow aqueous solution. The fluid flowed freely out of the vein but trickled out of the ureter. Later he injected the renal vein with a blue dye. On section of the kidney he observed the radial arteries and countless masses of attached glomeruli prominently dyed yellow. The veins of the cortex were dyed blue.

Next he cut the kidney into pieces each consisting of a papilla and its covering of cortex. The papillary blood vessels were filled with dye, but not the uriniferous tubules. He blew air into the tip of the papilla and: '... immediately countless silver ducts filled with air right up to the fornix appeared before the naked eye. It was a most beautiful sight.' Microscopically he observed his serpentine ducts (our convoluted tubules):

'Each opening in the pit of the papilla is continuous with a tube that is short and thick. It separates into two trunks which are smaller but still cylindrical in shape. These in turn after traversing some distances bifurcate into two other branches which are just barely reduced in diameter. It is amazing how different and how much larger these ducts are than blood vessels ... along the way they double and multiply continually right up to the base of the papilla. As they pass through the cortex [in the medullary rays] they are in lateral contact with the cortical arch and enter into it one above another and move independently of one another ... their topmost parts turn off to the sides so that each can meet up with its source.

Finally, I was sick of the painstaking effort and the stench of the organ (the fifth day now ending) and I was completely prepared to drop the matter. Yet regretting my fruitless expense of effort, I was given new incentive. And so I exercised the greatest patience on the whole piece that was left. It had been exposed continually for 5 hours to the burning heat of the sun and as a result it was an easy and pleasant task to cut it through the middle. I then blew air into the face of the papilla ... I repeated this procedure. The air moved according to my design and filled the medullary extensions up to their ends, although on the lacerated surface it bubbled up here and there and leaked out. But now I perceived something of unusual whiteness in the pulpy part of the cortical arch. I heated and reheated this pulpy matter blowing fresh air into it, forcing the air along from the outside

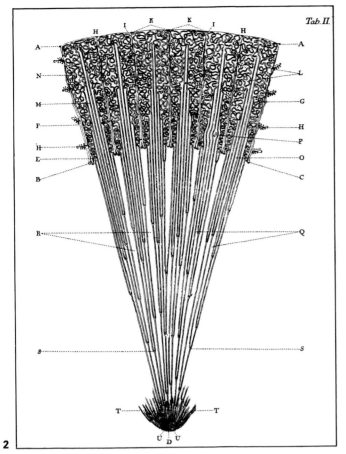

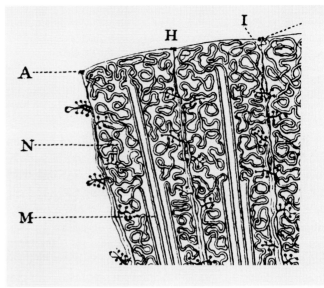

3

Fig. 2. Schumlansky's diagram of the uriniferous tubules and malpighian corpuscles in the human kidney. Note the absence of the loops of Henle, which were yet to be described.

Fig. 3. Enlargement of a portion of figure 2. Note that the glomeruli are drawn much too small and the lack of detail regarding the glomerular-tubular connection.

2

with a small tube and wetting the tissue with saliva. As a result of this treatment a white space appeared ... with a microscope I was pleased to observe in this same area the convolutions of serpentine ducts ... These serpentine tubes after gradually turning off to the side away from their companion straight tubes, which comprise the medullary extension, entered into the cortex ... They go off into their varying convolutions. Always retaining their cylindrical shape they are continuous with the straight tubes and they coil themselves and roll themselves into circles and semicircles everywhere. Ultimately each and every one of these serpentine ducts terminates in its own glomerular body (still dyed yellow) ... Therefore there are as many serpentine ducts as there are vascular glomerular bodies and they differ very little in nature from straight ducts except in respect of their convolutions which perhaps retard the excretion of urine.'

Schumlansky's plate illustrating these findings (fig. 2) contains 2 serious structural errors. One, not recognized at the time, is the absence of the loops of Henle [1], which were not discovered until 74 years later, and the consequent division of the convoluted tubules into proximal and distal segments. The other error, a serious disproportion between the diameter of the malpighian body and the

tubules, was obvious at the time and even led to the accusation that the plate was not drawn from nature. His plate shows the glomeruli to have a smaller diameter than the tubules, when in fact their diameter is much greater than that of the tubules. In addition, the plate is not convincing regarding the nature of the glomerular-tubular connection, even when a portion of the figure is enlarged (fig. 3). A few glomeruli are at the beginning of a tubule, but most are not and in fact there is no detail on this most important point.

The famous German physiologist-histologist Johannes Müller rejected Schumlansky's contention and was most positive in his assertions that there is no connection between the malpighian bodies and the uriniferous tubules [10]. In his book of 1830 on *The Fine Structure of the Secreting Glands*, Müller states:

'In mammals and man, the urinary ducts arising from the papillae proceed directly through the medulla, bifurcate again and again up to the cortical substance, where they spread laterally, and taking a serpentine course, so as to be twisted one among the other; the cortex consists of nothing but the convolutions of ducts. All of these ducts terminate in slightly attenuated blind extremities without any direct communication with the blood vessels or malpighian bodies. The urinary ducts are much larger in diameter than the smallest blood vessels, nor do they ever in any animal communicate with them; the blood vessels rather form a network between the urinary ducts; therefore the urinary ducts themselves secrete the urine' (author's translation).

It was only 9 years later in 1842 that William Bowman [3] in his brilliant paper *On the Structure and Use of the Malpighian Bodies of the Kidney* proved Schumlansky correct and Müller wrong, and in so doing provided the anatomic basis for the filtration theory of urine production. Using a double-injection method described by others, Bowman examined microscopically at $200-300 \times$ magnification preparations from a variety of species. He precisely described and illustrated the details of the glomerular capillaries and the attached afferent and efferent arterioles, and showed the expanded initial portion of the tubule, now known as Bowman's capsule, enveloping the capillary tuft. As Bowman stated:

'It would indeed be difficult to conceive a disposition of parts more calculated to favor the escape of water from the blood, than that of the malpighian body.'

It remained for the genius of Carl Ludwig to propose later that year that the mechanism for the escape of water and dissolved solutes was ultrafiltration, driven by physical forces [11].

It is appropriate to close with the final paragraph of Schumlansky's treatise:

'I have set forth the results of my investigations. If only these results would open up a path for explaining and more readily understanding the separation of the urine. But I leave this vast field of investigation to sharper intellects. Yours is the task, good reader, to determine whether my work has produced accurate results and whether nature imitates the same pattern in other creatures as in this [i.e. the pig] in the structure of the organs or behaves differently and what limitations it has placed on analogy in these matters. But now I must furl the sails which have carried me here to my goal.

No one thing pleases everyone.

One collects thorns, another roses.

If the thorns which I have perchance collected put forth blossoms exceeding the expectation of botanists and bloom advantageously for those who are friends of medicine, they will give me the first fruits of my labor. This is my ultimate hope.'

Acknowledgement

The author wishes to thank Mark Possanza for his careful translation from Latin into English of Schumlansky's *De structura renum*.

References

1 Henle J: Zur Anatomie der Niere. Göttingen, Abh Ges Wiss Math Physik Kl 1862, pp 223–254.

2 Schweigger-Seidel F: Die Nieren des Menschen und der Säugethiere in ihrem feineren Baue. Halle, Buchhandlung des Waisenhauses, 1865.

3 Bowman W: On the structure and use of the Malpighian bodies of the kidney with observations on the circulation through that gland. Philos Trans R Soc Lond (Part 1) 1842;57–80.

4 Malpighi M: De Viscerum Structura Excercitatio Anatomica. Bononiae, J Montij, 1666.

5 Hayman JM Jr: Malpighi's 'Concerning the structure of the kidneys'. Ann Med Hist 1925; 7:242–263.

6 Hirsch A: Bibliographisches Lexicon der hervorragenden Ärzte aller Zeiten und Völker, 2nd edn. Vienna, Leipzig, Urban und Schwarzenberg, vol 5, 1929–1934.

7 Schumlansky A: De structura renum tractatus physiologica-anatomicus. Argentorati, JG Treuttel, 1788.

8 Dudchenko MA: Aleksandr Mikhailovich Shumlyansky. Klin Med (Mosk) 1983:114–116.

9 Gusakov NI: For the two hundredth anniversary of AM Shumlyansky's work on the kidney 1782–1982. Sov Med 1983:117–118.

10 Müller J: De glandularum secernentium structura penitiori earumque prima formatione in homine atque animalibus. Lipsiae, L Vossii, 1830.

11 Ludwig C: De viribus physicis secretionem urinae adjuvantibus. Marburg, Elwert, 1842.

Am J Nephrol 1994;14:325–329

Francesco Paolo Schena

Chair and Division of Nephrology,
Dialysis and Transplants,
University of Bari,
Polyclinic, Bari, Italy

Domenico Cotugno and His Interest in Proteinuria

Key Words
Cotugno
Proteinuria
Nephrotic syndrome
Nephrology

Abstract
Cotugno (1736–1822) was the first to describe the presence of albumin in the urine of a patient with nephrotic syndrome, though he did not place much emphasis on this discovery, which is buried in his many other observations in anatomy, physiology, medical pathology and therapy. Cotugno was a well-known scholar of his time, though he came from a humble background and was largely self-taught. He gained a medical degree from the Salerno School of Medicine at the age of 20 years. He was a prolific researcher and writer, conscientious practitioner of medicine, and a collector of books and antiquities. Much of his library was lost after his death or burned by his wife for unknown reasons.

Introduction

Domenico Cotugno (fig. 1) was one of the early contributors to nephrology, as he was the first to describe the presence of albumin in the urine of a patient with nephrotic syndrome. Unfortunately, it is not easy to find much data on this important discovery, because Cotugno did not place much emphasis on this particular clinical observation. It is enclosed in a myriad of his other observations and discoveries in the fields of anatomy, physiology, medical pathology and therapy, which were published throughout his first 20 years of intensive scientific and clinical activity.

Because the subcutaneous edema of subjects who died with anasarca contained coagulable substances, Cotugno believed that these substances should also be present in the urine. He therefore performed a special experiment which consisted of heating the urine of a patient with nephrotic syndrome. The case report, described in chapter 17 of *De Ischiade Nervosa Commentarius*, was published in 1764 and follows here:

'A 28-year-old soldier who was on garrison duty in Baia Domizia, a very humid and sandy place on the Tyrrhenian Sea, in the month of June had intermittent fever and after 5 days hydrops. He was hospitalized in the Ospedale degli Incurabili in September for the presence of intermittent fever, anasarca, very little thirst and even less urine. Therapy: an emetic (root of ipecacuanha) as expectorant and china bark as antipyretic were given on the first day. The patient had disappearance of fever but persistence of hydrops. For this reason a small dose of scilla as cardiotonic and a decoction of sassafras as diuretic were administered. Since hydrops persisted a cream of tartar as diuretic was given. This decoction reduced oedema and increased diuresis.'

Cotugno observed the formation of a white coagulum, similar to the albumen of a hard-boiled egg, and described this phenomenon as 'albam massam tenerrimo iam coacto ovi albumine persimilem' (a dense white body like albumen of boiled eggs was found in the urine after heating). The same experiment was also performed on the urine of patients with diabetes, and he noticed a lesser amount of coagulable substance. This clinical and laboratory observation demonstrated for the first time the occurrence of albuminuria in nephrotic syndrome and in patients with diabetic nephropathy.

F. Paolo Schena, MD
Division of Nephrology
Polyclinic
Piazza G. Cesare 11
I-70124 Bari (Italy)

© 1994 S. Karger AG, Basel
0250-8095/94/0146-0325
$8.00/0

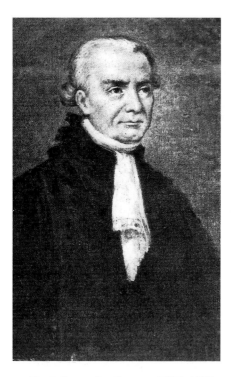

Fig. 1. Domenico Cotugno (1736–1822).

This discovery was cited in books of medical pathology and therapy by many authors, including Bartels, Brault and Senator, and in the *Thesaurius Dissertationum* of Sandifort, published in Rotterdam and Lyon between 1768 and 1778. *De Ischiade Nervosa Commentarius* was also published in English by Wilkie, an editor from London, in 1775 and in German by Schneider, an editor from Lipsia, in 1792. Fifty years later, in 1827, Richard Bright, from Guy's Hospital, London, showed the relationship between albumin and renal lesions and defined this as an important symptom of nephrotic syndrome.

Cotugno: The Scientist

In the 18th and 19th centuries, 3 men enlightened medical science: Morgagni, Cotugno and Virchow. While Morgagni was in his 80s, Cotugno, still only 25 years old, was emerging in all his greatness in anatomy and pathology. In the year of Cotugno's death, Virchow, who was to become the first investigator of cellular pathology, was born. Due credit must be given to Morgagni and Cotugno, who brought new insights into the anatomic alterations of organs in various diseases.

Domenico Cotugno, a man of Ruvo, a physician of Naples, and a scientist of the world, dedicated his life to research of undeniable historical and scientific merit. He was a well-known medical scholar of the time, so much so that he was described by Morgagni as 'il dottissimo' (the most learned person).

The Life and Writings of Cotugno

Domenico Cotugno was born on 29 January 1736 in Ruvo, a small town near Bari in southern Italy. He came from a family of very simple people of Neapolitan origin, who moved permanently to Ruvo in 1713 in the reign of Philip of Aragon. His father Michele, a modest farmer, married twice; his 1st wife, Angela Fiore, gave him 3 children, Luca, Antonia and Victoria. By his 2nd wife, Chiara Assalemme from Terlizzi, he had 3 other children, the first being Domenico Felice Antonio Cotugno, followed by Vincenzo and Donato. Domenico was adopted by his aunt Anna Antonia, his mother's sister.

Cotugno lived in Ruvo until he was 9 years old and there he learned the basics of Latin. He was then sent to a Catholic seminary in Molfetta, under the headship of Canon De Sanctis, where he remained until he was 12 years old (1748) studying arts and Latin, which he spoke fluently and elegantly.

On his return to Ruvo, he studied logic and metaphysics under the guidance of the Capuchin Piccinno, but he also taught himself mathematics and Greek. This solitary study was typical of Cotugno throughout his life. In a letter written to his nephew Peter he stated:

'We can get the best only from ourselves, without any support from others. Our mind strengthens, and becomes stronger, when it dedicates itself to an end and thus begins to appreciate its own value.'

Cotugno was a self-taught man and impatient of the authority of any teacher. He himself said:

'Great men cannot be created by a school; at the best, they can be trained. In fact, everybody should be the teacher of himself. The greatest minds of different arts had teachers of poor ability or none at all.'

Cotugno first studied anatomy, performing accurate dissections on domestic animals. He began his studies of medicine in Ruvo, with doctor Domenico Azzariti from Bisceglie, a practitioner. At the age of 17 years, in December 1753, he left for Naples to attend the university, where he followed the lessons of the well-known Francesco Serao at the Chair of Practical Medicine. During that period a brother of his uncle Vito Paolo (the Capuchin Paolo) sent him a monthly allowance. The following year, by chance, while he was going to visit two friends of his at the Ospedale degli Incurabili, one from the city of Bitonto and another from his home town, he was informed of a competition for a position of medical assistant in that same hospital. He participated and was classified 18th out of 29 participants. He presented a thesis in Latin on pleurisy; he surprised the examiners, who thought that he had memorized his dissertation. In doubt, they asked for another test, and chose a piece from Tacitus. The Governor of the Ospedale degli Incurabili, Don Gaetano Albertini, was fascinated by the clarity and elegance with which Cotugno explained Tacitus' thought in Latin, and became an admirer and patron of Cotugno.

At the age of 18 years (September 1754), Cotugno was appointed as a medical assistant at the Ospedale degli Incurabili, which was then one of the most important hospitals in Europe. The following year he received from the Governor an appointment to teach anatomy, because the Chair was vacant due to the regular professor's illness. In 1756, at the age of 20 years, he obtained a degree in medicine from the Salerno School of Medicine.

Cotugno had a room at the hospital and a small salary, and for 8 years he devoted himself to studying cadaveric anatomy, to consulting books in the library and to curing the patients. He remembered with great pleasure and fondness that period of time until the last years of his life. They were years of intensive work, when he made important discoveries in anatomy which gave him worldwide fame. In a conference at the Teatro Anatomico of the same hospital in 1772, he said:

'The spirit of real medicine is to be found only in facts; it searches any object for facts; it requires practice in any of its multiple aspects; medicine needs facts and not reasons.'

These words were the result of years of intensive anatomic dissections and clinical observations, devoted to the search for truth. They had also been stated 8 years earlier in a letter sent to Bianchi of Rimini in which Cotugno argued against the observations of the anatomist Albrecht von Haller from Göttingen on the discovery of the aqueduct of the internal ear. He formulated the role of the cochlea in hearing, an observation which was opposed and forgotten for some time. In 1862 it was definitely accepted by the scientific world, but as Helmholtz's theory and not as Cotugno's, though Cotugno had published the discovery in 1761 in *De Aquaeductibus Auris Humanae Internae Anatomica Dissertatio*. He made his discov-

eries known by sending copies of his paper to Bianchi of Rimini, to Caldani of Padua and to von Haller of Göttingen; he also travelled all over Italy, as reported in his *Iter Italicum Patavinum*, visiting Morgagni and Caldani. In 1777 the famous Strasburg anatomist, Meckel, performed an extensive series of studies, confirming all that Cotugno had declared earlier in his paper.

In 1762 he made some discoveries on the function of the nasal nerve, described as the parabolic incisive nerve (later known as Scarpa's sphenopalatine nerve), thus explaining the mechanism of the sneeze, and wrote a short autobiographic note *(De Sternutamenti Physiologia)* to Macri, which was only published in 1804 in Cotugno's annotations to Calvani's textbook of physiology.

In 1764 Cotugno published the commentary *De Ischiade Nervosa,* much appreciated by Vanswieten, chief physician in Vienna, whom Cotugno had the opportunity to meet during his trip to Vienna with the royal family of Naples. In *De Variis Diaphragmatis Affectionibus* he showed with much insight and originality the pathophysiology of the diaphragm. In *De Signis Morborum ex Abdominus Tactu Excipiendis* he laid the foundations of modern semiotics. In *Meccanismo del Moto Reciproco del Sangue per le Interne Vene del Capo* he outlined the principles of the circulation of the blood in the human brain found later in Mosso's studies. In *De Sedibus Variolorum Syntagma* he explained his observations regarding diagnosis, prognosis and therapy of smallpox, and instilled in parents the duty of vaccination for their children.

At the age of 40 years, in 1776, Cotugno was elected to the Chair of Anatomy in Naples, after an open competition; he held this Chair until the age of 85 years (1821), when he appointed Folinea as his successor. Because of his reputation, he was invited to the Chair of Anatomy of Pavia and later of Pisa, but he refused both in order to remain in Naples. When he was 52 years old, in May 1778, he went to Rome for 24 days and stayed at the French Locanda, across the street from the Church of San Carlo. On that occasion he visited many Roman dignitaries, prelates and cardinals, including Monsignor Borgia and Monsignor Cesari who later became cardinals, and the Cardinal of Jore.

In 1783 Cotugno saved the Duke of Calabria from certain death and in 1789 (at the age of 53 years), after the death of Vairo, physician of the Royal House, he was invited to accompany the Royal Family of Naples (King Ferdinand and Queen Maria Carolina, their two daughters, one of whom married the Royal Archduke Francesco, the Crown Prince, and the other the Archduke Ferdinando, Grand Duke of Tuscany, both sons of the Emperor

Leopold) on a trip to Vienna. He thus became physician of the Royal House. At that time he discarded the wig he had always worn and decided to dress his own hair for the rest of his life.

At the age of 58, in 1794, he married Ippolita Ruffo, Duchess of Bagnara, widow of the Duke of Bagnara, who had been under Cotugno's care for 2 years. He was introduced into the duke's house by the Neapolitan physician Vincenzo Napolitano, surgeon of the Ospedale degli Infermi. The marriage did not produce any children, but Cotugno maintained a close relationship with his nephew Peter, who lived with him for 42 years at Largo delle Vergini in Naples.

In his writings, Peter stated:

'This woman that my uncle took as wife was not at all suitable for a man of his quality. It is not that she was dishonest. She had a peculiar mixture of bigotism, prodigality and stupidity, that made her detestable.

All men in their life must, sooner or later, pay their tribute to humanity. This Domenico Cotugno, who was considered a genius by everybody, and indeed he was, this kind of man lost himself for a woman who did not deserve the least attention.

The great man, such that he was, recognized his error but there was nothing he could do to make up for such an error. He therefore tried to live with inimitable prudence so as not to expose himself to malicious gossip.'

In his family life, Cotugno was very reserved. He did not receive people in his house for conversation or idle talk, or for consultations. Instead, he preferred to stay alone, reading and writing continuously. After his marriage, he attended Mass every day; he took communion every Sunday in the Paolotti Fathers' Church of La Stella. His diet was composed mostly of vegetable soups (mainly of green chicory), simple meat soup, always without bacon or salted pork, boiled or broiled meat or fish, sometimes fried fish.

At the age of 63 years, in 1799, he went to Palermo in answer to a summons from King Ferdinand IV, who had moved to Sicily with his family after the French occupation of Naples. He later returned to Naples when the court was restored. At the age of 67 years, in 1803, he went to Barcelona by sea, with the Crown Prince who later became King Francesco I.

At the age of 82 years, at 17.00 hours on 29 November 1818, while he was in the Church of La Stella of the Paolotti Fathers, he had a transient cerebral ischemic attack with loss of consciousness, and from then on his health began to decline. Four years later he had another cerebral episode while in a carriage on the Chiaja riviera. He returned home, never to leave it until his death. In July of that year (1822) he lost his intellectual faculties and did not know how to write his own name. At the end of August he was so weak that he was unable to walk. At 23.00 hours on 5 November 1822, he died peacefully while sleeping on his right side. He was buried 2 days later in the Monastery of the Fathers of the Mission of the Virgins, beside his own home.

Cotugno, the Man

Much has been written on Cotugno's great medical talent, but little is known of the man Domenico Cotugno, who was known to his descendants as 'Il Signor Zio', an affectionate name given to him by his nephew, Peter Cotugno (son of Domenico's brother Vincent), in his biography published in 1828, 6 years after his uncle's death. Peter lived with the famous scientist in his house, a silent and discreet presence, observing the everyday activities of his uncle. It is he who recorded what is known of the man, Domenico Cotugno, who lived in extreme simplicity helping others, and by his exceptional ability putting himself in other people's shoes and understandig them. Peter wrote:

'These are qualities that make a man great in any era, ours included, distinguishing him from his peers.'

Domenico Cotugno lived for 86 years, a dedicated scientist, a great anatomist, a distinguished physiologist, an enlightened clinician, a philosopher, a man of letters, an artist and an esthete. His nephew Peter again wrote:

'He was one of those men that Nature sometimes produces in the world so that one can admire it and see where its power can reach, and to this, art had joined to form a very unique person.'

Cotugno received numerous appointments and honours (table 1). His profession allowed him to accumulate wealth that was partly donated to charity. He was so generous as to believe that he had never given enough. His house was always open. His feelings towards the Ospedale degli Incurabili, which had been the place of his training, were very strong and the hospital was the center of all his affections. Once, when he discovered that the hospital needed sheets, he gave the Governor 2000 ducats. On another occasion, while visiting the women's ward of the hospital, he noted that glass was missing from the windows, thus exposing the patients to further diseases. He immediately gave the Governor 300 ducats. On his death he bequeathed over 80,000 ducats to the hospital.

The ideals of liberty, equality and fraternity, which permeated Europe, had repercussions in the kingdom of Naples, where the marriage between King Ferdinand, a good and liberal patron of the arts and sciences, and Maria Carolina of Austria, a domineering and despotic woman, caused such a shift of the political course as to justify the statement that the government of Naples was the negation of God. The arrival of French troops in Naples breathed life into a democratic republic, which unfortunately did not last very long. The reaction following restoration was terrible: many distinguished men lost their lives, including Cirillo, a close friend of Cotugno. Cotugno, however, lived away from any political movement, in the sublime and serene world of science, in the laborious quest for truth. His word was moderate, in a historical setting of violent passions.

Cotugno was a fervent admirer of Plato, preferred Lessing's Laocoönte in archaeology and marvelled at the paintings and marble sculptures of Michelangelo and Raphael. He loved books, and his library was filled with books on various subjects, perhaps the first in Naples adorned with the most beautiful editions. He had a beautiful collection of consular, imperial and antique medals. He collected Greco-Italian vases, antique bronzes and marble sculptures. He had a collection of quite good paintings. During the last few years of his life, and particularly after his death, those in his service despoiled his house in every way. Many *confessors,* during the last years of Cotugno's life, used to carry away works of art when visiting him. The famous Neapolitan surgeon Leonardo Santoro, on leaving after visiting Domenico Cotugno, realized that the gallery where the scientist's manuscripts were kept was at the mercy of thieves, and recommended that Cotugno's wife should safeguard all those papers. She answered with an apparent lack of interest, and on leaving the surgeon said: 'Ah Domenico Cotugno, you have been magnificent in everything, only in one thing you have wrongly acted, in choosing this woman as wife'. His wife,

Table 1. Appointments and honours of Domenico Cotugno

Date	Age (years)	
1764	28	Member of the Academy of Bologna
1802	66	Member of the Council for the Improvement of the Royal Library
		Member of the Council for the Reform of Public Studies
1806	70	President of the Institute for Encouraging Natural Sciences
1808	72	Chief of the Health Council and of the Central Committee for Vaccination
1809	73	President of the Science Academy of the Royal Bourbon Society
1812	76	Member of the Council for the Reform of the Royal University
		Senior member of the Faculty of Medicine
		Twice President of the University
1815	79	Member of the Council for the Reform of Public Schools
1817	81	Member of the Copenhagen Academy
1818	82	Honorary President of the Academy of Physicians of Naples

after the death of the scientist, burned many of his papers and manuscripts for unknown reasons. A list of many of Cotugno's books was contained in a catalogue named *Catalogo di una Biblioteca Vendibile* which included about 4000 titles with prices, sold by the Printer Trani of Naples in 1828.

Further Reading   Cotugno P: Memorie su Domenico Cotugno. Rotary International Club di Molfetta, 1985.
Iurilli A: Opere. Manduria, Lacaita Editore, 1986.
Satta M: Domenico Cotugno e l'Albuminuria. Rassegna Pugliese di Scienze, Lettere ed Arti 1907; 23:70–74.

Am J Nephrol 1994;14:330–336

Mario Umberto Dianzani

Department of Experimental Medicine and
Oncology, Section of General Pathology,
University of Turin, Turin, Italy

Bizzozero and the Discovery of Platelets

Key Words

Bizzozero
Platelets
Blood clotting

Abstract

Bizzozero was born in 1846 and graduated in medicine at the age of 20 years. After working in Pavia for some years he was appointed Professor of General Pathology in Turin. Here he collaborated with many famous scientists in Italy and abroad. His interest in hematopoietic cells culminated in a description of platelets and their essential involvement in the blood clotting mechanism in vivo. Before Bizzozero's work, the description of platelets had been unclear, and both red and white cells were thought to be required for formation of blood clots. Although Bizzozero's discovery was disputed vigorously for several years, he was finally vindicated in 1892, unfortunately 1 year after his death. Apart from his extensive work, he bequeathed to science the benefit of his logical descriptions and rigorous experimental approach.

Introduction

Important scientific discoveries seldom result from the observations of single investigators. More often, they are preceded by several partial discoveries by different scientists. The real discovery, however, occurs when one scientist has the final intuition of the real meaning of previous fragmentary observations and collates them to provide clear evidence on a particular problem. Such was the case with the discovery of platelets. The scientist with the intuition, who provided clear evidence of their importance in blood clotting and in thrombosis, was Giulio Bizzozero, professor of general pathology at the University of Turin (fig. 1).

The Life of Bizzozero

Bizzozero was born in Varese on 20 March 1846 and first studied in Milan in a classical lyceum. At 16 years of age he was already studying medicine at the University of Pavia. He became greatly interested in experimental work and frequented the Laboratory of Experimental Physiology, which was directed by an Italian scientist of Viennese origin with a German name: Eusebio Oehl. Oehl introduced Bizzozero to positivism and experimental work. As early as 1862 the young scholar published his first paper in *Archivio per la Zoologia*, the subject being the distribution of vascular canals in the long bones of the frog.

Bizzozero graduated in medicine on 5 June 1866, when he was 20 years old, having already published several papers and acquired a good knowledge of histology, a science that did not have many followers in Italy at that time. The same year, Bizzozero became assistant to Paolo Mantegazza, who was already famous as Professor of General Pathology in Pavia. Mantegazza had considerable insight into pathophysiology and introduced his young assistant to the discipline with enthusiasm. In 1861 Mantegazza had founded a laboratory of experimental pathology in his institute, and he left its direction to Bizzozero as early as 1867. There, Bizzozero developed several important research projects and had numerous en-

Mario Umberto Dianzani, MD
Department of Experimental Medicine and Oncology
Section of General Pathology, University of Turin
Corso Raffaello 30
I–10125 Turin (Italy)

© 1994 S. Karger AG, Basel
0250–8095/94/0146–0330
$8.00/0

thusiastic collaborators. The most famous among them was probably Camillo Golgi, who became Professor of General Pathology in Pavia and was awarded the Nobel Prize in 1906, together with Ramon y Cajal, for the discovery of the 'black reaction' that led to a great increase in knowledge of the structure of nervous tissue and its cells. Other important collaborators were: Foà, who became Professor of Pathologic Anatomy first in Modena and then in Turin, where he started an important school of this discipline; Bozzolo, who became Professor of Clinical Medicine in Turin and founded the Turinese clinical school; Griffini, who became Professor of Pathologic Anatomy in Modena, and then Professor of General Pathology in Genoa; Manfredi, who became Professor of Ophthalmology in Pisa; and Bassini, Professor of Clinical Surgery in Padua.

Bizzozero's education in Pavia was strongly influenced by his frequent visits to and continuous contact with the laboratories of Virchow in Berlin, Frey in Zurich and von Kölliker in Basel. With the last 2 scientists in particular he developed friendly relationships and a continuous exchange of ideas occurred. Bizzozero deputized for Mantegazza as teacher of general pathology in Pavia in 1869 and 1872, when his professor left his chair to devote himself to anthropology; Mantegazza finally became professor of anthropology in Florence.

In 1873, Bizzozero left Pavia when he won the competition for the Chair of General Pathology in the University of Turin. He was only 27 years old at that time, full of vigor and enthusiasm. The Faculty of Medicine of Turin was divided at that time into 2 opposing groups: the 'conservative' group, which was opposed to all new things; and a group that was interested in a new style of scientific work.

The group of innovators was strongly influenced by Moleschott, a Dutchman who had graduated in Heidelberg and was then dismissed from his teaching position in that university because of his philosophic and scientific ideas. Moleschott was a follower of Feuerbach and introduced positivism and scientific materialism into Turin and Italy in general. Moleschott had been Professor of Physiology in Zurich when he met De Sanctis, formerly Professor of Humanities in Turin and then in Zurich. When De Sanctis became Minister for Education in Italy, he invited Moleschott to Turin as Professor of Physiology in 1861, where he remained until 1879, when he moved to Rome. Moleschott assisted Bizzozero and strengthened his scientific positivism.

Other important positivists were: Timermans, Professor of Clinical Medicine; Giacomini, Professor of Normal

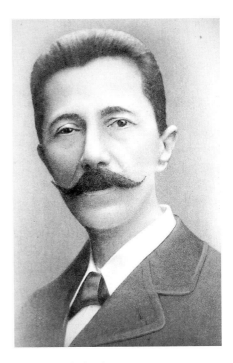

Fig. 1. Giulio Bizzozero.

Human Anatomy; Giacosa, Professor of Pharmacology; Mosso, Professor of Pharmacology and then Professor of Physiology after the departure of Moleschott; Pacchiotti, Professor of Propedeutic Surgery; and Pagliani, first assistant of Moleschott, like Mosso and Giacosa, and then Professor of Hygiene. With these friends, Bizzozero was able to produce a positivistic revolution in Turin, which started what could be called the 'golden half-century' of that university.

Timermans was Rector when Bizzozero started as a full professor and helped him to find 2 small rooms in the Institute of Anatomy, where Bizzozero set up his laboratory of experimental pathology. When Timermans left the rectorship, Bizzozero lost his 2 rooms and was compelled to house the laboratory in his own private residence on the Via Nizza. There he received collaborators and students and pursued important scientific research. After a few years he succeeded in adding to this laboratory a few small rooms in a university building in Via San Francesco da Paola, where other scientific laboratories of the Faculty of Medicine were situated. Only in 1893 did the Institute receive its final accommodation in Corso Raffaello.

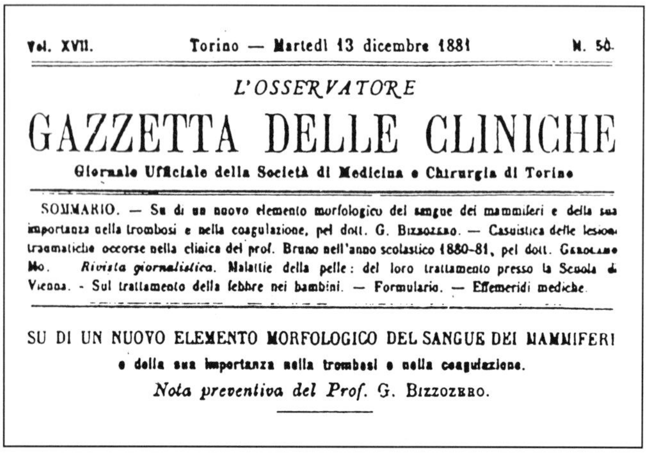

Vol. XVII.   Torino — Martedì 13 dicembre 1881   **N. 50.**

L'OSSERVATORE

GAZZETTA DELLE CLINICHE

Giornale Ufficiale della Società di Medicina e Chirurgia di Torino

SOMMARIO. — Su di un nuovo elemento morfologico del sangue dei mammiferi e della sua importanza nella trombosi e nella coagulazione, pel dott. G. Bizzozero. — Casuistica delle lesioni traumatiche occorse nella clinica del prof. Bruno nell'anno scolastico 1880-81, pel dott. Geronimo Mo. *Rivista giornalistica.* Malattie della pelle: del loro trattamento presso la Scuola di Vienna. - Sul trattamento della febbre nei bambini. — Formulario. — Effemeridi mediche.

SU DI UN NUOVO ELEMENTO MORFOLOGICO DEL SANGUE DEI MAMMIFERI

e della sua importanza nella trombosi e nella coagulazione.

Nota preventiva del Prof. G. Bizzozero.

Fig. 2. Preliminary note by Bizzozero on the discovery of platelets and their importance in clotting and thrombosis. Note the date of 13 December 1881. The oral presentation to the Academy of Medicine of Turin is dated 9 December 1881.

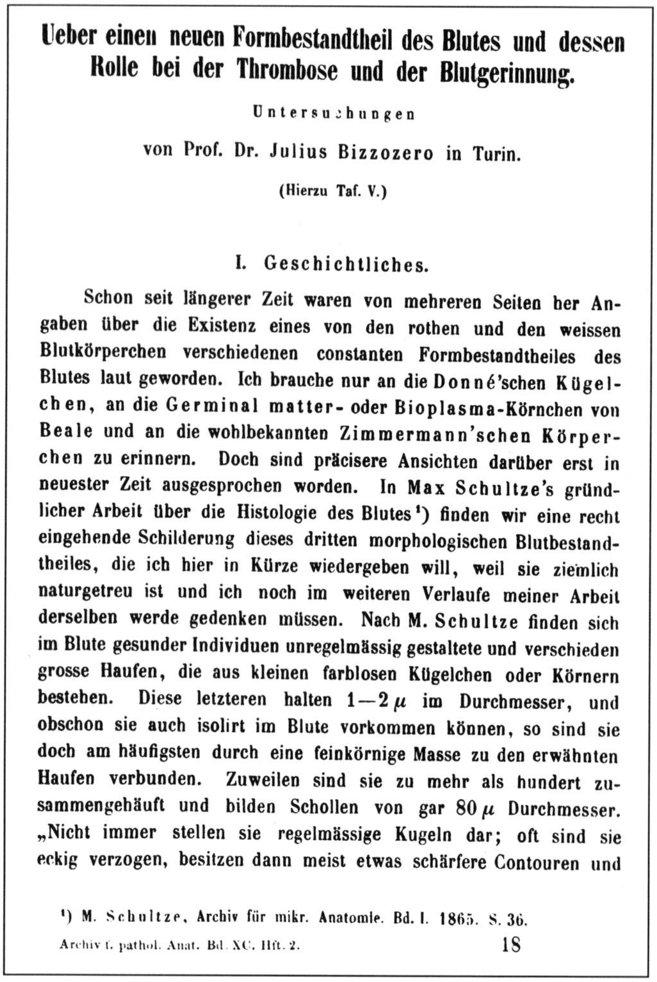

The Discovery of Platelets

Bizzozero had started to study the hematopoietic organs, particularly bone marrow and lymph nodes, as early as 1865 in Pavia. He continued this interest in Turin, at first with the collaboration of Guido Tizzoni, who subsequently became Professor of General Pathology in Modena, and then in Bologna. Their studies on the behavior of the hematopoietic organs after bleeding added considerably to knowledge of these subjects and the reputation of the Turinese school. Bizzozero also worked on regeneration and on the structure of epithelia and tumors, he was able to induce experimental tubercular granuloma in guinea-pigs after inoculation with material derived from tubercular lesions, and he studied the behavior of cells during their life cycle and their multiplication.

Bizzozero officially solved the problem of platelets in 1881. The first announcement of his discovery of platelets as the 3rd morphologic component of blood, particularly involved in blood clotting and thrombosis, was given at the Academy of Medicine of Turin on 9 December of that year. A preliminary note was published on 13 December in *L'Osservatore Gazzetta delle Cliniche* (fig. 2) [1]. The title of the article was very clear: 'Su di un nuovo elemento morfologico del sangue dei mammiferi e sulla sua importanza nella trombosi e nella coagulazione', and contained the bulk of the discovery.

On 3 March 1882, Bizzozero gave a more detailed talk to the Academy of Medicine of Turin. This text, together with that of the previous communication of 9 December

Ueber einen neuen Formbestandtheil des Blutes und dessen Rolle bei der Thrombose und der Blutgerinnung.

Untersuchungen

von Prof. Dr. Julius Bizzozero in Turin.

(Hierzu Taf. V.)

I. Geschichtliches.

Schon seit längerer Zeit waren von mehreren Seiten her Angaben über die Existenz eines von den rothen und den weissen Blutkörperchen verschiedenen constanten Formbestandtheiles des Blutes laut geworden. Ich brauche nur an die Donné'schen Kügelchen, an die Germinal matter- oder Bioplasma-Körnchen von Beale und an die wohlbekannten Zimmermann'schen Körperchen zu erinnern. Doch sind präcisere Ansichten darüber erst in neuester Zeit ausgesprochen worden. In Max Schultze's gründlicher Arbeit über die Histologie des Blutes[1]) finden wir eine recht eingehende Schilderung dieses dritten morphologischen Blutbestandtheiles, die ich hier in Kürze wiedergeben will, weil sie ziemlich naturgetreu ist und ich noch im weiteren Verlaufe meiner Arbeit derselben werde gedenken müssen. Nach M. Schultze finden sich im Blute gesunder Individuen unregelmässig gestaltete und verschieden grosse Haufen, die aus kleinen farblosen Kügelchen oder Körnern bestehen. Diese letzteren halten $1-2\,\mu$ im Durchmesser, und obschon sie auch isolirt im Blute vorkommen können, so sind sie doch am häufigsten durch eine feinkörnige Masse zu den erwähnten Haufen verbunden. Zuweilen sind sie zu mehr als hundert zusammengehäuft und bilden Schollen von gar $80\,\mu$ Durchmesser. „Nicht immer stellen sie regelmässige Kugeln dar; oft sind sie eckig verzogen, besitzen dann meist etwas schärfere Contouren und

[1]) M. Schultze, Archiv für mikr. Anatomie. Bd. I. 1865. S. 36.

Archiv f. pathol. Anat. Bd. XC. Hft. 2.   18

Fig. 3. The first page of the article Bizzozero published in *Virchow's Archiv für pathologische Anatomie und Physiologie* in 1882.

1881, were published in the March issue of the *Giornale della Accademia di Medicina di Torino* (this academy, founded by the King Charles Albert in 1846, is still in existence). In his March communication, Bizzozero gave more information that appeared in *L'Osservatore* about his rationale and the methods used, adding also new evidence about the involvement of platelets in blood clotting. In fact, he saw that a 'proplastic fluid' containing only fibrinogen and a 'thromboplastic substance' is made to coagulate by the simple addition of short pieces of thread coated with platelets.

The full description of the general problems of the experimental procedure and of the rationale of his discovery, as well as a thorough discussion of his own findings in comparison with other reports was published later [2] (fig. 3). This paper was 71 pages long, considerably longer than the preliminary notes in *l'Osservatore* and *Giornale della Accademia*, and also longer than a paper in French that appeared in *Archives Italiennes de Biologie* [3], the journal published by Angelo Mosso. Despite the fact that the Lancet carried a full-page report of Bizzozero's discovery in the issue of 22 January 1882 [4], where the exact 1881 reference was quoted, most people refer to 1882 as the year of the discovery of platelets. As Coller noted in this century [5], this was probably due to the lack of knowledge of Italian of most international scientists, as well to the length of the German article.

Bizzozero's interest in the problem of platelets, however, was born long before 1881. Mantegazza had studied the nature and the formation of white thrombi for a long time, and he published papers on this subject in 1869 and 1871 when Bizzozero was still in Pavia. It was only in 1878, however, that Bizzozero was able to buy a Hartnack microscope, which allowed further research possibilities. This microscope and its invoice for 1677 lire (a large sum of money for the time) are still preserved in the Institute of General Pathology in Turin (fig. 4). Thus the discovery communicated in 1881 may have taken at least 3 years of work. It is also important to remember that there were few communications on the subject between the first studies by Schmidt and others in the early 1870s and the papers by Hayem, who returned on the subject in 1878/1879. It seems possible that the papers by Hayem stimulated Bizzozero to study the topic himself.

Early Work

At the moment of Bizzozero's discovery the field was very confused. Several authors had reported their observations, but the descriptions they gave were far from clear and their interpretations were not convincing. Among the first to observe what might have been platelets were: Donné, who described small vesicles ('Kügelchen'); Beale, who described the presence of a 'germinal matter' in the blood, in addition to red and white cells (also described as 'Bioplasma Körnchen' (small nuclei)); and Zimmermann, who saw 'Körperchen' (small bodies). All these authors worked with blood samples withdrawn from the vessels, so it remains unclear whether what they saw were preexistant in the circulating blood, or artefacts formed in vitro. Moreover, their descriptions were rather vague and not consistent.

The first scientist to give a better description of the 'objects' was Schultze [6], who reported the common presence in extracted normal human blood of aggregates with differing, irregular sizes, which were formed by smaller particles or nucleus-like bodies with diameters of 1–2 μm.

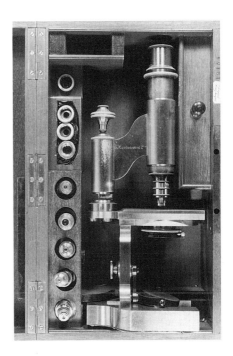

Fig. 4. The Hartnack microscope bought in 1878 by Bizzozero and used in the discovery of platelets. It is preserved in the Laboratory of General Pathology of the University of Turin.

As the diameter of the aggregates was about 80 μm, Schultze calculated that such aggregates were formed by at least 100 (perhaps several hundred) particles, or vesicles. He proposed that the vesicles mostly consisted of albumin-like material, similar to that present in protoplasm. The vesicles became swollen when suspended in water, but resisted for a longer time when exposed to dilute acetic acid. They disappeared after treatment with alkaline fluids and after exposure to lipid solvents. Schultze was also able to see many filamentous protrusions emerging from the periphery of some of the vesicles. Such protrusions were seen more often in coagulated blood. His opinion was that such particles, as well as their protrusions, might derive mainly from degenerated white cells, or at least that their formation occurred under the influence of white cells, which were abundant inside the clot.

The idea that the vesicles were related to blood clotting was strongly opposed by Riess [7], who considered that the presence of vesicles was a pathologic event, commonly encountered during infectious diseases, blood diseases, e.g. chlorosis, anemias and leukemias, diabetes and kidney diseases. Riess thought that the vesicles, which are rare in normal blood and decrease further in normal co-agulated blood, derived from the destruction of pathologically involved white cells. This opinion was accepted by Laptschinski [8].

Schmidt, a scientist with a great reputation, also studied blood clotting. He observed the common presence of vesicles even in normal extracted blood [9]. His opinion, however, was that these vesicles derived from the destruction of colorless blood cells, mainly produced by disaggregation of white cells. Osler and Schäfer, however, proposed that the vesicles were related to the presence in the blood of bacteria [10].

Another author who reported interesting observations on the vesicles was the famous Ranvier [11]. He studied blood clotting in vitro and saw that the vesicles were always connected with the fibrillar net of the clot. His opinion was that the vesicles were not derived from pre-existing white or red cells, but were related to the clot fibrils, where they might work as a coagulation nucleus, similar to a crystallization nucleus in a saturated salt solution seeded with a crystal of the same salt.

The Work of Hayem

Discussion of the vesicles then stopped until 1878/1879, when Hayem published his new observations obtained with instruments of greater definition [12]. He saw that the blood normally contains cellular elements other than red or white cells. Whereas these last cells did not undergo great changes when observed under the microscope, another component having at the beginning the appearance of a small red cell underwent rapid alterations. This component was described by Hayem as biconcave, sometimes changing to a round or to a long shape. Its diameter was reported as between 1.5 and 4.5 μm. Its color was yellowish or greenish but could become more intense by absorbing hemoglobin. Hayem thought that the new component was very similar to red cells and added that the formation of Schultze's aggregates was strictly related to the disintegration of this new component. The name used for this component was *hematoblast,* a name clearly pointing to a red cell derivation.

Hayem's papers renewed the discussion. Riess claimed that Hayem had not produced any clear evidence that his hematoblasts were the same as his own vesicles and insisted on the origin of vesicles from white cells in pathologic conditions [13]. Neumann claimed that hematoblasts were probably artefacts and nothing more than red cell stromata [14].

The Work of Bizzozero

This was the point at which Bizzozero's discovery arrived. Bizzozero's major experimental aim was to study circulating blood, and not blood extracted from the vessels as other authors had done. This he achieved by observing the mesentery or omentum of small rabbits or guinea-pigs, still attached to the living animal, under the microscope. These membranes were laid on a rather simple device placed on the flat table of the Hartnack microscope.

The device consisted of a glass surface 20 cm long, fixed by screws or weights on the microscope table. In the center of the plate, corresponding with the central hole in the table, he attached with Canada balsam a cork cylinder with a central hole. The cork cylinder was 15 mm high and 25 mm wide, the diameter of the central hole being 14 mm. On the upper part of the cylinder Bizzozero put a glass slide with a diameter of 18 mm, whose central part corresponded to the optical axis of the microscope. The omentum or the mesentery was laid on this slide, taking care to keep it moistened with saline. In this way, he could observe cells circulating inside the vessels by using different magnifications, and even an immersion objective lens, the immersion fluid usually being saline. Another precaution was the use of warmed fluids to keep the whole device at a physiologic temperature, as warmed microscope tables had not then been developed. He did not describe how he succeeded in achieving temperature control.

By using his immersion system, Bizzozero was able to observe what he defined as: 'the third circulating component of the blood', inside living vessels, close to white and to red cells. He defined this new component as 'piastrina', which he himself translated into German as 'Blutplättchen' and into French as 'petite plaque'; the English name became 'platelet'. Bizzozero's main finding was that platelets exist in circulating blood, and therefore they are not artefacts produced during clotting.

The platelets had a mean diameter 2–3-fold smaller than that of red cells. Their surface was generally flat, though sometimes lenticular, and their form generally round or oval. They were colorless and were randomly distributed inside the vessels, with no preference for either the center or the peripheral regions. They were present in both veins and arteries. When the circulation stopped due to death of the animal, platelets were still present inside the vessels for some time, but rapidly underwent alterations similar to those seen when a drop of blood was put under the microscope between two slides. Under these conditions, the platelets tended to form aggregates, sometimes including some white or red cells, which clearly corresponded to those described by previous authors. One of the most common changes of platelets described was the formation of filamentous protrusions (fig. 5). Bizzozero claimed that these protrusions were present before the formation of the clot and represented the start of the clotting process. There was no change in the appearance of either red or white cells during the platelet changes, which ended with the formation of a dense fibrillar net. Bizzozero thus definitely ruled out the hypothesis that platelets were derived from either white or red cells and they were clearly the 3rd physiologic cellular component of the blood, essential for blood clotting. Bizzozero also tried to stain the platelets with methyl violet, gentian violet, carmine, picrocarmine and hematoxylin, but concluded that the best observations were those done without any staining inside living vessels.

Bizzozero expanded his work to a study of the mechanism of thrombus formation, taking as his starting point the facts already established, mainly by the studies of Mantegazza, Virchow and Schultze and by the pioneering work of Cohnheim, Zahn, Weigert and Ranvier. Bizzozero's approach was again an in vivo one, in which he pricked a small vessel with a needle under the microscope. He observed that the first morphologic event was the attachment of platelets to the damaged internal surface. After attachment the platelets underwent rapid changes, mainly consisting of the formation of protrusions, as other authors had seen in extracted samples of blood. Almost immediately after this change, a net of fibrils appeared, so that the degenerating platelets became enmeshed in a fibrillar network. Inside this network the platelets degenerated further, until their disappearance as morphologically distinct cellular elements. The network sometimes also involved white and red cells, the number of red cells being important for the final color of the thrombus. Both white cells and red cells, however, remained as distinct entities for a long time without any evidence of degeneration. There was thus no proof of their participation in the formation of the thrombus. This discovery ruled out the hypothesis, accepted even by Montegazza, that white or red cells participated actively in the formation of the thrombus.

In another section of his paper, Bizzozero gave a full description of the experiments already communicated to the Academy of Medicine of Turin concerning the participation of platelets as an essential active element in the formation of thrombus. He prepared a 'proplastic fluid', consisting only of a fibrinogenic and a fibrinoplastic substance (which would today be called fibrinogen and

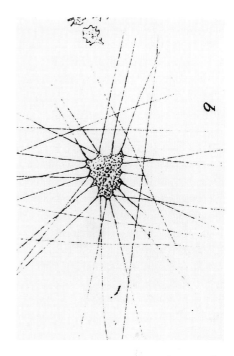

Fig. 5. A platelet drawn by Bizzozero for his article in *Virchow's Archiv* (see fig. 3).

thromboplastin). This fluid was unable to form a clot until the addition of single short segments of thread previously coated with platelets by agitation for 1 min in a small amount of freshly extracted blood; the red cells were then removed from the segments by repeated washings. Coagulation started immediately after the addition of the platelet-coated segments. Addition of washed red cells to the 'proplastic fluid' was without any effect. No effect was also observed after addition of slices of spleen, lymph nodes, or small amounts of bone marrow, which were used as a source of white cells as methods for the separation of white cells had not then become available. It was thus clear that only platelets were important for clot formation in the experimental system used.

Bizzozero was unable to establish the site of formation of platelets. He had long experience in studying the hematopoietic system, starting at Pavia in 1868 [15], and tested the possibility that this 3rd morphologic component of the blood was formed in bone marrow, like the other cellular components. He also studied spleen and lymph nodes. He was unable, however, to see a sufficient number of platelets in any organ to exclude the possibility that the observed presence was due to contamination with blood. In these investigations Bizzozero had the intuition, but not the proof. He clearly stated his failure with regret. The discovery that megakaryocytes were the site of platelet formation arrived much later.

Bizzozero's discovery provoked active discussion. The first report in the *Lancet* elicited 2 replies, by Neale and Norris, which were published in the *Lancet* 1 week after Bizzozero's report [16, 17]. Neale claimed priority, saying that he had observed the small bodies referred to as platelets by Bizzozero as early as 1854. Norris also claimed to have seen platelets before Bizzozero and to have understood their importance in blood clotting. Bizzozero replied immediately [18, 19] that both scientists had observed platelets in extracted blood and not in vivo, so they had no proof of the existence of platelets in the living animal; moreover, there was no evidence that what they observed were really platelets, and not artefacts. In the case of Norris' report, there was the serious probability that what he described were only altered red cells.

The most intense discussion, however, concerned the participation of white cells in blood clotting. Schmidt had insisted on the origin of platelets from white cells. Although Bizzozero was finally triumphant, after having convinced his friends Kölliker and Frey with his evidence, the problem was still open in 1892. Bizzozero asked his young collaborator Salvioli (formerly assistant in physiology with Moleschott, then Professor of General Pathology in Padua after a long training with Bizzozero) to study again the participation of white cells in addition to platelets. Salvioli's paper was communicated to the Academy of Medicine of Turin on 13 May 1892 [20], and his conclusion supported the views of Bizzozero and definitely excluded the participation of leukocytes in the blood clotting mechanism. Bizzozero did not live to enjoy his victory, however, and he died of pneumonia on 8 April 1901, at the age of only 55 years.

Conclusions

The influence of Bizzozero on the development of science in Italy was immense. It is sufficient to remember that at least half of Italy's current general pathologists, about two-thirds of the pathologic anatomists and about half of the professors of hygiene have been directly or indirectly influenced by him. His interest, however, was not restricted to the academic field and was much stronger in the development of experimental medicine. The results of most of his studies, not only those on bone marrow and platelets, remain unchallenged. The numerous examples include: the discovery of tonofibrils in skin epithelial cells and their behavior in epitheliomas; studies on cell division and on nuclei; and particularly studies on the different biologic behaviors of growing cells. What is astonishing in reading his papers, especially that in *Virchow's Archiv*, is the totally logical description of his ideas and of his experimental rationale, as well as his scientific rigor. One of the positivistic sentences he often used was:

'I trust only in what I succeed in demonstrating.'

His demonstrations were always clear-cut, all the possibilities in explaining a phenomenon being seriously discussed, so that the final interpretation was the only one tenable after thorough discussion. This procedure is the best inheritance he left to his students.

References

1 Bizzozero G: Su di un nuovo elemento morfologico del sangue dei mammiferi e sulla sua importanza nella trombosi e nella coagulazione. Osservatore Gazzetta delle Cliniche 1881;17:785–787.
2 Bizzozero G: Über einen Formbestandteil des Blutes und dessen Rolle bei der Thrombose und der Blutgerinnung. Virchows Arch Pathol Anat Physiol 1882;90:261–332.
3 Bizzozero G: Sur les petites plaques du sang des mammifères, deuxième note. Arch Ital Biol 1882;1:1–4.
4 Anon: A new blood corpuscle. Lancet 1882;1:111–112.
5 Coller BS: Bizzozero and the discovery of the blood platelets. Lancet 1984;i:804.

6 Schultze M: Arch Mikrosc Anat 1865;i:36.
7 Riess L: Zur pathologischen Anatomie des Blutes. Arch Anat Physiol 1872;8:237.
8 Laptschinski M: Zur Pathologie des Blutes. Zentralbl Med Wiss 1874;12:657.
9 Schmidt A. Pflügers Arch 9:356.
10 Osler W, Schäfer A: Über einige im Blute vorhandene bacterienbildende Massen. Zentralbl Med Wiss 1873;11:577.
11 Ranvier. Gazette Med 1873;93–94.
12 Hayem MG: Recherches sur l'évolution des hématies dans le sang de l'homme et des vertébrés. Arch Physiol Norm Pathol 1878;10:692.
13 Riess. Berlin Klin Wochenschr 1879;653.
14 Neumann. Z Klin Med 111:411.

15 Bizzozero G: Sulla funzione emopoietica del midollo delle ossa. Gazzetta Medica, 14 November 1868.
16 Neale. Lancet 1882;i.
17 Norris. Lancet 1882;i.
18 Bizzozero G: Le piastrine del sangue e la coagulazione. Giornale della Accademia di Medicina di Torino 1882;45:9.
19 Bizzozero G: Les petites plaques du sang et la coagulation. Arch Ital Biol 1882;1:276.
20 Salvioli I: Della compartecipazione dei leucociti nella coagulazione del sangue. Giornale della Accademia di Medicina di Torino 1892;40:371–376.

Am J Nephrol 1994;14:337–343

Giovanni Federspil[a]
Nicola Sicolo[b]

[a] Cattedra di Medicina Interna, and
[b] Cattedra di Endocrinologia, Istituto di Semeiotica Medica, University of Padua, Padua, Italy

The Nature of Life in the History of Medical and Philosophic Thinking

Key Words

History of medicine
Atomism
Vitalism
Naturalism
Mechanism

Abstract

The vitalistic doctrine of Aristotle and Galen, in which the soul is an indissoluble part of the body, was undisputed throughout most of the Middle Ages. The first radical change came with Telesio, who developed philosophic naturalism in which the soul has a reality of its own, though it is connected to the body. The definitive change came with Descartes, who believed that all biologic phenomena can be explained by the laws of mechanics, and only man is distinguished by the possession of a soul. For the next 300 years, this mechanistic view would be challenged by a new vitalism, in which the 'vital force' has an existence in its own right.

Introduction

The problem of the nature of life is an ancient and complex matter, which not only spans the entire history of philosophic thought but also runs through the whole history of biologic and medical cognition. The problem was born very early in Western thought, and since the very beginning, it irrevocably blended the reflections of biologists and physicians with those of philosophers. The former were forced to reflect on the phenomenologic reality they faced every day, and in some ways attempted to dominate it. The latter were also forced to include within their own speculative approach the part of reality represented by life.

The Classical View

Perhaps the first doctrine on the nature of organisms was elaborated by the Greek atomist philosophers and was later revisited by the Epicurean school. According to Democritus (460–? BC) nature consists of atoms, by which was meant invisible, incorruptible and ungenerable particles endowed with only local movements, which attract or repel according to an absolute need. Human beings are no exception to this general rule, as the soul also consists of atoms forming, where there is life and heat, a more refined matter supported by respiration. This short description illustrates the fact that Democritus' thought was governed by absolute determinism: in nature there cannot be any finalistic purpose.

The view of Aristotle, who represents the first vitalistic doctrine, was opposed to that of Democritus. According to Aristotle (384–322 BC), natural bodies consist of a primordial entity, the substance, itself composed of two elements: the matter, with no specific determination; and the form, an element capable of giving a specific determination to the matter and of transforming it into one or another specific thing. Thus, living organisms are natural bodies constituted of matter, meant as the physical body itself, and of a form, named by Aristotle soul or *endelechia*.

Giovanni Federspil, MD
Istituto di Semeiotica Medica
Via Ospedale 105
I–35100 Padova (Italy)

© 1994 S. Karger AG, Basel
0250–8095/94/0146–0337
$8.00/0

To clarify Aristotle's view, which is still often misunderstood, it is necessary to underline that his is not a properly dualistic doctrine that establishes the presence in living beings of two distinct and separable realities. Enrico Berti, an expert on Aristotle's philosophy, once stated [1]:

'The soul is not something added to the living body, but it is a whole with it, it is its very life, considered not as an action aiming towards realization of the different functions, but on the contrary as the capability of performing them as their principle ...

There is no duality between the soul and the body, since they are not two different substances, but they are constitutive and insoluble elements of a unique substance which is the living being.'

The second fundamental point of Aristotle's philosophy, which is closely related to the first, is represented by the existence of final causes. Relying on the doctrine of the four causes, Aristotle stated that in the world of life every single thing has an appropriate aim to which it spontaneously tends, and that no single item of knowledge of living beings can be exempted from the knowledge of their aim.

It is well known that Aristotle's doctrine had an enormous influence over biologic and medical thought, mainly through the work of Galen. Galen (129–189 AD) acquired from Aristotle a vitalism chiefly founded on a finalistic view of the physiologic phenomena, which constituted a heuristic principle able to clarify the function of different living organisms. In Galen's words [2]:

'Owing to the great discordance among the ancient physicians and philosophers about the usefulness of the parts – in fact some of them declare that our bodies are made without any finality, without any project, while others, on the contrary, think they have an extent and have been made according to a project ... I have tried first to find a standard of judgement of such a discrepancy, and later to set up a universal and unique method which enables us to find the usefulness of each of the parts and of the things that happen to them ...

What he [Hippocrates] says is this: 'All the parts of the body are sympathetic one to the other, i.e. all collaborate in the same activity ...' The abdomen, mouth, tongue, feet and hands, which we are going to consider, are made in this way. Nobody ignores their 'activity'. In fact it is clear they (hands) have been made to catch ... If the activity of the thorax, lungs and heart and of all the other parts were as clear as that of the eyes, hands and feet, we would not have many differences to discuss about the usefulness of the parts.

Now, since the activity of the majority of the parts is obscure, and without knowledge it is impossible to find the usefulness of a particular one, it is clear that all those who were wrong about the function of the organs were wrong about the usefulness of the parts.'

In this fundamental passage of Galen, two extremely important ideas are expressed: the first is that the parts of living beings are built according to a project and have a purpose in the preservation of life and of the species; the second is that finalism, when it is not founded on knowledge of the function, constitutes nothing more than an a priori conviction, a metaphysic theory. In modern epistemologic terminology, finalism represents for Galen the metaphysic nucleus from which a heuristic principle or a research program can be generated.

Theories of Life in the Middle Ages

The theories of Aristotle and Galen on living organisms achieved rapid success and were dominant, almost undisputed, throughout the the Middle Ages. The first radical change appeared only in the 16th century with Bernardino Telesio (1509–1587) and the so-called philosophic naturalism. Living beings, in Telesio's opinion, could be sharply distinguished from lifeless entities, because while the latter are generated from the ground or from the sun and are lower beings, the former generate from themselves or from their seeds and are, in this way, superior beings. For Telesio, plants and animals are made by combining the body and the soul, but the soul is no longer, as Aristotle and Galen suggested, the shape of the body, indivisible from it and constituting with the body a unique substance. Now the soul is considered as a reality substantially different from the body but connected with it by the seed, which influences the body itself and its parts by giving to it movements and modifications. Such 'spirit', which is a characteristic of non-human living beings, is an extremely slight corporeal substance included in the body.

Telesio's doctrine is extremely important, because it represents a fundamental departure from the classical theory of Aristotle and Galen. The living being is no longer made of two inseparable realities connected in a unique substance, but of two realities of the same order – the corporeal order – which coexist and reciprocally influence each other. In Telesio's philosophic naturalism the ancient vitalism disappeared, but was not replaced by true naturalism; its place was occupied by a different sort of vitalism, founded on a partially dualistic concept, which recognized an essential finalism of organic entities and in which two principles, different but of the same nature, body and soul, coexisted.

Development of a Modern View of Life

René Descartes
Although the first clear differentiation of modern thought from classical thought emerged through Telesio, the radical and definitive change took place with René

Descartes (1596–1650). According to him, no souls other than the rational soul, which is characteristic of men, exists, and consequently the life of the human body and of other living beings has to be described without any consideration of substantial forms or lower souls. In this way, organisms are nothing more than machines and the entire complex of phenomena they manifest – biologic phenomena – must be entirely explained by the laws of mechanics, i.e. of physics. Even sensations can be related to the movement of material particles and in this way to the material world.

Descartes stated [3]:

'In fact it is known that all these movements of muscles as well as all senses, depend on nerves which are small strings or tubes coming all from the brain and contain – like the brain – a certain gas or very light wind called 'animal spirits'.'

The expression 'animal spirits' should not be misleading, however, as the philosopher explained, because:

'... what I call 'spirits' are nothing more than bodies which have no other properties than to be extremely small and to move at a very high speed like the parts of the flame which come out from an oil lamp.'

Descartes' point of view was absolutely mechanistic and represents the root of all modern reductionism. Once the distinction between matter and form has been denied, any possibility of a vegetative soul for a living being is ruled out, and all biologic phenomena must be related to the movements of the *res extensa* and thus to the laws regulating inanimate nature. Thus, if Telesio's naturalism preserved the idea of reason in organic activities, with Descartes living beings, with the exception of man, cannot be distinguished from machines and can only act by the intervention of the 'proximal causes' without any finality.

The ideas of Descartes had a great influence on biology and medicine and initiated two different research programs: iatrophysics, considered to explain all biologic and pathologic phenomena by the laws of mechanics; and iatrochemistry, supposed to explain the same phenomena though chemical mechanisms.

Leibnitz
Gottfried Wilhelm Leibnitz (1646–1716) was the first, in redefining the *philosophia perennis*, who reintroduced the substantial matters called by Aristotle 'primary endelechias', indicating them with the name 'primitive forces'. Leibnitz began by asserting that the principles of physics are not sufficient to adequately and fully explain nature's phenomena. In fact, in living beings a finalism can be clearly recognized as part of a wider finalism of the world, in which everything has been made by God for the good of man.

The philosopher said [4]:

'I suggest to those who are fond of true philosophy, to beware of the statements of those spirits who say we are able to see since we have eyes, and not since our eyes are made to see.'

Leibnitz clearly distinguished the proximal causality from the final one and assigned to each of the two a well-defined role in the comprehension of nature. Such a position, often forgotten in subsequent discussions, is extraordinarily important because it permits a solution to many of the controversies born later.

'To reconcile those who hope to explain mechanically the formation of the first tissues of an animal and all of the mechanism of the parts, with those who justify the existence of these structures appealing to the final cause, it is necessary to make this observation: both could be good methods, both could be useful, not only to admire the work of the Great Creator, but also to find something useful in physics and medicine. So the Authors who follow these different ways should not mistreat each other ... For it would be better to combine the two considerations ... Notwithstanding, I think that the way of the efficient causes, which is deeper, more immediate and a priori, is more difficult when one goes into the detail, and I believe that our philosophers, in most cases, are yet very far from it. The way of the final causes is, on the contrary, easier and often does not stop being useful in order to imagine important and advantageous truths which would otherwise require a longer time to be found by another more physical way, as anatomy can show with considerable examples.'

Thus, according to Leibnitz, the body is connected with an *endelechia* or 'soul', and the complex of these two realities constitutes the living being.

New Vitalism
According to G.E. Stahl (1660–1674), a physician of the University of Halle, living beings are made of 'aggregates' which differ from inorganic aggregates by virtue of the fact of being made to accomplish a number of functions. The organic aggregates, however, are distinguished not only from inorganic inert bodies but also from man-made machines, because although these work passively animal bodies work continuously, modifying their own function constantly and adapting it to the achievement of their goals. Such a finalistic and intelligent activity of living organisms is identified with their souls, according to Stahl, i.e. with a metaphysic and immaterial matter added to the body, preserving it from being corrupted, as it

would have done if it could have acted according to its own material nature.

At this point it is not difficult to understand that the vitalism that asserted its authority during the 18th century was profoundly different from that of Galen and Aristotle. In the ancient concept the soul constituted a form indissolubly related to the matter, thus permitting the latter to be characterized. Stahl's vitalism, as well as that of his followers, saw the soul as an external principle which adds to or even penetrates into the inert body, transmitting to it movement, i.e. a kind of activity, and in some way vivifying it. In this sense, the vitalism of the 18th century is close to the naturalism of Telesio, according to which a soul, still material, adds to the body and envelops it in a metaphysic dualism in which a material reality coexists with a spiritual one.

Stahl's ideas exerted an extremely important influence on the biomedical thought of the 18th and early 19th centuries. In fact, the idea that a living organism is a reality substantially different from inorganic matter started taking shape in this period. Between the many types of vitalism of that time it is possible to distinguish two doctrines quite different from each other. According to the first, the living being was not moved by any immaterial principle, even if this could not be explained by the same principles able to justify inorganic phenomena. According to the second, living beings were characterized by the presence of an entity which was joined to the body but was not corporeal itself.

Giacomo Andrea Giacomini (1796–1849), a physician of Padua University and an extremely vigorous exponent of vitalism in the 19th century, wrote [5]:

'The living being is controlled by a power in opposition to the physicochemical laws, and during lifetime, this power opposes physicochemical influences; the vital strength is not secondary to the organization or to the result of the general forces but it is primary and determines the organic milieu in opposition to external influences.'

Such a biologic viewpoint cannot fail to have a deep impact even on medical theories; in fact, Giacomini continues:

'It is nature that cures disease. And by the term 'nature' we mean an activity, a force within the living organism, called by different people mediating force, organic resistance, autocracy, and considered in different ways ... To deny an activity of the organism which counteracts disease and keeps the body healthy against thousands of hazards is intellectual blindness. The mediating force of nature is the same force that renders this organism alive, develops it and maintains it; it is the force which establishes and maintains the organic milieu and makes it no longer susceptible to nature's laws, but to laws

in opposition to these, which by modification of it in different tissues and organs enables them of their characteristic actions.'

According to the vitalists of the 19th century, life does not develop through an ordered association of physical and chemical phenomena, but in opposition to them by the intervention of a force that has nothing in common with already known forces, and which has its own laws that can only be observed and described but not explained by more elementary phenomena.

Obviously, the vitalism of the first half of the 19th century was opposed by a reductionism deriving directly from iatrophysics and iatrochemistry. The opposition to vitalism was first of all founded on the uselessness of a concept like 'vital force', which added nothing new to what was already known on the basis of observable phenomena, and furthermore on the absence of satisfactory proofs in favor of the vital activity of which the vitalists were speaking. On the contrary, all vital phenomena, if adequately studied, could be explained according to common physical and chemical knowledge.

Maurizio Bufalini (1787–1875), physician at Florence University and a ferocious antagonist of Giacomini, wrote in 1844 [6]:

'It must be stated that the terms 'vital force' or 'vitality' are nothing else than the whole of the properties belonging not only to the organic compound, but are characteristic of all of the bodies uniquely existing in this.'

In the general cultural atmosphere of the 19th century, the quarrel with romantic vitalism naturally gave rise to a reaffirmation of the reductionist thesis. That period's reductionism, however, in many instances had the features of a rigid and simplifying metaphysic concept, which excluded any finality in vital processes and reintroduced biologic phenomenology into a universal deterministic vision.

In a brief essay dedicated to the 'Vital Force' and published for the first time in 1848, Emil DuBois-Reymond (1818–1896) illustrated in the following words the idea of vital phenomena dominating the biomedical world at that time [7]:

'In our opinion the force is the measure and not the cause of the movement ... It is quite clear that in these conditions it makes no sense to consider the force like a separate entity which maintains an existence independently from the matter ... A particle of iron is and remains the same thing whether it crosses the cosmos inside a meteorite or screeches on a rail, or if it passes inside a red blood cell through the temple bone of a poet. Just as in manmade machines nothing is added, and nothing is removed from the material particles. Such properties are eternally inalienable, non-transferable. At this point it is vain to ask whether the difference we recognize ... between the processes of dead and living nature really exists. Such a difference is imaginary. In the organism the particles do not possess new forces which could be considered as vital. The difference between so-called organic and inorganic nature is arbitrary.'

Thus, as:

'... a vital force does not exist ... the effects ascribed to it must be subdivided in those which came from the forces of elementary particles.'

Claude Bernard

The rigorous contrapositions of vitalists and mechanists found a harmonic composition in the concepts developed by the French physiologist Claude Bernard (1813–1878). Far from endorsing the excesses of either of the parties, Bernard reaffirmed the existence of a finality of the living being's internal units, but held that biologic finalism rises to its full extent only when the organism is considered as a whole. Simply because the cooperation of many units represents a fundamental element for comprehension of the human being, the organism appears to the physiologist and to the physician as something more than a simple assemblage of the parts constituting it. In such a case, both the metaphysic vitalism of the systematics and the rigid reductionism of mechanists are insustainable, and only a moderate vitalism, able to recognize the differences of living beings from the inorganic world, can represent an acceptable biologic doctrine.

Bernard wrote [8]:

'The physiologist who is outside the animal body he sees like a whole, has to take into account this whole ... It follows that while the physicist or the chemist can reject any finalistic component in the phenomena they observe, the physiologist must recognize a harmonic and pre-established finality in organic bodies in which all manifestations are combined with one another and depend one on the other. In fact, if the true value and sense are to be given to a certain physiologic property, this property has to be always referred to the whole ... It follows that in physiology the knowledge of the properties of isolated elementary units cannot give anything more than an incomplete synthesis; ... in a word, when physiologic elements are combined new properties, which could not be appreciated in each single element, appear ... This shows that the elements, although different and independent, do not simply associate with one another, but their unification expresses something more than the simple addition of their separate properties.'

On another occasion, analyzing the significance of vital forces, Bernard wrote [8]:

'Among naturalists, and even more among physicians, there are some who in the name of vitalism formulate the most erroneous judgements ... They consider life a mysterious and supernatural force which acts arbitrarily and releases itself from any determinism, and consider as materialists all those who try to lead all vital phenomena to causes determined organically or physicochemically ... The vitalistic ideas, in the sense we have discussed, are nothing more than faith in the supernatural ... I would agree with vitalists only if they limited themselves to admitting that living beings present manifestations absent in the inanimate world and, for this reason, constitute a peculiar character of it.'

The position of Bernard is extremely important, because it clarifies the extent of the differences between vitalism and mechanism.

In its self-evaluation, vitalism had progressively abandoned its initial Aristotelean position in which shape and matter coexisted in a unique substance, the living body. Beginning with the naturalism of the 16th century, the vegetative soul was considered as a material reality which 'added' to the body and 'inhabited' one or another part of the body. Thus, if in Aristotelean philosophy the soul was a substantial form, beginning with Stahl it became an 'entity' with an autonomous existence, an 'entity' completely independent of the body and capable of transferring to it movements and activities. The vital principle constitutes the deep and immeasurable reality responsible for all the phenomena of living beings; to it can be attributed all those biologic phenomena which at a certain moment cannot be explained through the identification of a proximal cause.

The radical modification of perspectives that took place in 18th century vitalism explains the profound hostility of many biologists and physicians, then and now, to a concept that to most people appears as a convenient verbal shift or as an excuse to avoid engagement in research for the cause of biologic phenomena.

Bernard recognized all this, but recognizing also the complexity and specificity of biologic phenomena, refuted simplistic reductionism and defended the idea of moderate vitalism which, without invoking supernatural entities, contemplated a reality in the living being characterized by an interior finality and substantially different from that of non-living things.

A 20th Century View of the Nature of Life

After this long, though incomplete, journey through the main doctrines on the nature of living beings developed over the centuries, it is now possible to draw some general conclusions.

When each individual doctrine is considered, it is evident that they are all a mixture of scientific and philosophic theses. This is not surprising: the complexity of the subject, which can be seen from quite different viewpoints, the knowledge that the philosophic and scientific approaches represent two completely different ways of reflecting reality, and finally, the difficulty of defining a unique criterion for differentiating science from philosophy, all justify the confusion and the superimpositions of the past. Indeed, the terms vitalism and mechanism point to two different metaphysic theories on the nature of living beings.

Although in the 19th century it was common to accuse the vitalists of using a metaphysic approach, and although this is sometimes repeated today, it is necessary to emphasize that from an epistemologic point of view both vitalism and mechanism are metaphysic doctrines, and that neither of them can be submitted to experimental control. From this standpoint, the dispute between these two approaches will surely continue in the future, depending on the swing of general philosophic ideas.

Apart from their metaphysic meaning, however, mechanism and vitalism have in the present century assumed a weaker position, becoming concepts with a purely methodologic meaning. Ludovico Geymonat, speaking about mechanism, stated [9]:

'The mechanistic thesis underwent many developments and profound modifications from Descartes to nowadays, from the fundamental field of metaphysics to the experimental one of scientific research. Today mechanism does not point to an affirmation that the biologic laws can be deduced from those of physics, but rather to supporting the idea that the only way to improve our knowledge of biologic phenomena is to use the same methodology as physics and chemistry.'

In fact, the same principle can be applied to vitalism. Today's vitalistic thesis no longer defends the existence of a 'vital principle' which inhabits the body and opposes and modifies physicochemical phenomena, directing them to a predetermined goal; it is now less simplistic and can be mainly seen in research on the morphology and physiology of individual organs or the biologic behavior of the organism in all its complexity. The main assumption of this 'methodologic vitalism' is that a satisfactory and complete knowledge of biologic phenomena can be gained only when each single acquisition obtained by physical or chemical methods is integrated into a unifying vision of the living being, and can be interpreted as phenomena adapted to preserve and transmit life.

What today distinguishes a vitalist from a mechanist is a methodologic behavior, rather than a metaphysic thesis. Reductionists, according to Evandro Agazzi, believe that the behavior of the parts explains the behavior of the whole, and minute analysis of the parts tends towards giving explanations that 'look at the bottom'. In contrast, the vitalist views the behavior of the organism as a system and:

'... contemplates the scientific explanation as 'looking up' towards principles capable of embracing as a whole a great variety of individual facts, among which the occurrence which has to be explained can be found' [10].

To the type of biologist who studies the higher levels of organization, the English-speaking world has given the name 'life-oriented physiologist'.

The situation was perfectly described in 1931 by Fulton, one of the most important physiologists of the 20th century [11]:

'Two kinds of opposite physiologists can be distinguished. There are physiologists who believe that the true object of their studies is the organism 'in toto'. There are also others who want to constitute a group aside ... Their method is physical and quantitative; they want to study life phenomena with methods derived from physics and physical chemistry. In many instances their interest, instead of being turned to the whole organism, is limited to the liquids of the body and to the substances which can be obtained from organs. It would be better if they could recognize that they are not at all physiologists, but rather biophysicists or electrochemists or even protein chemists. The contribution to chemistry and physics of the living beings due to this group of physiologists has been extremely important, but we should wish that physiology could return to consider the organism like a whole.'

If, as has been suggested on methodologic grounds, reductionism and mechanism retain their importance and function, what can be said today about metaphysic problems? The dualistic vitalism born with Stahl's doctrine and spread during the 18th and 19th centuries has surely declined forever. Today, nobody believes that living beings are inhabited by a soul or by a vital force that opposes the physicochemical forces and is even capable of altering their effects. The death of this kind of vitalism, however, does not remove all vitalistic concepts, nor does it necessarily means the victory of mechanistic metaphysics.

The quarrel, which in the last 3 centuries has set mechanism and dualistic vitalism against each other, leaves untouched the older vitalism born with Hippocrates and Aristotle, which originates from a finalistic vision of biologic processes. If it is true that a soul that goes in and out from the organism, that inhabits one or another part, and that opposes and suspends the physicochemical laws does not really exist, it is equally true that in the whole we call organism, where an enormous number of cells exchange their messages and react in a coordinated way with the purpose of preserving themselves, there exists a common principle, i.e. a unitary and finalistic organization of the vital functions. It is to just such a kind of principle that Aristotle gave the name of soul.

Acknowledgements

The authors are grateful to Professor A. Borsatti and Dr. E. Photiou for translation and revision of such an unusual text as the present one for biomedical literature.

References

1 Berti I: Profilo di Aristotele. Rome, Edizioni Studium, 1979, p 180.
2 Galeno C: Opere Scelte. Torino, Edizioni Utet, 1978, p 327.
3 Cartesio R: Le Passioni dell'Anima. Torino, Edizioni Utet, 1951.
4 Leibnitz GW: Scritti di Metafisica. Torino, Edizioni Paravia, 1969, pp 48–49.
5 Giacomini GA: Trattato Filosofico-Sperimentale dei Soccorsi Terapeutici. Padua, Tipografia del Seminario, 1833–1841, pp 69–70.
6 Bufalini M: Saggio sulla dottrina della vita. Forli. 1813, in Opere di Maurizio Bufalini. Florence, Gabinetto, 1844, p 26.
7 DuBois-Reymond E: I Confini della Conoscenza della Natura. Milan, Editione Feltrinelli, 1973, pp 95–96.
8 Bernard C: Introduzione dello Studio della Medicina Sperimentale. Milan, Edizioni Piccin, 1994, pp 92–93.
9 Geymonat L: Problemi metodologici e filosofici suggeriti dall'opera di Antonio Vallisneri, in Il Metodo Sperimentale in Biologia da Vallisneri ad Oggi. Padua, Accademia Patavina di Scienze, Lettere ed Arti, 1962.
10 Agazzi E: La teoria dei sistemi ed il problema del riduzionismo, in I Sistemi tra Scienza e Filosofia (a cura di E. Agazzi). Torino, Società Editrice Internazionale, 1978.
11 Fulton J: Physiology. New York, Clio Medica, Hoeber, 1931.

Am J Nephrol 1994;14:344–354

Klaus Hierholzer

Department of Clinical Physiology,
UK Benjamin Franklin,
Free University of Berlin,
Berlin, Germany

Carl Ludwig, Jacob Henle, Hermann Helmholtz, Emil DuBois-Reymond and the Scientific Development of Nephrology in Germany

Key Words
History of nephrology
Theories of urine formation
Endoscopy
Renal anatomy

Abstract
Medical science in the 2nd half of the 19th century proceeded in a stepwise fashion, when the development of new techniques permitted the evaluation of living processes by direct microscopic or endoscopic inspection, as well as by quantitative measurements of the underlying physical and chemical forces. Ludwig, Henle, Helmholtz and DuBois-Reymond all contributed in different ways to the evolution of medicine and physiology into natural sciences, freed from romantic, philosophic speculation. Nephrology benefitted from this development and from the contributions of the non-nephrologists to natural science.

Introduction

In 1959 Pitts predicted that the major developments in nephrology would depend on 3 factors [1]:

'First, the gradual accumulation of a critical mass of basic information; second, the new concept or way of viewing the problem; and third, the new method, or adaptation of the old, which permits a more precise testing of the concept.'

This prediction must be set against the situation in the 19th century, when natural sciences and medicine emerged from romantic natural philosophy. Was it this 3-step interaction of new data, new concepts and new methods that catalyzed progress? In nephrology in particular, what led to the realization that the apparently mysterious capacity of the kidneys to excrete poisonous material did not require a vitalistic power, but could simply be explained by underlying physical and chemical forces?

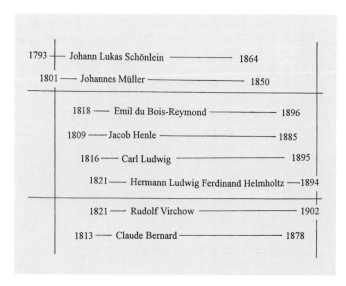

Fig. 1. Historical context of the scholars discussed in the present paper.

The author wishes to thank Ms. A. Kliesch and Professor R. Winau for expert help in researching the literature.

Klaus Hierholzer, MD
Department of Clinical Physiology
UK Benjamin Franklin, Free University of Berlin
Hindenburgdamm 30
D–12200 Berlin (Germany)

Table 1. Emil DuBois-Reymond (1818–1896)

1818	Born in Berlin, son of a government employee, immigrant from Switzerland (Neuchâtel)
1837	Studied science and arts, then medicine in Berlin, friendship with Hallmann and Brücke, buys microscope
1840	Assistant to Müller, electrophysiologic studies, construction of galvanometer, student of Schönlein
1841	Foundation of *Jüngerer Naturforscherverein*
1841	Examination as surgeon
1843	Promotion to MD (electric fish), in disputation takes an antivitalistic standpoint, contact with Humboldt
1845	Foundation of Berlin Physical Society
1846	Habilitation (muscle physiology), meets Helmholtz, publication of *Studies on Electricity of Animals*
1850	Travels to Paris
1852/1855	Travels to London
1858	Müller dies, DuBois-Reymond Professor of Physiology in Berlin
1867	Permanent Secretary of Academy of Science
1869/70 and 1882/83	Rector of the University
1875	Publication of collected studies on general muscle and nerve physics
1877	1st Institute of Physiology in Berlin opened
1896	Died in Berlin

Assistants and friends: Helmholtz, Ludwig, Henle, Brücke, Meyer, Heymanns, Munk, Bernstein, Heidenhain, Boll, Bezold, Herrmann, Kühne, Pflüger, Rosenthal, Virchow and others.

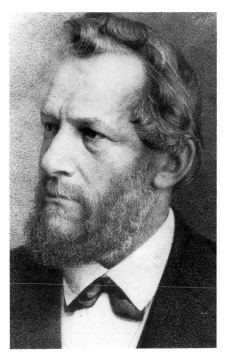

Fig. 2. Emil DuBois-Reymond (1818–1896).

The answer to this question can be elucidated by studying 3 leading scientists: Carl Ludwig, Jacob Henle and Hermann Helmholtz, who made basic contributions to science in general and to nephrology, without being nephrologists in the strict sense. Emil DuBois-Reymond can also be included, as he particularly influenced the development of physiology and medicine in that century. These figures are put into their historical context in figure 1, a context that includes Johann Lucas Schönlein and Johannes Müller, the scientific fathers of the other scholars listed. Claude Bernard lived in Paris at the same time; he was another leading figure with an important influence on the scientific development of medicine in the 19th century.

Emil DuBois-Reymond (1818–1896)

The contribution of DuBois-Reymond (fig. 2) to nephrology was rather indirect. He was a neurophysiologist, but also a central figure in freeing physiology from romantic, idealistic philosophy. The important dates in his life are given in table 1. He was the most outspoken advocate of modern physiology in its own right, which he considered to be organic or applied physics and chemistry. He learned to completely resist vitalism, to which he was exposed in Johannes Müller's department.

'All forces in living and non-living nature are similar and mechanical' [2].
'We do not need a mysterious servant to sneak in and to perform the job, the challenge is to explain everything by natural forces, matter and energy.'   Defence of his thesis, 1842

DuBois-Reymond was an electrophysiologist; it was he who developed the essential equipment, e.g. a 'Multiplikator' (galvanometer) and instruments for electrical stimulation, in order to measure action potentials and current flow in nerves and muscles. Although DuBois-Reymond's impact on nephrology was indirect, it was not unimportant. Apart from the general influence of his physical and mechanistic approach on all experimental disciplines, it

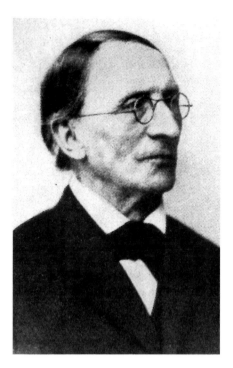

Fig. 3. Carl Friedrich Wilhelm Ludwig (1816–1895).

was he who strongly encouraged Carl Ludwig to write and publish his *Lehrbuch der Physiologie des Menschen* [3, 4], in which the filtration theory of urine formation was extensively discussed.

It was also in his laboratory that Rudolph Peter Heinrich Heidenhain (1834–1897) was trained, and eventually became another pioneer nephrologist, though a strong opponent of Ludwig. Heidenhain injected indigo carmine into hypotensive rabbits to show the successive blue staining of convoluted tubules: first of the cells, then of the lumen. He derived a 2-step secretory model of urine formation, in which filtration was not possible. He calculated a 'monstrous volume' of about 70 l/day of filtrate, which would necessitate the reabsorption of at least 68 l/day!

Finally, DuBois-Reymond, with his demonstration of nerve action potentials and Helmholtz with his measurement of nerve conduction velocity, stimulated a young physician, Ernst Unger in Berlin, to undertake transplantation experiments with nerves and later with kidneys. DuBois-Reymond's laboratory was probably where Unger became acquainted with the experimental techniques that he applied soon after in animal experiments in order to transplant kidneys: first homologous kidneys in animals; then in 1909, a heterologous kidney from an ape *(Macacus nemestrinus)* to a human patient [5, 6].

Carl Friedrich Wilhelm Ludwig (1816–1895)

Ludwig (fig. 3) was a close friend of DuBois-Reymond. Together with Claude Bernard he was to become the leading physical physiologist of his time. Often quoted is the foreword to the *Lehrbuch der Physiologie des Menschen:*

'Physiology is the physics and chemistry of the processes of life and the only way which promises success is the reduction of the complex processes of the organism to physicochemical relations' [7].

Ludwig's contribution to physiology in general and to nephrology in particular are classic examples for Pitts' paradigm. Three examples of Ludwig's work are discussed here: (1) his habilitation thesis on the mechanism of urine secretion (1842–1843); (2) his relationship with Jacob Henle; and (3) his continuous interest in the kidney, i.e. his later experimental work, which is not generally recognized.

The life of Ludwig is reviewed in table 2 [7, 8]. Apparently, as a student Ludwig had to leave the university of Marburg for disciplinary reasons. After his return he worked with Robert Bunsen and, with the help of Ludwig Fick, he obtained a position in anatomy. Due to his political activities in the late 1840s (in 1847/1848 with Bunsen he was a member of the executive committee of the *Vaterlandsverein* and editor of a liberal newspaper *Neuer Verfassungsfreund*), he could not expect an independent academic position in his country, and he therefore accepted positions in Zürich (as did Schönlein and Henle) and in Vienna (Josephs-Akademie) before he returned to Germany. His institute in Leipzig was a charismatic place, which attracted people from all over the world, e.g. Henry Pickering Bowditch, Ivan Petrovitch Pavlov, Angelo Mosso, Friedrich Miescher and Julius Berstein.

The list of Ludwig's contributions is impressive, and some but not all are given in table 3. Those particularly relevant to the present discussion are: (1) the development of the kymograph, which for the first time permitted continuous recording of biologic parameters; (2) the inauguration of in vitro studies on isolated organs, for which he suffered considerably from attacks by antivivisectionists; and (3) the formulation of the filtration/tubular absorption theory of urine formation. Figure 4 shows the original kymograph and examples of simultaneous recordings of blood and intrapleural pressures.

Ludwig's habilitation thesis was published in 1842 in Latin as *De Viribus Physicis Secretionem Urinae Adiuvantibus* [9] and 1 year later in German as *Beiträge zur Lehre vom Mechanismus der Harnsekretion* [10]. In it, Ludwig

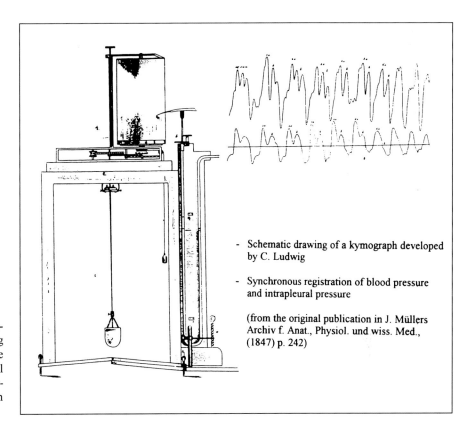

- Schematic drawing of a kymograph developed by C. Ludwig

- Synchronous registration of blood pressure and intrapleural pressure

(from the original publication in J. Müllers Archiv f. Anat., Physiol. und wiss. Med., (1847) p. 242)

Fig. 4. Schematic drawing of a kymograph developed by Carl Ludwig, allowing synchronous registration of blood pressure and intrapleural pressure. From the original publication in *Müllers Archiv für Anat. Physiol. und wiss. Med* (1847). With permission from Schröer [7].

Table 2. Carl Friedrich Wilhelm Ludwig (1816–1895)

1816	Born in Witzenhausen (Werra), father in army, later exchequer's officer
1835–40	Studied medicine in Marburg/Erlangen/Marburg
1840	Worked in Bunsen's laboratory
1841	Assistant at Institute of Anatomy, Marburg
1842	Delayed habilitation: *Mechanism of Urine Secretion* (antivitalistic approach)
1844	*Kidneys and Urine Formation* in Wagner's *Handwörterbuch der Physiologie*
1846	Kymograph, studies on blood circulation, a.o.
1846	Professor of Anatomy, Marburg
1849–55	Professor of Anatomy and Physiology in Zürich
1855	Professor of Physiology and Medical Physics, Vienna, formation of saliva, lymph, mechanics of circulation, blood gases
1865	Professor of Physiology, Leipzig, physiology of respiration, functions of central nervous system, etc.
1895	Died in Leipzig

Table 3. The contributions of Ludwig to physiology

Methodology	Scientific achievements
Kymograph for continuous autographic recording	Filtration theory of urine formation
Flow meter for quantitative blood flow measurement	Discovery of secretory nerves
In vitro techniques for the study of isolated organs	Hemodynamic studies (origin of 1st heart sound, organ circulation, 1st recording of capillary pressure, lymph formation) Studies of salivary gland and pancreatic secretion (secretion pressure) Studies on diffusion through membranes Neurophysiologic studies (description of nerve depressor, vasomotor centers in central nervous system)

pointed out that the force that drives urine excretion had not adequately been defined.

'One has considered a vital, a chemical and a mechanical force which accomplishes the separation of fluid through blood and glandular vessels.'

In order to analyze the problem he performed careful histologic studies, in vitro injection experiments with kidneys, which he perfused from the arterial or ureteral side (he extended these to kidneys from man, dog, rabbit, pig and horse), and model experiments with apparatus specially designed to imitate the flow pattern within kidneys. Furthermore, he acquainted himself with the field of hydraulics, apparently with the help of Eytelwein's *Handbuch der Hydraulik* [11].

Gottschalk has carefully reviewed these studies [12], but a few details from the original manuscripts can be added. Data accumulated at that time did not unequivocally show whether the glomerular capillaries branched, whether one or more efferent vessels existed, or whether tubules had direct contact with glomeruli. Ludwig settled these controversial issues once and for all. He also described for the first time 2 types of glomeruli in the human kidney: small deep ones and large superficial ones. On the basis of his and Krause's measurements of the diameters of renal vessels, he calculated that the total cross-sectional area of the glomerular vessels was larger than that of the afferent and efferent arterioles.

Ludwig also stressed that he had never observed: 'free ends of tubules ... however sometimes loops.' He did not specify in which section of the kidney, and the latter observation was not given any special attention; thus, tubules always had contact with glomeruli, but 'an open communication' between the capillary and the tubular lumen apparently did not exist. This he concluded because neither wax, protein, nor fat could penetrate from the arterial side. This of course was in clear contrast to Müller, who had denied a direct contact between glomeruli and tubules. Both Müller and Bowman had advocated tubular secretion as the primary process of urine formation. Ludwig concluded that pressure filtration of fluid was the primary process of urine secretion, i.e. a physical process as the underlying mechanism. Pressure in the vessels could force fluid through membranes, and increased pressure was thought to dilate the membranes, thereby enlarging pores:

'... the quantity of filtered fluid will therefore depend on the strength of the pressure, the [vascular] resistance, and the resistance within the membrane, as caused by pores, which opposes the effective [driving] force.'

Any vitalistic force, which was thought to attract and excrete poisonous material, was dismissed altogether, as was a chemical driving force, i.e. endosmosis, which was favored by several authors of that time. Ludwig, however, in contrast to Valentin [13] realized that pressure filtration could affect the rate of urine secretion but not vary its composition:

'By filtration through a thick membrane a concentrated solution can never be converted into a dilute one.'

The data collected by a number of authors whom he quoted (Berzel, Lecanu, Marcet, Lehmann and Becquerel), however, had unequivocally established that the composition of serum and urine could be different, which was not in accordance with simple filtration. Guided by further experiments with models and kidneys, he concluded:

'... downstream of the glomeruli, and in the blood therein, is ... an endosmotic force that would attract water and solutes ... concentration and composition of urine would therefore depend on the contact time within the kidney and the specific weight [Dichtigkeit] of plasma [in the peritubular vessels].'

There is much more to be learned from this small, 42-page thesis about the balance of the opposing hydrostatic and endosmotic forces, the site of the filtration barrier in the glomeruli, and the mechanism underlying the expulsion of tubular fluid into the renal pelvis. Ludwig's final statement in the thesis sums up his view – the view of a physical physiologist who was not a nephrologist:

'Thus we see in these arrangements a simplicity [simplicity in terms of pure physical forces], a harmony, which in its beauty is not surpassed by any natural process.'

Ludwig's thesis was not accepted at first by the Medical Faculty in Marburg. Perhaps it was too mechanistic, and Ludwig's reputation from his restless days as a student was an obstacle. Ludwig was not intimidated, however, and responded that he would publish the text himself with a note that it had been rejected. The paper was finally accepted.

Although Ludwig was not a nephrologist in the strict sense, he had a continuing interest in the kidneys. This is often overlooked, because in later years Ludwig stimulated his young coworkers to carry out renal research, which he supervised, but he did not participate in publishing the work. Pertinent examples are the studies of Loebell (1849), Goll (1857), Hermann (1861), Overbeck (1863) and Ustimovich (1870) [7, 14]. Using a variety of approaches these scientists could demonstrate experimentally that urine excretion is indeed dependent on blood pressure, as postulated in Ludwig's initial thesis, but also on venous pressure, renal blood flow, resistance of the drainage pathways and finally on the content of urea and other waste products in the blood. That he truly continued to be interested in the kidney is documented by another letter of Ludwig, in which he reported to Henle his latest microscopic observations in dog kidneys. Finally, it was one of Ludwig's students, Rudolf Metzner, who formulated the most complete yet largely ignored theory of urine formation by a 3-step process, which for the first time included filtration, reabsorption and secretion [15], certainly under the influence of Ludwig's continuous interest in the kidney.

For the present discussion, it is tempting to compare Ludwig with Jacob Henle and to recall the relationship between the two scientists.

Jacob Henle (1809–1885)

Henle (fig. 5, table 4) was perhaps the most respected German morphologist of the 19th century. In Bonn he became an assistant of Müller, who advocated 'observation and experiment' as the means to derive a synthetic philosophic understanding of the nature of life. In Müller's department he became acquainted with physiologic and histologic research techniques. With Müller he moved to Berlin in 1833. Refinement of microscopic techniques and histologic observation became his main field of interest.

In Müller's private laboratory he met and worked with Schwann and Brücke. He lived in the apartment of Hegel's widow '... in the furniture of professor Hegel ...' (letter to his parents 1833, see [16]) and he was regularly invited to Mendelssohn-Bartholdy's musical matinees: '... you should hear him play Beethoven's symphonies ... also his own works ...'.

Henle was the first ever to offer a course in general microscopic anatomy to students in Berlin. This was not easy, if it is considered, as Bidder reports [17], that initally the department of Müller had only 1 microscope. Interested students, e.g. Helmholtz, had to buy their own instruments. Henle's many contributions are listed in table 5. For the present discussion, his work on epithelia and his renal work are of particular interest.

The scientific exchange between Henle and Ludwig is very well documented [8, 14, 18]. In his habilitation thesis Ludwig had already expressed his admiration for Henle. At the end of the morphologic section he summarized:

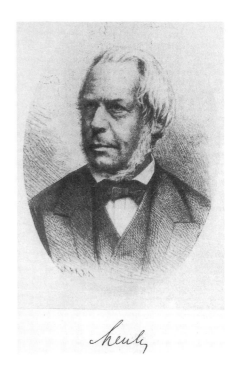

Fig. 5. Jacob Henle (1809–1885).

Table 4. Jacob Henle (1809–1885)

1809	Born in Fürth Studied medicine in Heidelberg and Bonn, assistant of Müller, study of causes of contagious diseases
1833	Moved to Berlin with Müller
1837	Habilitation in Berlin (delayed due to political difficulties as a liberal), prosecutor in Müller's department
1838	Offered first microscopy course to students
1840	Professor of Anatomy in Zürich, publication of Pathol *Untersuchungen (Contagium Animatum),* publication of *Handbuch der rationellen Medizin* and edited *Zeitschrift für Rationelle Medizin.* Influenced by Schwann's cell theory
1844	Professor of Anatomy in Heidelberg (also taught anthropology and physiology), postulated a 'natural scientific pathology'
1852	Moved to Göttingen, refinement of microscopy
1863	Described loop structure of renal medulla, reported findings to Ludwig
1885	Died in Göttingen

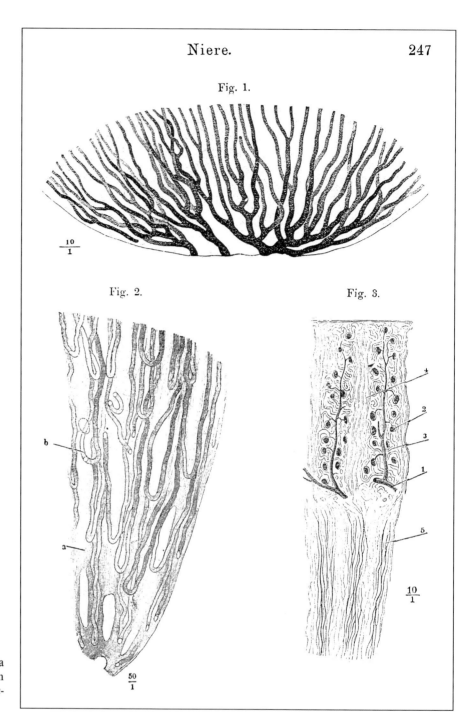

Fig. 1.

Fig. 2.

Fig. 3.

Fig. 6. Section through the papilla of a kidney, injected from the ureter. From Henle's *Grundriss der Anatomie des Menschen* [19].

'The basic structure of the kidneys [Nierenbestandteile] has been evaluated by Henle; up to now I have to endorse his findings, they seem to be outstanding.'

Henle, then in Heidelberg, had negotiated with the publisher Anton Winter about the publication of Ludwig's *Lehrbuch der Physiologie des Menschen*. From 1846

onwards there was an intensive correspondence between the two. During the course of his studies with physical models and biologic membranes, Ludwig again contacted Henle in 1849 to discuss his ideas about the role of water molecules in the permeability of biologic membranes. When Henle had made his landmark observation in the renal medulla (fig. 6) [19], he approached Ludwig immediately to inform him and to express the hope that the newly identified structure would soon be followed by an adequate functional interpretation. This, however, was too optimistic, and even almost a century later the loop of Henle was thought to be simply due to 'organogenesis' and was without any functional significance; the epithelium was so unimpressively developed that it would at best permit some diffusional equilibration. Even in Henle's time, however, it had become apparent that the medullary structure as earlier depicted by Bellini and by Schumlansky was no longer acceptable.

It is quite interesting to read how Ludwig responded. He immediately set out to confirm the surprising structural peculiarity, and after 3 months, he told Henle in a letter that he would not have detected the loops by himself, but that now he had succeeded and could confirm Henle's findings. Figure 7 shows part of the letter with Ludwig's drawing of Henle's loop. Ludwig in the same letter said:

'That your kidney segment [Nierenstück] is of great functional importance is obvious if one considers what will be caused by the mechanical peculiarities of the tubule. Also, comparative anatomy, particularly of animals with and without medulla and of animals which excrete dry or fluid urine, respectively, will now become important ...'

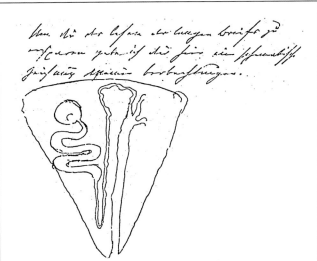

"Um Dir das Lesen des langen Briefs zu ersparen, gebe ich Dir hier eine schematische Zeichnung meiner Beobachtungen".

"In order to save you from reading the long letter, I give you a schematical drawing of my observations".

Fig. 7. From a letter of Carl Ludwig to Jacob Henle, 18 August 1863. With permission from Dreher [18].

Ludwig knew that one of Henle's main interests was comparative anatomy (table 5). He was confident that the new segment would permit him to adapt his original filtration theory of urine formation. He argued that the narrow loops are resistance elements which would affect filtration and permit exit of solutes into the surrounding capillary blood.

Disagreements between Ludwig and Henle eventually interrupted the contact. They strongly disagreed as to the primacy of functional versus morphologic interpretations. When the 2 volumes of the *Lehrbuch der Physiologie des Menschen* [3, 4] had appeared, which Henle had recommended to the publisher in Heidelberg, he strongly disapproved of the fact that it ignored structural aspects and stressed functional explanations at the expense of structure-function relationships. Ludwig responded with: '... what would you expect from a textbook of physiology?' The matter of the disagreements between Ludwig and Henle are discussed in Zupan [8] and in Lenoir [14]. For the present discussion it should be stressed again that methodologic developments – in this case refinement and skillful application of microscopic techniques – led to new insights.

Table 5. Scientific interests and contributions of Henle

Postulates *contagium animatum* (influence on R. Koch)

Description of *epithelia* (GIT, lymph vessels, blood vessels, others)

Analysis of histology of hair

Description of loop structure, renal medulla

Description of liver cells

Description of retinal elements, and macula lutea

Description of structure of cornea

Comparative studies on annelides and snails

Studies on origin and nature of sperms and ova ('cells')

Description of nucleus in muscle cells

Description of 'closed glands' without excretory ducts (i.e. endocrine)

Various publications: Original papers, text books, *Zeitschrift für Rationelle Medizin.*

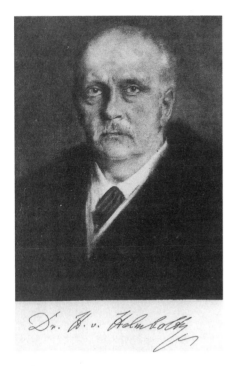

Fig. 8. Hermann Ludwig Ferdinand von Helmholtz (1821–1894).

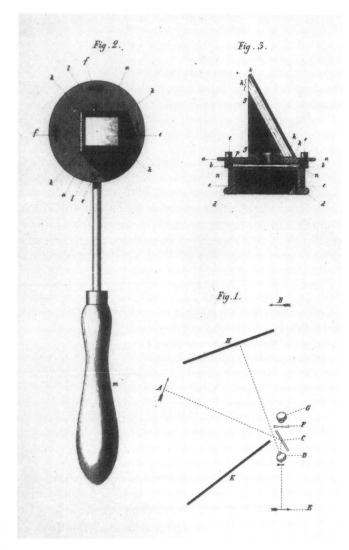

Fig. 9. Ophthalmoscope designed by Helmholtz in 1851. With permission from Bleker [22].

Hermann Ludwig Ferdinand von Helmholtz (1821–1894)

Together with DuBois-Reymond, Ludwig, Henle and Brücke, Helmholtz (fig. 8) was a major exponent of natural science and physical medicine in the last century. Helmholtz provided several examples that validate the Pitts paradigm. He started as a surgeon in Berlin and, after a detour through physiology – a happy and successful one, as far as physiology is concerned – became chairman of the most respected chair of physics in Germany, that of the University of Berlin. Some details of his life are given in table 6.

When he started his scientific career in Müller's department, it was general opinion that it should be possible to design a perpetuum mobile [20]. This tempted Helmholtz to evaluate the theoretic basis of such a possibility. His mathematic approach and treatment of the problem led him to formulate the law of conservation of energy, a landmark contribution to physics. At that time Helmholtz was a practising surgeon in Berlin and Potsdam, using his spare time to acquire the necessary mathematic tools for a quantitative analysis of the problem.

Microscopy was the second field in which Helmholtz became interested. As a student he had bought himself a microscope and had prepared a thesis on the nervous system of invertebrates. He succeeded in demonstrating that nerve fibers were directly connected with ganglion cells. The list of his methodologic inventions, his experimental measurements and his theoretic concepts in morphology, physiology (sensory physiology, color vision, acoustics) and physics (hydrodynamics, electrodynamics, etc.) is almost endless. Helmholtz as a natural scientist certainly has the same stature as Newton, Leibnitz and von Humboldt.

Table 6. Hermann Ludwig Ferdinand Helmholtz (1821–1894)

1821	Born in Potsdam, son of high school teacher
1837	Intention to study physics, instead studies medicine in Berlin Military surgeon, exposed to J. Müller
1842	Promotion to MD on *nervous systems of invertebrates*, practising surgeon at Charité Berlin, then Potsdam, concentrates on mathematics and physics, 'physical physiologist'
1847	Derivation of *Law of conservation of energy* in order to prove falsification of *perpetuum mobile* concept
1848	Teacher of anatomy at Art Academy in Berlin, assistant in J. Müller's Department
1849	Professor of Physiology and General Pathology in Königsberg
1851	Develops ophthalmoscope, stimulates field of endoscopy
1853	First trip to England (Tyndall, Faraday, Thomson)
1855	Professor of Anatomy in Bonn, conduction velocity of nerves Works in physiol. optics (colour vision), *Handbuch der physiologischen Optik*
1858	Professor of Physiology in Heidelberg, theory of sound perception, hydro- and electrodynamic measurements and calculations
1871	Professor of Physics in Berlin, physiological physicist (free energy, resolution of light microscopy, electric balance, meteorology)
1888	President of 'Physik.-Techn.-Reichsanstalt'
1893	Trip to USA (Chicago)
1894	Died in Berlin

From the viewpoint of nephrology, one particular methodologic development deserves mention. The observation that under certain conditions the eyes of animals (particularly cats and owls) and of humans gleam with reddish color had attracted attention. Various tentative explanations had been given. Helmholtz, then a young professor in Königsberg, asked whether the explanation was not simply that the retina, in the back of the eye, reflected light straight back into the observer's eye? Perhaps an answer would not only explain the phenomenon but also help in the analysis of amaurosis. Helmholtz set out to try to direct light into eyes directly from the position of the observer's eye. In his own words:

'... Therefore I undertook to glue together an instrument out of lenses and glass plates for microscopic purposes ... After 8 days or so I had the great pleasure to be the first one to clearly see a living human retina in front of him' [21].

This birth of the ophthalmoscope was in 1851. The original instrument is shown in figure 9. It soon became possible to test and describe the various segments and structures of the eye. The new instrument spread throughout the world, and 5 years after the invention of the technique the young physician Friedrich Moritz Heymann (1828–1870) described particular retinal lesions in Bright's disease. Only 7 years after the initial description the most esteemed ophthalmologist of Italy, Antonio Quaglino, published the first atlas in Milan *(Sulle Malattie Interne dell'Occhio),* and in 1859 Ludwig Traube (1818–1876) established a causal relationship between a certain retinopathy and hypertension in the aortic system [22]. At that time the Riva-Rocci technique for blood pressure measurement was not yet available.

This was not the only consequence of the newly discovered ophthalmoscope, however. Non-invasive endoscopy in general had been born, laryngoscopy was developed by Cermack in 1858, and urologists started to develop the first cystoscopes in Breslau and Berlin [23]. Thus, the 'ascending nephrologists', as urologists were called by James Israel [24], achieved access not only to the urinary bladder but eventually also to the renal pelvis. Helmholtz, without ever having dealt with the kidneys, had made a basic contribution to several aspects in the field of nephrology.

References

1 Pitts RF: Introduction: intrarenal sites of salt and water exchange. Symposium on salt and water metabolism (1959). Circulation 1960;21: 859–860.

2 Boruttau H: Emil DuBois-Reymond. Vienna, Verlag von Julius Springer, 1922.

3 Ludwig C: Lehrbuch der Physiologie des Menschen. Heidelberg, Winter, vol 1, 1852.

4 Ludwig C: Lehrbuch der Physiologie des Menschen, 2nd edn. Leipzig, Winter, vol 2, 1856.

5 Unger E: Über Nierentransplantation. Berlin Klin Wochenschr 1909;1:1057–1060.

6 Unger E: Nierentransplantation. Berlin Klin Wochenschr 1910;2:573–578.

7 Schröer H: Carl Ludwig. Begründer der messenden Experimentalphysiologie 1816–1895; in Degen H (ed): Grosse Naturforscher, Bd. 33. Stuttgart, Wissenschaftliche Verlagsgesellschaft mbH, 1967.

8 Zupan P: Der Physiologe Carl Ludwig in Zürich 1849–1855. Inaugural Dissertation. Aus dem Medizinhistorischen Institut der Universität Zürich. Zürich, Juris Druck Verlag, 1987.

9 Ludwig C: De Viribus Physicis Secretionem Urinae Adiuvantibus. Marburg, Elwert, 1842.

10 Ludwig C: Beiträge zur Lehre vom Mechanismus der Harnsekretion. Habilitationsschrift. Marburg, Akademische Buchhandlung Hrsg. N.G. Elwert, 1843.

11 Eytelwein JA: Handbuch der Mechanik fester Körper und der Hydraulik. 3. Aufl. Leipzig, Fleischer, 1842.

12 Gottschalk CW: A history of renal physiology to 1950; in Seldin DW, Giebisch G (eds): The Kidney. 2nd edn. New York, Raven Press, 1992, pp 1–29.

13 Ludwig C: Nieren und Harnbereitung; in Wagner R (ed): Handwörterbuch der Physiologie. Göttingen Bd. 2, 1844, pp 628–640.

14 Lenoir T: Politik im Tempel der Wissenschaft; in Raulff H, Raulff U (eds): Edition Pandora Bd. 2. Frankfurt, New York, Campus Verlag, 1992.

15 Thurau, K, David JM, Häberle DA: Renal Blood Flow and the Dynamics of Glomerular Filtration: the Evolution of a Concept from Carl Ludwig to the Present Day; in Gottschalk CW, Berliner RW, Giebisch GH (eds): Renal Physiology: People and Ideas. Bethesda, Maryland, American Physiological Society, 1987, pp 31–62.

16 Hoepke H: Jacob Henles Briefe aus seiner Berliner Zeit 1832 und 1833. Heidelberger Jahrbücher VII. Berlin, Göttingen, Heidelberg, Springer Verlag, 1963.

17 Morawitz P: Vor hundert Jahren im Laboratorium Johannes Müller. Von weil. Prof. Friedrich Bidder, Dorpat. Münch Med Wochenschr 1934;81:60–64.

18 Dreher A: Briefe von Carl Ludwig an Jacob Henle aus den Jahren 1846–1872. Heidelberg, Medical Dissertation, 1980.

19 Henle J: Grundriss der Anatomie des Menschen. Atlas. 2. Auflage. Braunschweig, Druck und Verlag von Friedrich Vieweg und Sohn, 1883.

20 Ebert H: Hermann von Helmholtz. Grosse Naturforscher. Bd. 5. Stuttgart, Wissenschaftliche Verlagsgesellschaft, 1949, pp 1–199.

21 Sigerist HE: Grosse Ärzte (Geschichte der Heilkunde in Lebensbildern). München, Lehmanns Verlag, 1958, pp 292–298.

22 Bleker J: Die Geschichte der Nierenkrankheiten. Mannheim, Boehringer Mannheim GmbH, 1972.

23 Winau R: Aspekte der Entwicklung der Urologie in Berlin. Uro Imaging 1991;1:120–124.

24 Bloch P, Israel J, Schultze-Seemann P: James Israel 1848–1926; in Winau R (ed):Wiesbaden, Franz Steiner Verlag, 1983.

Further Reading

Bowditch HP: The School of Physiology at Leipzig. Boston Med Surg J 1870;82:304–306.

Boylan JW: Founders of Experimental Physiology. Biographies and Translations. Munich, JF Lehmanns Verlag, 1971.

Brinkmann R: Romantik in Deutschland: ein interdisziplinäres Symposium. (Deutsche Vierteljahrsschrift für Literaturwissenschaft und Geistesgeschichte; Sonderbd.) Stuttgart, JB Metzlersche Verlagsbuchhandlung, 1978.

DuBois-Reymond E: Vorläufiger Abriss einer Untersuchung über den sogenannten Froschstrom und über die elektromotorischen Fische. Ann Physik Chemie (Pogg Ann) 1843;58:1–30.

DuBois-Reymond E: Untersuchungen über thierische Electricität. Berlin, von Veit, vols 1 and 2, 1848–1884.

DuBois-Reymond E: Gesammelte Abhandlungen. Vol II. Leipzig, von Veit, vol 2, 1877, p 623.

DuBois-Reymond E: Der Physiologische Unterricht sonst und jetzt. Rede bei Eröffnung des neuen Physiologischen Instituts der Königl. Friedrich-Wilhelm-Universität zu Berlin. 6 November 1877. Berlin, Verlag von August Hirschwald, 1878.

DuBois-Reymond E: Über den Neo-Vitalismus; in DuBois-Reymond E (ed): Reden von Emil DuBois-Reymond, 2nd edn. Leipzig, von Veit, vol 2, 1912, pp 492–515.

DuBois-Reymond E: Zwei grosse Naturforscher des 19. Jahrhunderts. Ein Briefwechsel zwischen Emil DuBois-Reymond und Karl Ludwig. Leipzig, Verlag von Johann Ambrosius Barth, 1927.

Eckart W: Geschichte der Medizin. Heidelberg, Berlin, Springer Verlag, 1990.

Ellinger PH: Theorien der Harnabsonderung; in Adler A, Ellinger PH, Fürth O, Jordan H, Lichtwitz L, v. Möllendorf W, Mond R, Rothman S, Schmitz E, Schwenkenbecher A, Seyderhelm R, Strasburger J, Trendelenburg P, Verzár F (eds): Handbuch der normalen und pathologischen Physiologie. Resorption und Exkretion. Berlin, Verlag von Julius Springer, 1929, p 451.

Eulner HH, Hoepke H: Der Briefwechsel zwischen Rudolph Wagner und Jacob Henle 1838–1862. Arbeiten aus der Niedersächsischen Staats- und Universitätsbibliothek Göttingen Bd. 16. Göttingen, Vandenhoeck und Ruprecht, 1979.

Groeben C, Hierholzer K: Emil DuBois-Reymond (1818–1896), Anton Dohrn (1840–1909): Briefwechsel. Berlin, Heidelberg, Springer Verlag, 1985.

Heidenhain R: Versuche über den Vorgang der Harnabsonderung. Pflügers Arch Gesamte Physiol Menschen Tiere 1874;9:1–27.

Helmholtz H von: Natur und Naturwissenschaft. Bücher der Bildung Bd. 11. München, Albert Langen.

Helmholtz H von: Die Tatsachen in der Wahrnehmung. Zählen und Messen. Darmstadt, Wissenschaftliche Buchgesellschaft, 1959.

Henle J: Zur Anatomie der Niere. Abhandlungen der Gesellschaft der Wissenschaften. Göttingen, Mathematisch-physikalische Klasse 1862;10:223–254.

Henle J: Handbuch der rationellen Pathologie. Braunschweig, Vieweg, 1847.

Hirschberg J: Geschichte der Augenheilkunde. Bd. 3. Italiens Augenärzte 1800–1850. Leipzig, Verlag von Wilhelm Engelmann, 1915.

Kübler G: Geprüfte Liebe. Jacob Henle und Elise Egloff in Familienbriefen (1843–1848). Zürich, München, Artemis Verlag, 1987.

Lübbe H: Wissenschaft und Weltanschauung. Ideenpolitische Fronten im Streit um Emil DuBois-Reymond; in Krings H, Oeing-Hanhoff L, Rombach H, Baruzzi A, Halder A (eds): Philosophisches Jahrbuch. Freiburg, Munich, Verlag Karl Alber, 1980.

Mann G: Naturwissen und Erkenntnis im 19. Jahrhundert: Emil DuBois-Reymond. Hildesheim, Gerstenberg Verlag, 1981.

Metzner R: Die Absonderung und Herausbeförderung des Harnes; in Nagel W (ed): Handbuch der Physiologie des Menschen. Braunschweig, Vieweg, vol 2 part 1, 1906, pp 207–335.

Rijlant P: The coming of age of electrophysiology and electrocardiography. Schriftenr Gesellsch Naturwiss Technik Med Leipzig 1980;171:108–123.

Rothschuh KE: Physiologie. Der Wandel ihrer Konzepte, Probleme und Methoden vom 16. bis 20. Jahrhundert. Orbis Academicus Bd.11/15. Freiburg, München, Verlag Karl Alber, 1968.

Rüdiger W, Schubert E, Flemming B, Schmerbach HJ (eds): 100 Jahre Physiologisches Institut. Das Physiologische Institut der Humdoldt-Universität 100 Jahre nach seiner Gründung. Berlin 1977. Wissenschaftliche Schriftenreihe der Humboldt-Universität zu Berlin, 1977.

Schubert E: Die Physiologie an der Berliner Universität zwischen Universitätsgründung und Ende der nationalsozialistischen Herrschaft 1945. Charité-Annalen, Neue Folge, Band 7, 1988.

Wiedemann HR: Briefe grosser Naturforscher und Ärzte in Handschriften. Lübeck, Verlag Graphische Werkstätten, 1989.

Winau R: Medizin in Berlin. Berlin, W de Gruyter-Verlag, 1987.

Am J Nephrol 1994;14:355–360

Evamaria Kinne-Saffran
Rolf K.H. Kinne

Max-Planck-Institut für molekulare
Physiologie, Dortmund, Germany

Jacob Henle:
The Kidney and Beyond

Key Words
Henle
Loop of Henle
Renal anatomy
Epithelium
Microscopy

Abstract
The progress in science made by Henle depended on the improvements in light microscopy achieved in the 19th century. The advent of achromatic lenses in particular made it possible for Henle and his contemporary and friend Schwann to uncover the typical structures of cells, thus bringing order at the microscopic level to the world of living tissues. Henle's 'comprehensive' approach – 4 basic types of tissue: epithelial, connective, muscular and nervous, contrasted with the accepted doctrine of Bichat of 21 different types of tissues that enter into different combinations in forming the organs of the body – together with rapid progress in chemistry and physics permitted the subsequent intimate probing of cellular physiology. Henle's work was not confined to the description of anatomic structures. After he had observed microorganisms in the excretions of diseased animals, he embraced the unpopular theory of 'contagion' as the source of infection, though he himself was not able to prove that microorganisms were the direct cause of diseases. His discovery of the renal tubule that now bears his name came comparatively late in his career, and although he described its structure in detail he offered no suggestions as to its function.

Introduction

The name of Henle is usually associated with a specific structure in the kidney, the so-called loop of Henle. This tubular segment plays a pivotal role in the urinary concentrating mechanism, which is based on the counter-current system [1]. The medullary and cortical thick limb of the loop of Henle have served as model epithelia for active transepithelial chloride transport and are the site of action of clinically important diuretics that interact directly with the sodium/potassium/chloride cotransporter, identified as the essential element in active chloride transport [2–4]. The thick ascending limb has also provided significant insight into the processes that link active ion transport and metabolism in an epithelium on the brink of hypoxia

[5]. Finally, this renal segment is the site of production of the Tamm–Horsfall mucoprotein. This synthesis and secretion of a protein in the tubule is unique among mammalian systems, but is often found in lower vertebrates [6].

Thus, there is ample reason to hail Henle's contribution to nephrology. Henle's scientific impact, however, reaches far beyond the kidney. He is considered to have been the first to describe epithelial cells in detail and to comprehend that, despite their diversity, epithelia belong to one system with morphologic and functional similarities – 'epithelial tissue'.

In this paper, therefore, the role of Henle in the development of the concept of the epithelial tissue will be discussed first, followed by an outline of the discovery of the

Evamaria Kinne-Saffran, MD
Max-Planck-Institut für molekulare Physiologie
Abteilung Epithelphysiologie
Postfach 10 26 64
D-44026 Dortmund (Germany)

structure in the kidney that carries his name and its importance for current understanding of renal function. This sequence reflects the historical time course of Henle's contributions to nephrology, as his observations on the kidney occurred rather late in his scientific career, at a time when his other contributions were already widely accepted.

Friedrich Gustav Jacob Henle: His Life

Friedrich Gustav Jacob Henle, now known simply as Jacob Henle, was born in 1809 to a merchant family in Fürth, a small town in southern Germany. Henle studied medicine in Bonn and Heidelberg, but was from the very beginning determined to enter research rather than practise medicine. He was particularly interested in studying the fine structure of human organs and tissues and their physiologic functions. This early decision was greatly influenced by the deep impression made on him by the great comparative anatomist and physiologist Johannes Müller, with whom he collaborated until the death of Müller in 1858. In 1832 Jacob Henle graduated from the University of Bonn. In his doctoral thesis *De Membrana Pupillari Aliisque Oculi Membranis Pellucentibus (On Pupillary Membranes and Other Translucent Membranes in the Eyes)* he described in a masterly manner the fine structures of the eye seen through the microscope. After the final medical examinations in 1833, which he had to take in Berlin, then capital of Prussia, he stayed on and worked for Müller, who had accepted the Chair of Anatomy and Physiology at what was then the Friedrich-Wilhelm-Universität. It is noteworthy that during these years Henle became a close friend of Theodor Schwann who was also working as a microscopist for Müller.

In 1838 Jacob Henle, after a hectic period and even imprisonment for his membership of an outlawed student fraternity, gained the qualification for lecturing at a university with his habilitation thesis *Symbolae ad Anatomiam Villorum Intestinalium Imprimis Eorum Epithelii et Vasorum Lacteorum (Contributions to the Anatomy of Intestinal Villi with Special Reference to their Epithelia and Lymph or Lacteal Vessels),* in which he describes his observations on the luminal membranes of the intestine and the membranes of the chyle-producing vessels. In the introduction to this thesis, Henle remarks:

'I owe the origin of this little work to the fortunate chance that during the winter of 1834–1835, when I happened to observe the intestine of a dead person, the chyle-producing vessels appeared completely filled with white chyle' [7].

Apparently the cold had helped to preserve the organs.

In 1840 Henle became Professor of Anatomy and Physiology at the University of Zürich. There he published in 1841 his *Allgemeine Anatomie (Comprehensive Anatomy),* the first systematic treatise of histology [8]. In the following years he continued to do research and to teach at the universities of Heidelberg (1844–1852) and Göttingen (1852–1885), where he died at the age of 76 years, still acting as Chairman of the Department of Anatomy and Physiology.

The reports of Henle's personality are varied. His son-in-law highlighted his deep emotional involvement in matters of science and daily life, whereas others, e.g. a fellow member of the department in Göttingen, were impressed by his cool intellect, his cautious behavior and critical evaluation of all matters with which he was concerned. In addition, he was admired for his capability of putting a vast number of individual microscopic observations coherently into the broader perspective of organ and body function. This last attribute probably reflects the influence of his mentor Müller, who outlined in his inaugural lecture *Physiology, a Science in Need of a Philosophic View of Nature* his approach to science, maintaining that the physiologist must combine empirically established facts with philosophic thinking.

The Concept of Epithelial Tissue

As mentioned above, Henle submitted his habilitation thesis in 1837. In this treatise he carefully described the microscopic appearance of the surface layer *(cuticula)* of the intestinal tract and noted that cellular elements can be found in the scrapings of the uppermost layers of the surface from all parts of the digestive tract. He defined this *cuticula* as free of blood vessels, blood components and nerve endings, but characterized by typical nucleated morphologic features, and which provided continuous cover from the oral cavity to the rectum. From these studies and his other investigations, he concluded that similarly to the skin, all mucous membranes are covered by a thin layer of cells and not simply by coagulated mucus without any further structure, as was contended by most of his contemporaries. In addition, he established 3 basic types of epithelium: *epithelium squamosum* (squamous epithelium), *epithelium cylindricum* (columnar epithelium) and *epithelium cylindricum vibratorium* (ciliated columnar epithelium). These different forms of the epithelial cell are characteristic for each of the segments of

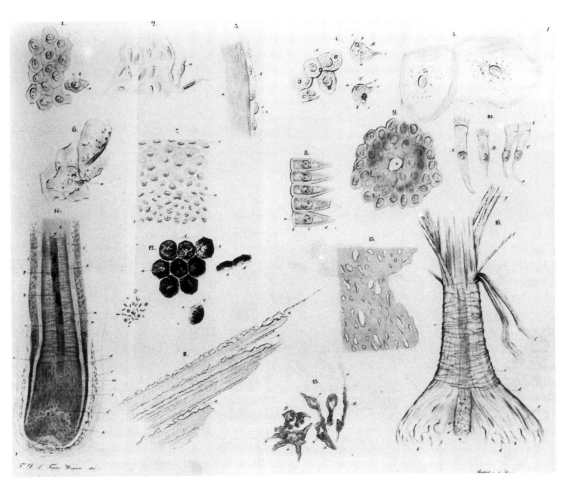

Fig. 1. These drawings were preceded by the following note from Henle: 'If not stated otherwise, the illustrations have been drawn at 410-fold magnification from deceased humans. Ocular no. 2 and objective lenses no. 4, 5 and 6 of a microscope manufactured by Schiek were used'. The following numbers as given in the figure represent epithelial cells from: (1) the peritoneum; (2) calf carotid artery; (3) valve of crural vein; (4) choroid plexus; (5) oral cavity; (6) epidermis, made translucent with acedic acid; (7) calf eye con- junctiva; (8) rabbit small intestine; (9) guinea-pig large intestine; (10) sheep nasal mucosa; (12) pigmented choroid plexus; (13) supra-choroid lamina (lamina fusca) of the sclera. Parts 11, 14, 15 and 16 show a longitudinal section through a nail and illustrations of the lower part of a single hair with its follicle, the inner layer of the hair bulb, and white hair of the head treated with acidic acid, respectively. (Some information of the original, very detailed legend to this figure has been omitted.) Reproduced from [8].

the intestinal tract. Furthermore, they are never inter-mixed:

'... but in the various regions of the intestinal tract cylindrical cells are succeeded by squamous cells and by cylindrical cells of both types – ciliated and nonciliated.'

Henle later extended this notion from the intestinal tract to the whole body and stated that all surfaces of the body are covered with a layer of nucleated cells of varying thickness that compose the 'epithelial tissue'. As illus-trated in figure 1, this tissue not only forms the outer skin but also lines all surfaces of the body cavities, i.e. the peri-toneum, the ventricles of the brain, the oral cavity, the surface of the small and large intestine, blood vessels, and the pharynx [8, 9]. Henle also offered some suggestions on the functional role of these epithelia in attributing to them, at least in the glands, an involvement in the secre-tion of fluids and in the modification of their final compo-sition either by:

'... pulling substances from the blood or by retrieving substances from the secreted fluid back into the cells and even transforming them somehow within the cells' [8].

These studies form the foundation of 'epitheliology', on which our current concepts of epithelial function are based.

The Loop of Henle

In the following years Henle applied the concept of epithelial tissue to glandular and tubular organs, including the kidney. In 1862 the epithelial nature of the convoluted and straight portions of the cortical tubule and of the medullary and papillary collecting tubules, the duct of Bellini [10], had been established. In January of that year Henle reported to the members of the Scientific Society at the University of Göttingen on an exciting observation he had made – that there exist 2 types of tubule in the medullary tissue [11]. One is the well-known ductus papillaris or papillary collecting duct with a diameter of 0.05–0.06 mm, lined with a uniform columnar epithelium in which the height of the cells increases continuously towards the opening at the papillary tip. The other type of tubule has a much smaller diameter of about 0.02–0.03 mm and is lined by small squamous cells. These latter tubules run parallel to the collecting ducts but return in a narrow hairpin loop into the medullary tissue. Henle further stated that these loop-like tubules are arranged in a circular fashion around the collecting ducts.

At that time it was quite popular to identify the fine structure of organs by injecting colored material into the vascular or ductal systems; this approach had failed, however, to reveal the medullary tubule system in its full extent. It occurred to Henle to take advantage of a kind of 'natural injection', i.e. the calcareous deposits commonly found in the renal medullary tissue of cadavers. The horseshoe-like aggregates in the tip region of the papilla provided the first hint of the presence of loop-like structures. The success of this approach led him to note in a letter to a friend:

'... that it is a great pleasure to have found something new in a thousand times studied and apparently fully exploited organ like the kidney.'

Furthermore it gave him great satisfaction that this discovery was based, albeit indirectly, on a kind of injection technique so that:

'... his colleagues no longer can look down upon him from the top of their injection syringes.'

Henle called his observations preliminary because at this point he had not been able to show the connection between the tubular structures in the cortex and those in the medulla. This difficult task was achieved by Schweigger-Seidl 3 years later in 1865 [12]. Henle also did not offer any suggestions about the possible functional aspects of this peculiar anatomic feature. It is noteworthy, however, that he reported that the formation of the calcareous aggregates started in the tip of the papilla and then extended towards the cortex. In retrospect this seems to be the first description of the corticomedullary osmotic gradient. It took about another 100 years before these anatomic findings were incorporated into the concept of the counter-current mechanism for urinary concentration [13, 14].

In *Grundriss der Anatomie des Menschen (Compendium of Human Anatomy)* published in 1883 [15], Henle summarized the knowledge at that time about the structure of the renal tubule to which he had contributed so many details. Figure 2 shows a longitudinal section of a papilla in which, by a specific maceration technique, the loop-like tubules are highlighted. Figure 3 shows the connection between the cortical tubules and the collecting ducts via short and long loops of Henle, including the so-called *Schaltstücke* and connecting tubules. In this compendium Henle's systematic and thorough treatise of microscopic observations, their critical evaluation and compelling integration into a larger framework came to full fruition.

Conclusions

As in many other instances, the progress in science made by Henle depended on the development of a new technique and a scientist who realized its potential. Thus, before improvements in light microscopy were achieved most students of nature had to be content to classify living forms as best as they could, according to the morphology observed with the naked eye. During the 19th century new microscopes, and especially the advent of achromatic lenses, made it possible for critical observers like Jacob Henle and his contemporary and friend Schwann to lay bare the typical structures of cells, thus bringing order at the microscopic level to the world of living tissues. This 'comprehensive' approach – 4 basic types of tissue: epithelial, connective, muscular and nervous, compared with the accepted doctrine of the famous anatomist Bichat [16] of 21 different types of tissues that enter into different combinations in forming the organs of the body – together with rapid progress in chemistry and physics permitted the subsequent intimate probing of cellular physiology.

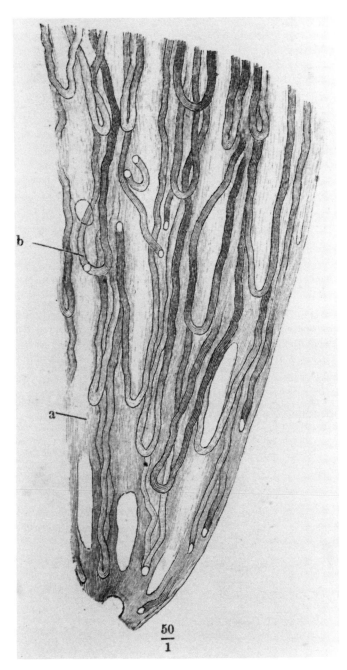

Fig. 2. Longitudinal section of the renal papilla. The collecting ducts (a) and the loop-like tubules (b) are visualized by treatment of the tissue with dilute potassium hydroxide solution followed by a rinse in water. Reproduced from [15].

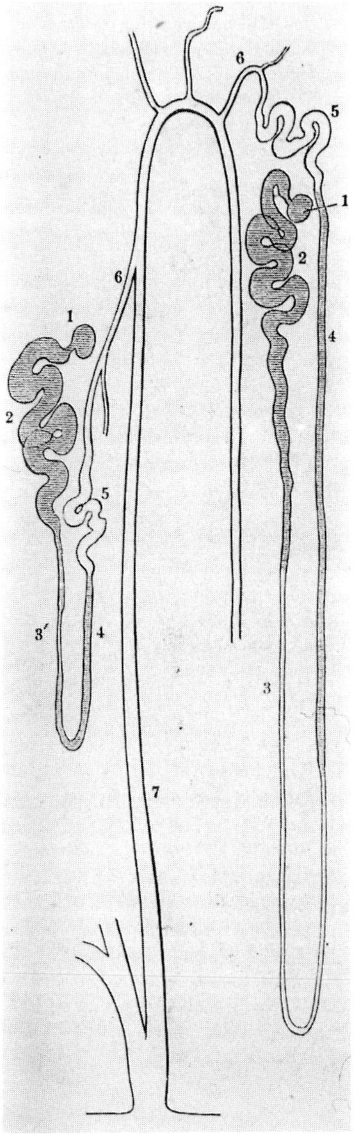

Fig. 3. Depiction of the renal nephron and its nomenclature according to Henle. (1) Glomerulus; (2) convoluted cortical tubule; (3) loop-like tubule or Henle's tubule; (4) dark tubule; (5) Schaltstück ('switching' segment); (6) connecting tubule; (7) collecting duct. Reproduced from [15].

Jacob Henle's work was not confined to the description of anatomic structures. After he had observed microorganisms in the excretions of diseased animals, he embraced the unpopular theory of 'contagion' as the source of infection, though he himself was not able to prove that microorganisms were the direct cause of diseases. Among his students at the University of Göttingen, however, was Robert Koch, who brought Henle's firm belief in the germ theory to fruition. Together with Louis Pasteur, Koch championed the most dramatic revolution of 19th century medicine by showing that bacteria did indeed cause many diseases, thereby paving the way for controlling some of the most horrifying maladies of mankind.

Acknowledgements

The authors dedicate this chapter to Professor Dr. med. K.J. Ullrich in gratitude and appreciation, as teacher, mentor and prominent nephrologist. They also gratefully acknowledge the help of Professor Irmgard Müller, head of the Department of History of Medicine, Ruhr-Universität Bochum, in the initial search for Henle's publications, and of Mrs Helga Wagner, librarian at the Max Planck Institute, in tracing the different locations at which they are kept. Special thanks go to Professor C.V. Gottschalk (Chapel Hill, North Carolina, USA) for pointing out the role of Schweigger-Seidl, to Mr Dominick delGuidice (Bar Harbor, Maine, USA), retired highschool teacher of Latin and Greek, for his substantial help in translating sections of Henle's habilitation thesis, and to Mrs Daniela Mägdefessel, Mrs Gesine Schulte and Mr Falk Sieland for help in preparing of the manuscript.

References

1 Kuhn W, Ryffel K: Herstellung konzentrierter Lösungen aus verdünnten durch blosse Membranwirkung. Ein Modellversuch zur Funktion der Niere. Hoppe-Seylers Z Physiol Chem 1942;276:145–152.

2 Schlatter E, Greger R, Weidtke C: Effect of 'high ceiling' diuretics on active salt transport in the cortical thick ascending limb of Henle's loop of rabbit kidney. Correlation of chemical structure and inhibitory potency. Pflügers Arch 1983;396:210–217.

3 Greger R: Ion transport mechanisms in thick ascending limb of Henle's loop of mammalian nephron. Physiol Rev 1985;65:760–797.

4 Kinne RKH: The Na-K-Cl cotransporter in the kidney. Ann N Y Acad Sci 1989;574:63–74.

5 Brezis M, Rosen SN, Epstein FH: The pathophysiological implications of medullary hypoxia. Am J Kidney Dis 1989;13:253–258.

6 Tamm I, Horsfall FL: A mucoprotein derived from normal urine which reacted with influenza, mumps and Newcastle disease viruses. J Exp Med 1952;95:71–97.

7 Henle J: Symbolae ad Anatomiam Villorum Intestinalium Imprimis Eorum Epithelii et Vasorum Lacteorum. Habilitationsschrift, Berlin, 1837.

8 Henle J: Allgemeine Anatomie. Lehre von den Mischungs- und Formbestandtheilen des menschlichen Körpers. Leipzig, Voss, 1841.

9 Henle J: Über die Ausbreitung des Epitheliums im menschlichen Körper. Mullers Arch Anat Physiol Wissensch Medizin 1838;103.

10 Mellini L: Exercitatio Anatomica de Structura et Usu Renum. Florence, ex typ. sub signo Stellae, 1662.

11 Henle J: Zur Anatomie der Nieren. Mittheilungen an die Göttinger Gesellschaft der Wissenschaften. Januarheft pp 4–12. Library of Georg-August-Universität, Göttingen, 1862.

12 Schweigger-Seidl G: Die Nieren des Menschen und der Säugetiere in ihrem feineren Bau. Halle, Buchhandlung des Waisenhauses, 1865.

13 Wirz H, Hartitay B, Kuhn W: Lokalisation des Konzentrierungsprozesses in der Niere durch direkte Kryoskopie. Helv Physiol Pharmacol Acta 1951;9:196–207.

14 Ullrich KJ, Kramer K, Boylan JW: Present knowledge of the counter-current system in the mammalian kidney. Prog Cardiovasc Dis 1961;3:395–431.

15 Henle J: Grundriss der Anatomie des Menschen. Braunschweig, Vieweg und Sohn, 1883.

16 Bichat MFC: Anatomie Descriptive. Paris, 1801–1803.

Am J Nephrol 1994;14:361–364

Vittorio Bonomini[a]
Claudio Campieri[a]
Maria Piera Scolari[a]
Marina Zuccoli[b]

[a] Institute of Nephrology, and
[b] Department of Astronomy, University of Bologna, Bologna, Italy

The Age-Old Spirit of Nephrology from the Oldest University in the World

Key Words
Nephrology
Multidisciplinarity
University of Bologna
Renal pathology

Abstract
The University of Bologna began teaching in 1088, and the Faculty of Medicine was granted the same rights as lawyers in 1288, largely due to the reputation and teaching skills of Taddeo Alderotti. Among the other famous names associated through the ages with the Bologna School of Medicine are Malpighi, Valsalva and Murri. From the earliest times in Bologna, nephrologists attempted to show an interaction of the kidney with the outer environment (astronomy and astrology) and with other organs (anatomy) and an integration of the sophisticated structures within the kidney itself (microscopy). At the turn of the 19th century, the biochemical frontier was reached, and a new teaching methodology emphasizing careful consideration of all possible differential diagnoses was developed.

Introduction

The University of Bologna, the oldest university in the world, started its teaching activity in 1088 AD [1, 2], though only in 1219 was medical teaching recognized by a Bull of Pope Honorius III. The regular course, based on a 4-year program, started in about 1260 and the first teacher was Taddeo Alderotti [3, 4], known also as the 'Protomedicus'. In 1288 the City granted the Faculty of Medicine the same rights as those previously granted to lawyers. This acknowledgement *(Privilegium Scholarium Magistri Tadei)* was the direct result of the high reputation and professional skill of Taddeo, who is mentioned by Dante in his masterpiece (Paradiso XII, 83). Pupils came from all over Italy to study under Taddeo, and later spread the knowledge they had acquired in Bologna [5].

Conscious of this illustrious past, the research for this paper was started in the libraries, museums and public institutions of the University of Bologna, and the authors efforts were rewarded by finding many miniatures, manuscripts, papers and experiments [6, 7]. This investigation started from the basic assumption that the age-old spirit of nephrology is research by correlation. From the beginning the practice of nephrology has shown a 'traditional spirit' of investigating the interactions of components around or within the kidney: the outer environment, the other organs and the sophisticated functions of the kidney itself.

Many early scientists were involved in the attempt to define possible correlations of the kidney with the outer environment, particularly with astronomy and astrology, to enable the kidney to be set free from the prison of theoretic rules derived from the classical view of the human body. Later on, links were found between the kidney and other organs or functions, as anatomy, autopsies and experimentation began to elucidate the basic functioning

Professor Vittorio Bonomini, MD
Director, Institute of Nephrology
S. Orsola University Hospital
I-40138 Bologna (Italy)

of the body. Later still, the age of microscopic observation gave more detailed insights into the kidney, until the biochemical frontier was reached and passed at the end of the 19th century.

The authors have found it gratifying to find that throughout the centuries there have been many points of similarity with today's multidisciplinarity concept of nephrology. Only the most relevant findings are discussed here: the kidney and the outer environment; the kidney and other organs; and the kidney and its structure. A final reference to 'the biochemical frontier' of the end of the 19th century and to some methodologic approaches by Augusto Murri will complete the analysis.

The Kidney and the Outer Environment

From the beginnings of nephrology, examination of the urine was correlated with physical events, and therefore astronomy and astrology were often taken into account in the practice of medicine. Contacts with the outer environment signified a desire for more precise explorations of physical phenomena that would go beyond the simple interpretations of the kidney in the classical models of Hippocrates and Galen. There was an exchange of teachers between astronomy and medicine, and the *Liber de Urina Non Visa* (1219) by William of England was read during the 4th year of the astronomy course.

Taddeo Alderotti's *Consilia Medica de Mictu Urine cum Sanguine* (1250) is a contribution in which advice was given to disciples and doctors about the appearance of the urine. The difference between *permixtio* or the mixing with an abnormal component and *alteratio* depending on a pathologic event was analyzed in detail. Pietro Torriggiano, the most outstanding pupil of Taddeo, wrote *De Ypostasis*, a fine analysis of the various patterns of urinary sediment.

The *De Secretis Humanae Dispositionis per Urinam Dignoscendis* (1447) by Ferdinando of Cordoba, the *Libellus Posthumus de Urinarum Differentis Causis et Indicis* (1557) by Cesare Oddone and the *De Urinis Liber I* (1570) by Girolamo Cardano are other contributions from an era spanning over 400 years in which urine examination constituted a public aspect of practising medicine. In many miniatures the red-dressed physician is represented examining a urine sample. Tables or schemas were also available for physicians to help them in interpreting the physical findings in the urine and in evaluating their appearance in comparison with the character of the patient, defined as 'sanguineus, colericus, phlegmaticus' or 'melancolicus' according to Galen's theory of the 4 humors. Even if the correlations with the outer environment were sometimes misinterpreted and condemned (as demonstrated by the burning of William of England's book in Paris in 1494 on a charge of black magic), historically speaking this approach was fundamental for more than 3 centuries.

The Kidney and Other Organs

Clinical observations focused on the functional correlations between the kidney and other organs. The anatomic study of human disease by autopsy was fundamental in achieving these results.

Guglielmo of Saliceto, a pupil of Taddeo and an outstanding surgeon, describes in his *Liber in Scientia Medicinalis* (1260) hard and diseased kidneys as the cause of fluid retention and edema: 'Signa duritiei in renibus sunt quid minoratur quantitas urinae' (the kidneys are smaller and harder and therefore the urine output decreases). Girolamo Mercuriali in *De Omnibus Corporis Humanis Excrementis Libri Tres* (1572) assessed the possibility of diagnosing pregnancy by urine examination.

Pellegrino Capponi [8] was a doctor who graduated in 1575 from the University of Bologna in medicine and philosophy. He treated diseases with mineral water from Porretta Spa and deserves special attention for his manuscript *Discorso dell'Orine (Discourse on Urine)* (1575), in which he defined the variations in urinary output according to water intake and the presence of diseases of the kidney. He gave details of the appearance of the urine according to the presence or absence in the diet of chromatic foodstuffs. He defined the increase in specific gravity as 'thickness' and the decrease as 'thinness', casting doubt on the term 'substance' as defined by the philosophers. He reported on a case of acute onset of polyuria with sudden death and focused on the role of the kidney in association with the liver in the elimination of toxins. Part of this manuscript was published for the first time in 1987 in the *Italian Journal of Nephrology* [9].

The Kidney and Its Structures

In 1649 the Senate of the City of Bologna established a new and more suitable seat for anatomic studies, which can be visited today in the Anatomic Theatre within the Archiginnasio Palace, formerly the site of the University of Bologna. The development of anatomic research was

Bonomini/Campieri/Scolari/Zuccoli   Age-Old Spirit of Nephrology facilitated by Marcello Malpighi and continued by his pupil (later the teacher of Morgagni) Anton Maria Valsalva, who in 1697 received the appointment of Public Dissector from the Senate of Bologna.

Malpighi taught in Bologna from 1666 to 1691 when he went to Rome as doctor to Pope Innocent XII. In *De Renibus Dissertatio* (1666) he viewed the kidney as a complex of smaller units ('like smaller kidneys') defined as '... renal glands and with the appearance of fish eggs'. Injection with blue ink showed that these glands were 'wrapped by vessels like climbing tendrils' and were interposed between the arteries and veins. His *Anatomica Sive in Cadaveribus Sectis Observationes* (1687) is a fine example of a pathologic report complete with personal drawings, where terms like 'nephritic' and 'calculi' recur together with the description of polycystic and abnormal kidneys [10, 11]. The report on the autopsy of Gaspare Mazzoni performed on 6 October 1687 described a monstrous-sized kidney: 'Renes in monstruosam excreverant mole', secondary to acute obstructive renal failure which caused the death of the patient.

At this time public dissections were performed and anatomy was also taught by means of wax models. One of the experts in this latter technique was Ercole Lelli, who was appointed in 1742 as anatomy modelist by Pope Benedict XIV, formerly Cardinal Prospero Lambertini. Many of his masterpieces, which can be admired in the university anatomy museum, dealt with renal pathology, e.g. horseshoe kidneys, and a fine study of the renal vasculature with injections of two different colors into the arteries and veins. From clandestine research in the early days, anatomy of the body had become pivotal in medical teaching, with a recognized need for what were at the time sophisticated didactic tools.

The Biochemical Frontier and New Methodology in Teaching

Augusto Murri is representative of the attempt at the end of the 19th century to define the more sophisticated functions of the kidneys and their biochemical nature. Beginning his career as a family doctor, he was then called to join the staff of the Medical Clinic in Rome. In 1876 he achieved the highest academic and clinical position in the Bologna School of Medicine as Chairman of the Medical Clinic. In his *Intorno alla Genesi Renale dell'Urea (On the Renal Genesis of Urea)* (1873) [12] he gave a precise description of hyperfiltration of the solitary kidney and of alterations in the urinary pattern of urea excretion in renal diseases. This paper was an accurate review with personal experimental work on a topic initially debated by Professor Rosenstein from Groningen and Professor Primavera from Naples. The 'bristle' pattern of urea crystals in the urine of renal patients returns to the normal 'plate' pattern if albumin is precipitated by nitric acid instead of by heating. This was the fundamental conclusion reached by Murri on the basis of his experimental work. The hypothesis that in renal diseases the kidney increases filtration and eliminates toxins to the point of altering the qualitative appearance of urea excretion was experimentally tested and contributed to highlighting the point of contact between apparently opposite theories. To him we owe the term 'dialyzer' for the glomerulus, which he used in his *Emoglobinuria da Freddo* (1880) *(Cold Hemoglobinuria)* [13].

Murri's humanity in treating patients and his clinical skill were associated with a precise methodology [14] in teaching medicine, characterized by deep critical consideration of all possible differential diagnoses. He believed that the most important aim of teaching is to guide the student '... not only to cognition but above all to recognition' of the diseases. This 'technique of thinking should become a methodologic habit for every medical teacher', and not only a methodologic declaration. His faith in the capacity of thought was not always appreciated by his colleagues, but his confidence in his own methods became even stronger after a prolonged absence from teaching. He managed to forge reciprocal ties between the academic profession and private practitioners.

Conclusions

From its simple past the multidisciplinarity of nephrology has become consolidated over the centuries and today is a complex but fascinating reality that every nephrologist has to face daily. Analysis of the contributions made by the great physicians of the past can help, side by side with the study of more recent methodologic approaches, to conserve the quality and some of the satisfaction of a profession that is destined in the near future to be faced with further surprises and challenges. This cultural dimension reinforces the lesson of multidisciplinarity as a constant feature of nephrology in its evolution across the centuries.

References

1 Sorbelli A: Medioevo. Secc. XI-XV, in Storia dell'Università di Bologna. Bologna, Zanichelli, vol 1 and 2, 1944.

2 Simeoni L: L'età moderna. 1500–1888, in Storia dell'Università di Bologna. Bologna, Zanichelli, vol 2, 1947.

3 Tordi D: Il Protomedico Taddeo Alderotti (1215–1295). Estratto dagli Atti della Società Colombaria. Florence, Stab. Tip. già Chiari succ. C. Mori, 1930 – VIII.

4 Siraisi NG: Taddeo Alderotti and His Pupils. Princeton, Princeton University Press, 1981.

5 Cristiani A: I Lettori di Medicina allo Studio di Bologna nei Secoli XV e XVI. Bologna, Analisi, 1990.

6 Pazzini A: Modernità e tradizione nella storia della Facoltà Medica di Bologna Studi e Memori, in Storia dell'Università di Bologna, Nuova Serie. Bologna, 1956, pp 391–415.

7 Forni G: L'Insegnamento della Chirurgia nello Studio di Bologna dalle Origini a Tutto il Secolo XIX. Bologna, Cappelli, 1948.

8 Fantuzzi G: Notizie degli Scrittori Bolognesi, Bologna, Stamperia S. Tommaso d'Aquino, 1781–1789. Reprinted Bologna, Forni, 1965.

9 Bonomini V: Pellegrino Capponi e la Nefrologia Bolognese. Giornale Italiano di Nefrologia 1987;4:99–102.

10 Celebrazioni Malpighiane. Discorsi e Scritti Azzoguidi-Soc. Tip. Editoriale, Bologna 1966.

11 Minelli G: All'origine della biologia moderna, in Celebrazioni del Nono Centenario dell'Università di Bologna. Editoriale Jaca Book, Nuova Timec Albaraite 1987.

12 Murri A: Due Nuovi Argomenti Intorno alla Genesi Renale dell'Urea. Florence, Lo Sperimentale Anno XXV, 1873.

13 Murri A: Della Emoglobinuria da Freddo. Bologna, Tipografia Fava e Garagnani, 1880.

14 Murri A: Quattro Lezioni ed Una Perizia. Bologna, Zanichelli, 1972.

Am J Nephrol 1994;14:365–370

J. Stewart Cameron

Renal Unit, Guy's Campus, United Medical and Dental Schools, London, UK

John Bostock MD FRS (1773–1846): Physician and Chemist in the Shadow of a Genius

Key Words

Bostock
Uroscopy
Dropsy
Albuminuria
Uraemia

Abstract

John Bostock has a reasonable claim to being one of the first chemical pathologists. Most of his work was done before that of William Prout, with whom both he and Bright were in contact. Bostock's work was done about the same time as that of his friends and colleagues Marcet and Wollaston. Although others, notably Cruickshank, Wells and Blackall had previously studied the chemistry of normal and pathological urine, the breadth and detail of Bostock's observations were unprecedented, and he and Wells were the first to relate findings in the urine in disease to findings in the serum. Bostock, however, was the first to realize the relationship between the diminution of urea in urine as it rose (or in his terms, appeared) in the blood, while the albumin in the blood fell as that in the urine increased.

Introduction

Everyone working in the field of the history of nephrology knows the name and works of Richard Bright, who is correctly revered as one of the founders – if not *the* founder – of the discipline of nephrology. Despite the fact that Bright himself was a modest and generous man, his very eminence has tended to obscure the work of his colleagues and contemporaries, and even of his predecessors. This is particularly true of those concerned with advances in the chemistry of renal disease made about his time, mainly in France and Britain. None has suffered more than his elder colleague and collaborator, John Bostock (fig. 1). Bright thought sufficient of Bostock's work on the blood and urine of the patients he had studied clinically and post mortem to quote his letters detailing these findings verbatim in his *Reports of Medical Cases*. Some of the crucial

observations in the description of what would now be called nephrotic syndrome are to be found in these letters.

No study of Bostock has been published previously, though an MSc thesis dealing with his scientific contributions can be found in the University of London library [1]; however, this says almost nothing about his contributions to the study of renal disease. Other published sources of information are the entries in the Dictionary of National Biography [2] and Dictionary of Scientific Biography [3] and obituaries [4–6]. Some details of Bostock's family are given in the Bickerton manuscripts [7], a collection of papers dealing with the history of Medicine in Liverpool, and held in the Liverpool Reference Library. Finally, there is an extensive entry in Pettigrew's *Medical Portrait Gallery* of 1844 [8], which is particularly valuable in giving details of Bostock's medical education.

Professor J.S. Cameron, MD, FRCP
Clinical Science Laboratories
17th Floor Guy's Tower
Guy's Hospital
London SE1 9RT (UK)

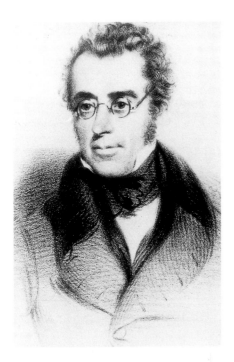

Fig. 1. John Bostock. Lithograph by WD Drummond after an engraving of J Partridge, 1836. With permission from the Wellcome Institute Library, London.

Biography of John Bostock MD FRS

John Bostock was born in the busy port of Liverpool in 1773. His father, John Bostock the Elder (1740–1774) [9], also of Liverpool, had studied medicine in Edinburgh under William Cullen (1710–1790), the leading teaching physician of his day, and graduated as a doctor in 1769. He travelled and studied in Europe, taking an honorary degree in Leiden. Bostock Senior's only medical publication was his graduating thesis, a rather unoriginal description of gout, *De Arthritide*. In 1770 he returned to Liverpool and became a physician at the Royal Infirmary in Liverpool. In 1771 he married Elizabeth Ashton, daughter of one of Liverpool's principal families, her father John Ashton being a merchant who had been responsible for the construction of the first navigable canal in England (the Sankey canal). Tragically, Bostock Senior died of an acute illness at only 34 years of age, only 1 year after Bostock Junior was born [10]. His mother remarried the Reverend John Yates, a dissenting Unitarian minister in 1779, by whom she had two half-brothers for John Junior, both of whom had distinguished careers and acquired national reputations: James Yates, who was one of the

founders of London University; and Joseph Brook Yates, to whom Bostock later dedicated a major work.

John Junior's medical education commenced at the age of 19 years in 1792, when he went to London to study with Joseph Priestley at the New Hackney College, at that point a ferment of new advances, and thus received a first-hand education in the contemporary chemical theories of respiration. The following year, after apprenticeship to an apothecary, he worked in the very busy Liverpool General Dispensary. The notable physicians James Currie and Matthew Dobson (died 1784), who first described sugar in the blood and urine of diabetic subjects [11], were among his teachers there. Then he followed his father's path to Edinburgh (as a dissenter he could not attend Oxford or Cambridge). Interest in the new science was particularly high among the non-conformist community, and the medical school of Edinburgh was then at its apogee. There, Bostock's tutors included Black (1728–1797) and Munro Secundus, and he also attended Andrew Marshal's course in anatomy in London during the winter of 1795–1796 – 'the best teacher of anatomy in his day' [8].

Bostock returned thereafter to Edinburgh, and after studying chemistry with Hope and physiology with Allen, which influenced him strongly, he graduated in medicine in 1798 with a thesis *On Secretions*. This dealt mostly with bile [12], including studies on the formation of an artificial bile; he dedicated this, his first work, to his friend the famous radical Roscoe, who was at that time attacking the slave trade, one of the sources of Liverpool's prosperity – as it was of Bright's family, and much of Bristol where Bright was born. A number of letters between Bostock and Roscoe are held in the Roscoe papers in the Liverpool Library [13]. Bostock then returned to Liverpool to become assistant to Currie, who was at that time the senior physician at the Infirmary. Among other duties was helping with the design of fever wards, opened in 1800.

During this period Bostock was very active in the cultural life of Liverpool, helping with Roscoe and Rutter to set up the Botanic Gardens [14], which opened in 1802, and the Natural History Society; he also assisted in re-starting the Literary and Philosophical Society [15]. Together with fellow chemist and amateur Egyptologist T.S. Traill, he helped to found the Royal Institution in 1814 and became its first professor [16]. Initially he lived in the centre of the city at 9 Clayton Square, later moving south to the Dingle at Knotts Hall Bank. In 1812 he married a Miss Whitehead from London and had several children.

In 1817, 'having made a secure fortune' [4], Bostock moved to London to pursue his interests in science, particularly chemistry, and gave up the practice of medicine [3]; in 1827 he was living at Upper Bedford Place, at that time near the northern edge of London and very near to the present London University buildings. In 1818 he was elected to the Royal Society and proposed Bright for membership in 1820; later (1832) he was to become Vice-President of that august body. In London he was on familiar terms with Alexander Marcet (1770–1822) [17] (who had been a fellow-student in Edinburgh), Roget (another fellow student, whose *Thesaurus* of the English language brought him lasting fame), along with de la Rive (1770–1834), Young, Wollaston and Davy. He became tutor in chemistry at Guy's Hospital on Marcet's unfortunate death in 1822, a post he held for several years. Thus, he and Bright were in regular contact at least from 1820 onwards; although they had a medical education in Edinburgh in common, Bostock had left more than a decade before Bright went there in 1810.

As in Liverpool, Bostock was active in many societies in London apart from the Royal Society. He was Treasurer of the Medico-Chirurgical Society of London, as well as holding office in the Linnean, Zoological and Horticultural Societies, was President of the Geological Society (1826) and also served on the Council of the Royal Society of Literature. He remained based in London for the rest of his life, but travelled to France in 1830, staying in Paris 'chiefly for the purpose of the education of his children', remaining there for about 18 months.

His scientific output was enormous and very broad [1]: animal chemistry, forensic chemistry, pharmaceutical chemistry, physiology, botany and geology. His leisure activities included a translation of the 37 books of Pliny's natural history, 2 of which were published.

Bostock died on 1 August 1846 of cholera, aged 73 years, and was the subject of long obituary notice in the *Proceedings of the Royal Society* by the Marquis of Northampton [5], then president of the Society, in the *Lancet* [6] and in the *Gentleman's Magazine* [4].

Bostock's Work on Renal Disease

Bostock was well prepared to study animal chemistry, being qualified in medicine and having studied chemistry extensively. He published his first paper on the composition of urine in 1803 [18], when Bright was still at school, only 5 years after William Cruickshank's seminal paper [19] and some time before the presentations of the work of William Wells (1757–1817) work [21]. Bostock followed this with much more detailed analyses of the chemical composition of various normal and pathological body fluids [23] published in 1805 and 1813.

Bostock's observations on the urine of the patients studied by Bright are contained in 3 letters to Bright dated 27 April, 28 May and 4 June 1827, headed *Observations on the Chemical Properties of the Urine in the Foregoing Cases. Dr John Bostock, MD* [24]. The histories and autopsies of the now famous unfortunates John King, Elizabeth Beaver, Mary Sallaway, Daniel Peacock, Hugh Thomas, Mary Ann Richardson, Elizabeth Stewart, William Bonham, a woman called Smith, Mary Castle, Henry Izod, Mr Galloway, Thomas Drudget, Leonard Evans, William Roderick, Mary Fitzgerald, Francis Fish, William Brooks, Robert Spooner, William Todd and Eliza Plume were all described in detail in the previous section, and the kidneys of King, Thomas, Sallaway, Stewart, Peacock, Thomas, Izod and Evans formed the basis for some of the most beautiful illustrations in medical publishing, then or since.

In the first letter Bostock reported on 28 urine samples from 13 patients, 9 in the above list. Bostock quoted both Cruickshank [19] and John Blackall (1771–1860) [25] when discussing the low specific gravity and presence of albumin in all these specimens. He coagulated the urine samples by heating them and applied various chemical tests (strong tannin, bichloride of mercury, muriatic acid, ferroprussiate of potash) because: 'it still remains for us to enquire whether the albumen in dropsical urine is precisely similar to the albumen in the serum'; he concluded it was, having 'every property' of that in blood.

He considered the effect of the degree of alkalinization (the pH) of the urine on the separation of the albumin, and the effects of bleeding on all the constituents, reaching no firm conclusions, which would not surprise us today. He quantified the albumin in the urine by evaporation, and the urea by redissolving an evaporated deposit in alcohol. He noted that although: 'it is commonly said that the presence of albumen in the urine is a morbid occurrence', even with his own urine: 'I have very seldom found the fluid to be entirely free from it'. He also studied urine during treatment with mercury, which Blackall [25] had indicated in 1814 might provoke coagulable urine (see Peitzman [26] for discussion), but drew no conclusions on this point.

In the second letter (page 83) he described 3 more urine samples, 1 of them from a dispensary patient of Hodgkin. This letter contains the important statement: 'I think I may venture to say that the serum in these cases contained less albumen than in health'. Bostock also found by analysis involving alcohol and sodium nitrate: '... an animal matter possessing peculiar properties, which seemed to approach that of urea', in several of the supernatants after precipitation of the albumin from the serum, particularly those of Roderick and West, the first time this had been noted. Bright remarked in a footnote that Prout (William Prout 1785–1850) [27] had also noted a substance similar to urea in a sample of blood provided by Bright. Prout had been a contemporary of Bright's in Edinburgh in 1810–1811 and the following year at Guy's Hospital; he was an important figure, along with Bostock in Britain and Andral in France, in the beginnings of clinical chemical pathology [28].

The third letter (page 84) described blood and urine from a single un-named dropsical patient, and having noted to his surprise that the amount of albumin in the serum (judged by specific gravity and heat) was scarcely different from that found in the urine, Bostock made the most important statement summing up his observations:

'We have here, therefore, an example of the blood exhibiting a very great deficiency in albumen, at the same time as we observe the mode in which it passes off from the system by means of the kidney, while this organ has its appropriate office of secreting the urea nearly suspended.'

This provides a very neat description of the functional changes of both massive proteinuria and advancing uraemia. These chemical observations were confirmed by Robert Christison (1797–1882) who published an excellent paper with clinical and chemical data in 1829 [29]. Surprisingly, in view of their close personal and professional relationship, there is only one other joint publication by Bostock and Bright [30]. Bostock published only two further papers on the composition of the urine [31, 32] which summarized the data he had obtained on normal and abnormal urine samples. He did, however, work on the 'uncombined alkali' in the blood [33], published as letters between himself and Marcet [17] on the subject, eventually coming to the conclusion that this was soda and not potash, i.e. sodium and not potassium bicarbonate. He also studied the urine and blood of a young woman taking very large quantities of bicarbonate as a treatment for tuberculosis, noting that the plasma contained an unusual quantity of uncombined alkali, and that this appeared in the urine in quantity, unlike in health [34]. Finally, Pettigrew [7] notes that in 1804 Bostock was awarded an honorary medal by the Medical Society of London for a paper on Two Cases of Diabetes, in one of which (diabetes mellitus) the urine contained glucose and urea, while in the case of diabetes insipidus there was a 'deficiency of urea' in the urine. This study does not appear to have been published.

Other Scientific Works of Bostock

Bostock's principal early work was on the field of respiration [35], a very active area at that time. This activity arose partly from theories about disease and the quality of air, but also from the increase in the understanding of chemistry in relation to animal heat. Some of his early enquiries arose out of observations made in the fever hospital in Liverpool.

Perhaps Bostock's best known contribution to medical science, apart from his work with Bright, is his description of his own case of hay fever in 1819 [36, 37]. Finn [38] recently put this paper in context, repeating the early suggestions of Elliotson [39] and others that this complaint was rare until the pollution introduced by the industrial revolution. Finn [38] also draws attention to Bostock's lost paper presented to the Liverpool Literary and Philosophical Society in 1817 on *The Best Means of Obviating the Nuisance Arising from the Smoke of Steam Engines.* Perhaps he had suffered himself from these!

Bostock was also very interested in the classification of plants after the work of Linnaeus, but it must be admitted that his criticism and revision of the nomenclature used in the London pharmacopoeia of 1807 by Powell [40] had little or no permanent effect. He did, however, describe and name a number of plants for the first time; Lee [41] has written extensively on Bostock's work in the field of botany.

In the field of forensic chemistry, Bostock studied means of detecting arsenic [42] and mercury [43] in body fluids. He experimented, unsuccessfully, with what he called electrochemical separation of substances. In chemistry, he studied the efflorescence of bricks in old buildings [44] and showed that this was magnesium sulphate, a compound not present in the original material. He was asked in 1826 to investigate the purity of Thames water as a supply for drinking [45]. He notes, not surprisingly:

'... the water of the Thames ... is in a state of considerable purity ... but as it approaches the metropolis it becomes loaded with a quantity of filth, which renders it disgusting to the senses and improper to be employed in the preparation of food.'

He found that alumina could be used as a flocculant to purify the water, leading indirectly a century and half later to the terrible epidemic of dialysis-related dementia. He turned his attention to perfecting writing ink [46], suggesting that the best ink is obtained by diluting the fluid in strong coffee which: 'improves its colour and adds to its lustre'.

In physics he worked on voltaism [47] and was one of the first to realize the enormous significance of Faraday's experiments of 1832 [48]. He studied variations in the boiling points of fluids [49] and noted that these could be reduced by adding particulate matter and increased by using specially clean glassware [50]. He was interested in meteorology and published a description of an improved barometer [51]. Finally, like Bright [52], Bostock was a keen geologist, but he seems to have communicated only 1 paper to the Geological Society [53] (of which he became President), though an earlier paper on a geological subject exists [54].

While at Guy's Hospital during the 1820s, Bostock wrote the first comprehensive textbook of physiology in English, the *Elementary System of Physiology* [55], which ran to almost 900 pages; this book was popular for 2 decades and ran to 3 editions. It covered all the usual physiological topics, but also contained chapters on the connection between mind and body: 'of volition and passions'; 'of cranioscopy and physiognomy'; 'of sleep and dreaming'; and last of all, 'of the decline and dissolution of the system'. This work was eventually superseded by Müller's textbook. Bostock also published a brief history of medicine in 1835 [56], which had originally been the preface to the *Cyclopaedia of Medical Practice*, to which he contributed a number of sections [1, 8]. This essay was dedicated to Richard Bright [54].

Summary

John Bostock has a reasonable claim to being one of the first, if not the first, chemical pathologist [26]. Most of his work was done before that of William Prout [27], with whom both he and Bright were in contact [24] as Prout had been a contemporary and friend of Bright. Bostock's work was done about the same time as that of his friends and colleagues Marcet [17] and Wollaston [57]. Although others, notably Cruickshank [19], Wells [20] and Blackall [25] had previously studied the chemistry of normal and pathological urine, the breadth and detail of Bostock's observations were unprecedented, and he and Wells [20, 21] were the first to relate the findings in the urine in disease to findings in the serum. Bostock, however, was the first to realize the relationship between the diminution of urea in urine as it rose (or in his terms, appeared) in the blood, while the albumin in the blood fell as that in the urine increased.

What sort of a man was Bostock? It must be confessed that he was probably famous in his day more because of his industry than his originality, as the *Dictionary of National Biography's* waspish review [2] suggests. Nevertheless, his observations on hay fever [36, 37] and his insight into nephrotic syndrome assure him of a place in medical history, as Pettigrew recognized by including him in his series of medical portraits [8] of the great physicians of his and previous eras. On his death in 1846, a colleague writing under the pseudonym of Athanaeum wrote in the *Gentleman's Magazine* [4]:

'In private life he was respected and beloved. He was at all times equally ready to impart the overflowings of his sensitive and affectionate heart, and the varied stores with which his intelligent mind abounded.'

References

1 Smith SG: The Contributions to Science of John Bostock MD FRCS 1773–1846. MSc thesis, presented 1953, accepted 1954–1955. University of London Library.
2 Bostock, John the Younger, in Dictionary of National Biography. London, Smith Elder, vol 2, 1908, pp 885–886.
3 John Bostock, in Gillispie CC (ed): Dictionary of Scientific Biography. New York, Scribner, vol 2, 1976, pp 335–336.
4 Obituary: Dr Bostock FRS. Gentleman's Magazine. December 1846, p 653.
5 Northampton, Marquis of: John Bostock FRS. Proc R Soc 1846;5:636–638.
6 Obituary. Dr J Bostock. Lancet 1846;ii:222.
7 Bickerton manuscripts. Liverpool Reference Library.

8 Pettigrew TJ: A Medical Portrait Gallery. London, Whittaker, vol 3, 1844, pp 4–20.
9 Bostock, John the Elder, in Dictionary of National Biography. London, Smith Elder, vol 2, 1908, p 884.
10 Letter from Dr Norton to Dr W Withering, in Bickerton manuscripts, vol B, Liverpool Reference Library.
11 Dobson M: Experiments and observations on the urine in diabetes. London, 1776.
12 Bostock J: Dissertatio Physiologica Inauguralis, Quaedam de Secretione in Genere, et Praecipue de Formatione Fellis Complectens. Edinburgh, 1798.
13 Roscoe Papers. 920 ROS 348, 349–352, 5743, 1464. Liverpool Library.

14 Subscription List and Lists of Proprietors: 1800, 1805. 580BOT p 1–3. Liverpool Reference Library.
15 Minute Book 1812–1817. Literary and Philosophical Society of Liverpool. O60 LIT. Liverpool Reference Library.
16 Liverpool Royal Institution Reports. Liverpool, 1822, p 12.
17 Coley NG: Alexander Marcet (1770–1822), physician and animal chemist. Med Hist 1968; 12:394–402.
18 Bostock J: Observations on the urine. London Med Phys J 1803;9:349–355.

19 Cruickshank WV: Observations on the urine by Mr Cruickshank, in Rollo J (ed): Cases of Diabetes Mellitus. London, J Dilly, 1798, pp 443–451. (Cruickshank, chemist and surgeon of Woolwhich, characterised carbon monoxide and assisted Crawford in the discovery of Strontium. He is often confused (including by myself in the past [58]) with his namesake and contemporary WC Cruickshank (1745–1800) who was assistant to John Hunter and published the important 'The anatomy of the absorbing vessels of the human body' (London 1786). See Partington Ann Sci 1941–7;5:157.)

20 Wells WC: Observations on the dropsy which succeeds scarlet fever. Trans Soc Improvement Med Surg Knowledge 1812;3:167–186.

21 Wells WC: On the presence of the red matter and serum of the blood in the urine of dropsy which has not resulted from scarlatina. Trans Soc Improvement Med Surg Knowledge 1812;3:193–240.

22 Bostock J: Essay on the analysis of animal fluids principally with the view of ascertaining their definite characters. Edinb Med Surg J 1805;1:257–266.

23 Bostock J: On the analysis of animal fluids. Medico-Chirurg Trans 1813;4:53–88.

24 Bright R: Reports of Medical Cases. London, Longmans Green, 1827, pp 75–84.

25 Blackall J: Observations on the Nature and Cure of Dropsies, and Particularly on the Presence of the Coagulable Part of the Blood in Dropsical Urine. 3rd edn. London, Longmans Green, 1818.

26 Peitzman SJ: Richard Bright and mercury as the cause and cure of dropsies. Bull Med Hist 1978;52:409–434.

27 Brock WH: The life and work of William Prout. Med Hist 1965;9:101–126.

28 Foster WD: The early history of clinical pathology in Great Britain. Med Hist 1959;3:173–187.

29 Christison R: Observations on the variety of dropsy which depend upon diseased kidneys. Edinb Med Surg J 1829;32:262–291.

30 Bostock J, Bright R: Analysis of a specimen of cutaneous perspiration. Medico-Chirurg Trans 1828;14:424–436.

31 Bostock J: Morbid states of the urine, in Forbes J, Tweedie A, Conolly J (eds): Cyclopaedia of Practical Medicine. London, Sherwood Gilbert and Piper, vol 4, 1834, p 359.

32 Bostock, J: On the constitution of the urine. Medico-Chirurg Trans 1838;21:25–28.

33 Bostock J, Marcet A: A correspondence between Dr Bostock and Dr Marcet, on the subject of the uncombined alkali in the animal fluids. Nicholsons J 1812;33:147–151.

34 Bostock J: An account of chemical examination of the urine and serum of a person who had taken large quantities of soda. Med Chir Trans 1814;5:80–92.

35 Bostock J: An Essay on Respiration. Parts I and II. Liverpool, Longman Rees, 1804.

36 Bostock J: Case of a periodical affection of the eyes and chest. Medico-Chirurg Trans 1819;10:161–162.

37 Bostock J: On the catarrhal aestivus or summer catarrh. Medico-Chirurg Trans 1828;14:437–446.

38 Finn R: John Bostock, hay fever, and the mechanism of allergy. Lancet 1992;340:1453–1455.

39 Elliotson J: On hay fever. Lancet 1830;ii:370–373.

40 Bostock J: Remarks on the Nomenclature of the New London Pharmacopoeia. Liverpool, 1810.

41 Lee: Lancashire and Cheshire Naturalist 1923;17:126–129, 157–160, 198–200.

42 Bostock J: Observations on the different methods recommended for detecting minute portions of arsenic. Edinb Med Surg J 1809;5:166–174.

43 Bostock J: Experiments to ascertain how far the presence of albumen and muriatic acid interfere with the action of bichloride of mercury and protomuriate of tin upon each other. Edinb Med Surg J 1825;23:65–69.

44 Bostock J: Further experiments and observations on the efflorescence of walls. Nicholsons J 1803;6:109–114.

45 Report of HM Commissioners on the Supply of Water to the Metropolis. London, vol 2, 1828, 271–275, 305–308.

46 Bostock J: Writing inks. Trans R Soc Arts 1829;47:69–73.

47 Bostock J: Outline of the history of galvanism, with a theory of the action of the galvanic apparatus. Nicholsons J 1802;2:296–304; 1802;3:3–12.

48 Bostock J, Christie SH: Report on Prof. Faraday's paper. Proc R Soc 1832;3:113–121.

49 Bostock J: Variation of boiling points. Q J Sci 1825;19:148.

50 Bostock J: The boiling point of ether. Thomsons Ann Philos 1825;9:196–200.

51 Bostock J: Some observations on the imperfections of the barometer. Thomsons Ann Philos 1818;11:198–207.

52 Kark RM: The life, work and geological collections of Richard Bright MD (1789–1858); with a note on the collections of other members of the family. Arch Nat Hist 1981;10:119–151.

53 Bostock J: Notice respecting the pebbles in the bed of clay which covers the new red sandstone in SW Lancashire. Trans Geol Soc Ser 2 1826;2:136.

54 Bostock J: On the blue iron earth. Thomsons Ann Philos 1818;11:391–393.

55 Bostock J: An Elementary System of Physiology. London, Balwin Cradock and Joy, 1824.

56 Bostock J: Sketch of the History of Medicine from Its Origins to the Commencement of the Nineteenth Century. London, Sherwood Chilbert and Piper, 1835.

57 Wollaston, William Hyde, in Gillispie CC (ed): Dictionary of Scientific Biography. New York, Scribner, vol 14, 1976, pp 586–593.

58 Cameron JS: The history of the nephrotic syndrome, in Cameron JS, Classock RJ (eds): The Nephrotic Syndrome. New York, Marcel Dekker, 1988, pp 3–56.

Am J Nephrol 1994;14:371–376

Leon G. Fine
Jennifer A. English

Department of Medicine, University
College London Medical School,
London, UK

John Blackall (1771–1860): Failure to See the Obvious in Dropsical Patients with Coagulable Urine?

Key Words

Blackall
Dropsy
Albuminuria
Renal pathology
Mercury poisoning

Abstract

Despite his success in publishing a book which was widely read and which drew attention to the fact that some cases of dropsy are associated with coagulable urine, John Blackall failed to make the link between this phenomenon and disease of the kidneys. Thus, to Richard Bright must go the credit for providing the critical understanding of the phenomenon. The single most probable reason for Bright's success and Blackall's failure was that Bright carried out post mortem examinations of almost all of his patients. In addition, Bright was ruthlessly systematic in documenting his autopsy findings, and not least was the fact that he possessed the rare talent of being objective in looking at his data, without being influenced by the preconceptions of the times.

Introduction

Identification of the cause of dropsy, i.e. the accumulation of fluid in the serous cavities and in the interstitia of tissues, intrigued virtually all of the ancient and medieval medical writers. A careful search of the writings on dropsy of such luminaries as Hippocrates, Galen, Areteus, Aetius and Avicenna reveals sporadic case reports of hardened or scirrhous kidneys or kidneys which are altered from their normal appearances [1]. A diminution of the volume of the urine was similarly recognized. Similar reports are scattered throughout the literature of the 17th and 18th centuries and these have been elegantly catalogued by Rayer [2]. It is clear, however, that by the beginning of the 19th century it had not been realized that there could be a causal relationship between kidney disease and dropsy. Perhaps the single most important reason for this was the scarcity of post mortem examinations of the internal organs.

In 1790 Cotugno ushered in an innovative experimental approach to dropsy; he examined the urine of dropsical subjects and found that in some it coagulated on heating [3]. Others had shown that blood and serum may be present in the urine following scarlatina, but this was regarded as a form of bleeding into the urine. Noting that normal serous fluids did not coagulate on heating, Cotugno found that they did if the serous membranes were inflamed. Extending this principle he performed an experiment to test whether the dropsical fluid was excreted into the urine:

'It seemed best to settle this question by a definite experiment, heating the urine. For I had often conclusively shown that the fluid collected beneath the skin of such dropsical cadavers con-

---

Leon G. Fine, FRCP
Department of Medicine
University College London Medical School
5 University Street
London WC1E 6JJ (UK)

© 1994 S. Karger AG, Basel
0250–8095/94/0146–0371
$8.00/0

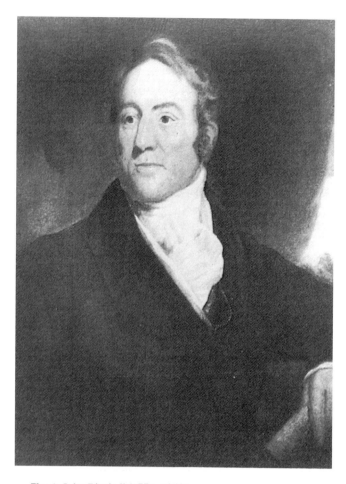

Fig. 1. John Blackall (1771–1860).

tained material capable of coagulation and I hoped that, if the sick man passed such fluid by way of the urine, coagulation would be seen if the material which flowed out were heated, which, as I had anticipated, was proved by experiment. For with two pints of this urine exposed to the fire, when scarcely half evaporated, the remainder made a white mass already loosely coagulated like egg albumen.'

Thus it was shown for the first time that urine, which is never coagulable in healthy people, can under some circumstances contain a coagulable substance.

Cotugno also found coagulable material in the urine of some diabetic subjects. He erred, however, in concluding that the presence of coagulable material signalled recovery of the disease in that it reflected passage of such coagulable material from the serous fluid of dropsy into the urine. Nevertheless, this seminal work involving genuine experimentation must be heralded as 'one of the first triumphs of chemistry applied to pathology' [2].

Cruikshank deserves the credit for being the first to attempt, in 1798, to separate those dropsies in which the urine is coagulable from those in which it is not [4]. Writing in Rollo's *Cases of Diabetes Mellitus* he suggests that the presence of coagulable material implies that the dropsy is dependent on 'morbid viscera', which at the time meant a diseased liver or spleen. Again the kidney did not merit a mention!

The foregoing remarks show that by the early 19th century there was a tenuous understanding that some cases of dropsy were associated with abnormal kidneys and that some cases were associated with coagulable urine. What now seems to be an obvious association, i.e. the relationship between diseased kidneys and coagulable urine, was obviously not intuitive at the time. It was arrived at, indirectly, through the writings of William Wells in 1812. In his paper to the Society for the Improvement of Medical and Surgical Knowledge [5], he not only demonstrated that the red colour of the urine in dropsies associated with scarlatina was due to the red matter of the blood (red blood corpuscles had not yet been discovered), but also that this urine contained the serous portion of blood, i.e. serum. Using both heat and nitric acid he showed that floccules appeared. To quantify the amount of serum in the urine, he mixed different proportions of serum and normal urine. Out of 138 cases of scarlatina he found 'serum' in the urine of 78. Importantly, he noted that when serum was added to urine, the urine may have a perfectly normal appearance, and indeed he found that 'serum' was present in the urine of 23 of 29 cases of dropsy not associated with scarlatina. Once again he was limited by his inability to examine the viscera of such patients after death. He records 1 case in which:

'... the kidnies [sic] were much harder than they usually are. The cortical part was thickened and changed in its structure from the deposition of coagulable lymph and there was a small quantity of pus in the pelvis of one of them. I do not conclude, however, from these appearances and those which were found in the former case that the kidnies are always diseased when the urine in dropsy contains much serum.'

Thus, no relationship between kidney disease and coagulable urine had been established in the early 19th century. In France, Fourcroy (1800), Nysten (1811) and Chapotain (1812) described coagulable urine in patients with dropsy, with Nysten even noting that it: 'foamed strongly on shaking and remained frothy for a long time', but none of these authors appears to have been drawn to the kidneys to explain the phenomenon [2].

2

The Doctor, in his obser-
vations on this case, is inclined to lay
great stress on the coagulability of the
urine by heat. He says,

"The extraordinary coagulability
of the urine forms a peculiar feature
of the complaint. It was principally
this circumstance which determined
me to bleed, notwithstanding the apparently hopeless condition of the patient and the obscurity of the pulse as
a guide. I have never hesitated,
when the urine coagulates, to bleed in
dropsies, and I have never yet had
reason to believe the practice injudi-
cious; and I cannot help expressing
here my opinion, that the profession
are highly indebted to Dr. BLACKALL,
for so pointedly directing our attention to this condition of that discharge.

I am not, indeed, prepared to ad-
mit, that the sensible qualities of the
urine form a principle upon which to
found a practical division of dropsies,
but I feel assured that the coagulability of the urine will almost invariably
warrant the practice of bloodletting.
The appearance of the blood drawn
incontrovertibly proved, in this instance, the inflammatory tendency,
and the propriety of the practice."

3

Fig. 2. Title page of the 1st edition of John Blackall's book on dropsy.

Fig. 3. Extract from a review of the book *Clinical Reports on Dropsies* by Robert Venables, which appeared in the *Lancet* of 18 December 1824. The recognition that was accorded to Blackall's work on dropsy is evident from the remarks of the reviewer.

John Blackall and *Observations on the Nature and Cure of Dropsies*

John Blackall (fig. 1) was born in 1771 in Exeter, England, and educated at Exeter Grammar School and Balliol College, Oxford. He received his BA degree in 1793 and his MD degree in 1797. He received a second MD degree from St. Bartholomew's Hospital in 1801. He gained his MRCP in 1814 and became FRCP in 1815. He worked as a physician in Totnes, Devon, from 1801 to 1807, after which he returned to Exeter. In 1812 he became physician to the Hospital for Lunatics. In 1813 he published his *Observations on the Nature and Cure of Dropsies* [6] (fig. 2) which went through 5 editions (1813, 1814, 1818, 1820, 1824) including an American edition in 1820 based on the 3rd London edition. This work was widely regarded as a significant contribution to the medical literature (fig. 3).

Blackall was highly regarded as a physician:

'His information on medical matters, singularly extensive and accurate, had been qualified by a wide and varied research from many departments of human knowledge; his diagnostic powers were of the highest order' [7].

He practised until the age of 80 years and died aged 88 years in 1860.

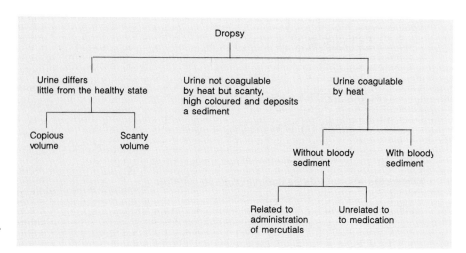

Fig. 4. Schematic overview of the categories of dropsy described by Blackall.

Blackall's single work (no other publications by him have been traced) has a title that raises the possibility that he may have made the seminal discovery for which Richard Bright later received the credit. This article examines whether this was the case or not. His book was fully titled *Observations on the Nature and Cure of Dropsies and Particularly on the Presence of the Coagulable Part of the Blood in Dropsical Urine* and contained 15 chapters and *An Appendix Containing Several Cases of Angina Pectoris with Dissections, etc.* Blackall indicates in the introduction that he was aware of previous reports of coagulable urine in dropsy and cites the writings of Fordyce, Darwin, Cotunnius (Cotugno), Vauquelan, Fourcroy and Cruikshank. His interest in the topic seems to have been stimulated by a single case under the care of his preceptor Dr Latham.

It is difficult to follow a simple pattern of thought through the book, so a simple description of its contents would be confusing. Figure 4 categorizes, in a simplified fashion, the different forms of dropsy that Blackall considered. What follows describes his experience with each.

Dropsy in Which the Urine Differs Little from the Healthy State

In this general category Blackall describes individual cases of anasarca without any unique or distinguishing features, in which the urine is described as pale, crude and apparently diluted. He notes that this is not very common in dropsy. In none of the patients was a coagulum produced by heat or nitrous acid but in 2 cases oxymuriate of mercury detected a small amount of 'albumen'. For no obvious reason, he concludes that this form of dropsy is connected with 'great and irretrievable injury of internal organs'. He regarded digitalis as being of little use in the treatment of these patients, and indeed felt that the polyuria was a very bad sign as it precluded the use of many diuretics.

He described another group of cases in which the only difference seems to be that the volume of urine was small. Here for the first time he alludes to the 'bad effects of mercury', which he regarded as being far more common than generally suspected, as is discussed below.

Dropsy in Which the Urine Is Not Coagulable, Is Scanty, High Coloured and Deposits a Sediment

Blackall includes a variety of cases of ascites, hydrothorax, pericardial effusion and anasarca in this category. He refers to the sediment in the urine as 'lateritious' (brick-coloured). The sediment in many cases was pink. Of the 21 case reports provided, most are very brief and in only 2 (cases 11 and 21) were autopsies performed. In 1 case the liver was hard and small.

Blackall attempted to define the nature of the sediment. It was precipitated by 'the infusion of galls' but not nitrous acid, suggesting that it was not protein. Oxymuriate of mercury occasionally produced a coagulum resembling the effect of heat. Blackall concluded that this was: 'in a great measure at least, albumen'. He further concluded that the pinkish material was: 'pure ammonia, the muriate of barytes and acetate of lead [and] a large proportion of saline matters'. Despite the fact that he paid such attention to this pinkish sediment, he is objective enough to conclude that it is not always present in dropsy associated with a scirrhous liver, as Cruikshank had proposed, nor did its absence allow any conclusions to be drawn about the cause of the dropsy.

Dropsy in Which the Urine Is Coagulable by Heat: Associated with Scarlatina

Blackall devotes almost 140 pages to this topic. In most cases the dropsy appeared weeks or months after the attack of scarlatina, and in half of these cases Blackall found a blood-stained urine sediment. Most were treated with digitalis; indeed, Blackall states: 'I know of no instance where digitalis has failed'. A few cases developed erysipelas of a limb at the time that dropsy was present.

In only 1 case was an autopsy done and in this:

'... the kidneys were rather soft and flaccid and more loaded with fat than could have been suspected after so long an illness, but in other respects quite natural.'

Of interest is the fact that this particular case, while included in the chapter on scarlatina, did not have scarlatina but an erysipelatous inflammation of the lower extremities. Couched in modern terms this case is likely to have been secondary infection of grossly oedematous legs, while the renal appearance is consistent with 'lipoid nephrosis'.

As far as the bloody urine sediment is concerned, Blackall had no doubt that this was true haemorrhage, as 'its appearance could hardly deceive'.

Dropsy in Which the Urine Is Coagulable by Heat: Associated with Administration of Mercurial Compounds

Throughout the book Blackall alludes to the potentially deleterious effects of mercury (calomel). He seems to have had little respect for a therapy which, if continued, led to the gums becoming sore and greatly debilitated the patient. The refrain: 'I cannot help fearing that mercury had some share in thus changing the type of disease' (chapter 4, case 8) is chanted in one form or another repeatedly. Blackall was impressed with the long-term adverse effects of mercurials, and when complicated by continued salivation, he believed the underlying disease to be more speedily fatal. One autopsy was performed on a patient who succumbed to general debility, severe oedema of the legs and a sloughing ulcer of the leg. The urine was coagulable by heat. Post mortem examination showed pleuropericarditis was present and the: 'kidneys [were] unusually firm'. Another autopsy was performed on a patient who received mercurials for treatment of diarrhoea, which turned out to be related to ileocaecal tuberculosis, and in this case: 'the kidneys [were] remarkably loaded with blood as if infected'.

Dropsy in Which the Urine Is Coagulable by Heat: Associated with Drinking Cold Water when Heated and Fatigued, Exposure to Cold, Intemperance, Cachexia and Scurvy

This is a heterogeneous collection of cases of anasarca, ascites, or leg swelling in which scanty, coagulable urine was found. No insight into involvement of the kidneys was provided.

Dropsy in Which the Urine Is Coagulable by Heat: Associated with Hydrothorax, Ascites and Hydrocephalus

It is not at all clear what this group of 9 patients with 'hydrothorax' represents, because examination of the chest using percussion and auscultation had not been described. In one case the autopsy revealed a unilateral hydrothorax, atelectasis of the underlying lung and the: 'kidneys [were] remarkably small and sound'.

Similarly, in an autopsy on 1 case of ascites with copious coagulable urine, a hardness and enlargement of the right lobe of the liver was found, firmly resisting the knife. The other viscera were sound: 'except the kidneys, which were remarkably solid and hard, their structure somewhat confused'. Blackall recognized this appearance of the kidneys to be very uncommon and remarks that he is not aware that: 'such a hardness approaching to scirrhous has ever been attributed to the use of mercury', but contradicts this statement by referring to 1 of the cases described above.

Blackall's Overview

In his defence it must be said that any failure of Blackall to recognize the association of coagulable urine with kidney disease can be attributed to the very small number of post mortem examinations which he performed on his patients. But he did fail to recognize the association! In attempting to summarize his findings, he is obtuse and vague in the extreme. Indeed, he indicates that coagulable urine: 'is not connected exclusively with any particular situation'. He did attempt to address the nature of the coagulable substance that he recognized as 'serum', noting that both heat and nitrous acid produced the coagulum. It appears that it was commmonly accepted at the time that oxymuriate of mercury could be used to detect very minute quantities of albumin, but Blackall considered this test to be unhelpful: 'since it acts on the urine in many other cases of dropsy', i.e. also those that do not have coagulable urine. This statement confirms that he thought that the coagulum was some component of serum other than albumin.

In some cases, he considered the urine to be deficient in urea (a substance isolated in 1797 by Fourcroy and Vauquelin [8]), acidic, 'unanimalized' and resistant to putrefaction. He was unable to determine from his experience whether coagulable urine ever precedes the onset of dropsy. He confirmed Wells' observation that a bloody sediment is found after an attack of scarlatina and suspected that the use of calomel aggravated this state.

Perhaps Blackall's single most important contribution, when viewed with hindsight, was his demonstration that mercurials were being abused and that the 'mercurial habit' caused irritation and inflammation, and also dropsy. He further ascribed some cases of fevers of children to the excessive use of calomel.

In reviewing the 9 autopsies that he described in his book, Blackall concluded that the urinary organs are often free from any appearance of unsound structure, despite the great fault in their secretion and that, in 2 mercurial cases, the kidneys were firmer than normal.

Finally, Blackall posed the obvious question: where does the coagulable part of the urine come from? He refered to the earlier contention of Erasmus Darwin that it enters the bladder by an inverted motion of the lymphatic system, but is quick to refute this by saying that it has: 'no kind of support from anatomy'. Could the dropsical accumulations supply the albumin in the urine, he asks? As it is hardly ever found other than with dropsy, and as the fluid is wholly unfit for the purposes of circula-tion, he concluded that it is appropriate that it should be discharged. He argued that the kidneys, from their 'comparative simplicity of secretion', are probably the 'glands' most suited for this purpose, as: 'they appear to be possessed of a sort of selective power capable of separating the blood from whatever is hurtful to it'. On the other hand, he contended that this understanding does not account for the presence of blood in the urine and noted that, occasionally, coagulated urine had been observed in patients without dropsy or in hydrocephalus where the amount of accumulated fluid was small. Most importantly, the excretion of the coagulable substance increased precisely when the disease was worst and decreased when relief was obtained, contrary to his expectation that recovery should be associated with an 'unloading' of the material into the urine.

Blackall was forced to conclude that he was uncertain about whether the serum found in the urine was derived from dropsical accumulations. At no point does disease of the kidney as a cause of the coagulable urine rear its head!

Acknowledgements

The authors are appreciative of having been provided with an unpublished English translation by Professor J.S. Cameron of Pierre Rayer's writings on the history of renal disease, which was invaluable in the preparation of this paper.

References

1 Southey R: The Lectures on Bright's Disease. Br Med J 1881;1:541–546, 587–589, 625–627, 669–672, 713–715.
2 Rayer P: Traité des Maladies des Reins. 3 vol with atlas. Paris, Ballière, 1839.
3 Cotugno D: De Ischiade Nervosa Commentarius. Vienna, R Graffer, 1790.
4 Cruikshank WG: Experiments on urine and sugar by Mr Cruikshank; in Rollo J (ed): Cases of Diabetes Mellitus. London, J Dilly, 1798, pp 443–451.
5 Wells WC: Observations on the dropsy which succeeds scarlet fever. Trans Soc Improvement Med Surg Knowledge 1812;3:167–186.
6 Blackall J: Observations on the Nature and Cure of Dropsies and Particularly on the Presence of the Coagulable Part of the Blood in Dropsical Urine. London, Longman, Hurst, Rees, Orme and Brown, 1813.
7 Harris JD: The Royal Devon and Exeter Hospital. Exeter, Eland Bros, 1922.
8 Fourcroy AF, Vauquelin N: Mémoire pour servir à l'histoire naturelle clinique et médicale de l'urine humaine. Mémoires de l'Institut 1797; 2:431–437.

Am J Nephrol 1994;14:377–382

Giovanni Aliotta[a]
Giovambattista Capasso[b]
Antonino Pollio[a]
Sandro Strumia[a]
Natale Gaspare De Santo[b]

[a] Department of Plant Biology,
University of Naples Federico II, and
[b] Chair of Nephrology, Department of
Pediatrics, Second University of Naples,
Naples, Italy

Joseph Jacob Plenck (1735–1807)

Key Words
Plenck
Diuretics
Botanical medicines

Abstract

Joseph Jacob Plenck (1735–1807) is considered to be the forerunner of modern European dermatology, who also compiled a list of about 800 plants with medicinal uses. Of these about 115 have diuretic properties and are currently included in various pharmacopeias. They were traditionally used to cure ascites of various causes, in urolithiasis, nephritis, cystitis, bladder ulcers, strangury, urinary retention and incontinence. Few of these plants have been fully investigated by modern medicinal chemists, and many are worthy of further study.

The Life of Plenck

Joseph Jacob Plenck (fig. 1) was born in Vienna on 18 November 1735. He graduated as *Magister Chirurgiae et Obstetriciae* in 1763 in the same city, after which he opened a surgical theater in the St. Mark's district. He had 2 wives, neither of whom survived him: at the age of 21 years he married Catherina Sophia Sartori and in 1763 he married Francisca Anthrath. At the age of 35 years, he was summoned by Empress Maria Theresia to teach of surgery and obstetrics at the recently founded University of Tyrnau (1770) in Hungary. Plenck later moved to the University of Buda and finally to the University of Pest. In 1783, Plenck was appointed Director of the Military Pharmacies in Vienna. In 1786, Emperor Joseph II founded the Military Medical Academy (figs. 2 and 3) at the urging of his surgeon, Professor Brambilla (fig. 4), to train surgeons to work in the military hospitals of the various provinces. In the Medical Academy, the so-called Josephinum, Plenck taught botany, mineralogy and surgery, and also discharged the duties attached to the highly satisfying post of life secretary of Academy. He worked hard for nearly 20 years, but had to give up his work because of poor health. He died in Wieburgasse on 24 August 1807.

Plenck's scientific activity was intense [1–8]. He is considered the forerunner of modern European dermatology. He usually wrote in Latin, but German translations exist of all his works, with occasional French and English ones; Italian editions can also be found in Venice and Naples. Editions from Paris, Nancy, Lisbon, Utrecht, St. Petersburg, Venice, Lyon, Strasbourg, London and Naples testify to the existence of an international market for Plenck's writings.

Plenck and the Use of Diuretics

In his book *Icones Plantarum Medicinalium Secundum Systema Linnaei cum Enumeratione Virium et Usus Medici Chirurgici et Diaetetici,* published in folio in both Latin and German from 1788 onwards, Plenck used the Linnaean classification to discuss plants to be used to cure

Professor G. Aliotta
Dipartimento di Biologia Vegetale
Via Foria 223
I–80100 Naples (Italy)

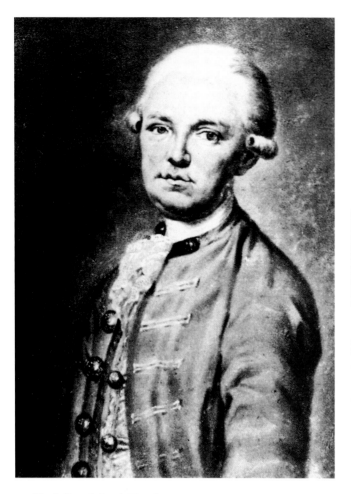

Fig. 1. Joseph Jacob Plenck.

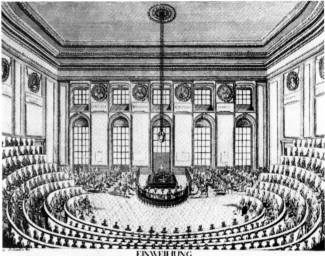

EINWEIHUNG
DER IOSEPHINISCHEN MILITAERAKADEMIE DER CHIRURGIE

Fig. 3. Interior view of the Military Medical Academy, Vienna.

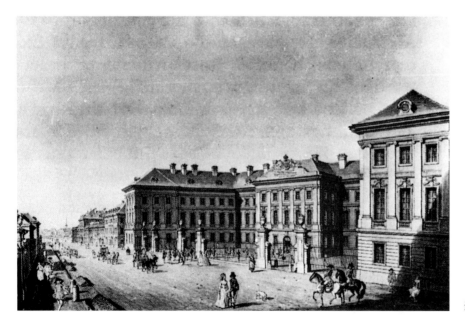

Fig. 2. Exterior view of the Military Medical Academy, Vienna.

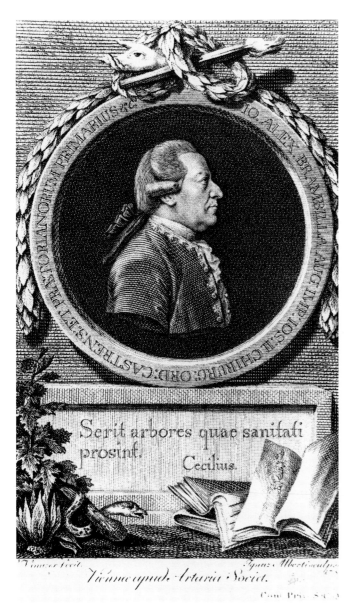

Fig. 4. Professor Alexander Brambilla, personal surgeon to Emperor Joseph II.

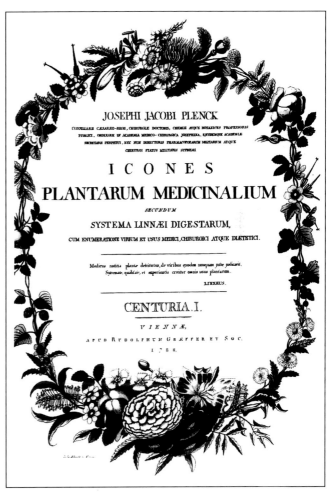

Fig. 5. Frontispiece of *Icones Plantarum Medicinalium* of Plenck.

diseases (fig. 5). The book is dedicated to Joseph II (fig. 6), and the request for official approval from the Emperor is of interest:

'Concede, therefore, O most August of Princes that this work may shine through your auspices.'

In the preface of the book, Plenck quotes the works of Zorn, Blackwell and Regnault, stressing that they were inadequate. No other quotations are given, and Plenck simply ignored other scientists and considered their contributions as a common inheritance of the scientific community.

In his book, Plenck reproduced the plants in their natural size and color. For each plant he reported the name, class, order, type, species, place of origin, pharmaceutical role, name in German, name in French, odour, taste, pharmacologic actions and medicinal use. From the approximately 800 plants included, about 115 have diuretic actions and are currently included in various pharmacopeias.

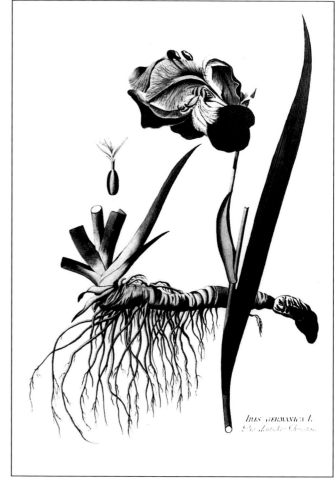

Fig. 6. Dedication of *Icones Plantarum Medicinalium* to Emperor Joseph II.	**Fig. 7.** Illustration of German iris used to treat hydrothorax.

Diuretic plants were used to cure ascites (garlic), ascites of alcoholism ('in hydrope spiritus vini abusus'; greater celandine), ascites and anasarca (sassafras) hydrothorax (German iris; fig. 7). Many of these plants were used for urolithiasis and were classified as follows: (1) plants of general use in urolithiasis (Mahaleb cherry); (2) plants capable of breaking up or dissolving calculi (Chinese lantern); (3) plants for removing very small calculi (*Erica* sp.) (fig. 8); (4) plants for removing gravel from kidney and bladder (meadow saffron); (5) plants for treating renal colic (giant fennel).

Diuretic plants were also used in nephritis (liquorice, sea onion), cystitis (common madder, sea onion), bladder ulcers (Galingale flat sedge, wild parsnip) and strangury (liquorice, sea onion, mountain ash), the last to be used in youngsters with 'stranguriam dolorosissimam juvenis sa-

nat'. Diuretic plants were also used to cure urinary retention, urinary incontinence, bladder paralysis and urinary suppression (sea onion).

Of these plants, special mention must be made of sea onion (*Scilla maritima* L.; fig. 9), which was a general remedy for kidney and lung diseases: 'specifice in renes et pulmones agens'.

An Attempt to Update Plenck

The attempt by the authors to update Plenck's book has produced 2 major findings. First, the names proposed by Linnaeus for many of the plants have been changed on the basis of modern taxonomy. For example, according to the International Code of Botanical Nomenclature, if a

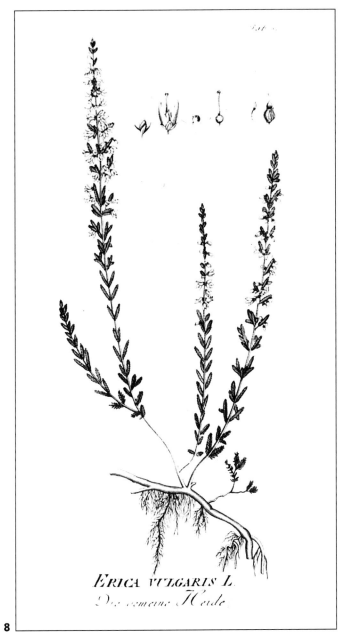

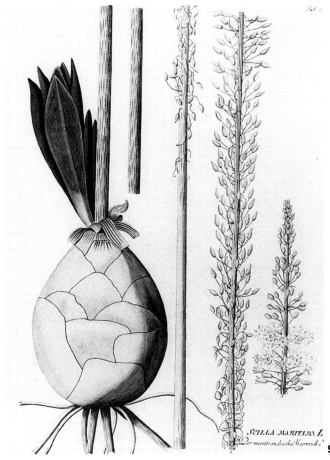

SCILLA MARITIMA L.

8

9

Fig. 8. Illustration of *Erica vulgaris* used to remove very small calculi.

Fig. 9. Illustration of sea onion used as a general remedy for diseases of the kidney.

species named by Linnaeus has been placed in a different genus, the second part of its name, the specific epithet, becomes the name of the new genus (e.g. *Apium petroselinum* L. has become *Petroselinum crispum* (L.) Miller; the author who proposed the invalidated name is placed in parentheses and is followed by name of the author who made the change. Secondly, the pharmacologic effects of many of the plants reported by Plenck are still not fully explored, though uses of many of the species are cited in the pharmacopeias of many countries.

Only a few of the plants traditionally considered to be diuretics have been screened for their chemical constituents, and these latter do not necessarily correspond to active substances used in renal therapy. For example, only a few reports concerning the flavonoids hesperidin and rutin have shown the diuretic effects of these substances. Flavonoids are phenolic compounds that occur in abundance in some plant families, e.g. Umbelliferae and Rutaceae. Experiments with rutin suggest that flavonoids may have important diuretic effects. In this respect flavonoids deserve the attention of medicinal chemists who have provided practising clinicians with a wide range of synthetic diuretics.

Modern Diuretics

Since 1919, when Alfred Vogl, a Viennese medical student, observed the diuretic properties of merbaphen, an organomercurial being used to treat syphilis, the development of diuretic drugs has passed through a series of distinct stages. The thiazide era was followed by the era of the 'high-ceiling' diuretics, the antikaliuretics, which was followed in turn by the era of the polyvalent agents that cause both natriuresis and uricosuria. During the course of this process, medicinal chemists have seldom referred to earlier listings of medicinal plants.

A resurgence of interest in the study and use of medicinal plants has taken place during the last 2 decades. The importance of plant-derived drugs is underlined by the following facts: (1) the World Health Organization has estimated that 80% of the world's population rely chiefly on traditional medicine; (2) Most traditional therapies involve the use of plant extracts or their active constituents; (3) 25% of all prescriptions in the USA between 1959 and 1980 contained extracts or active principles prepared from higher plants. Similar percentages (22–25%) appeared in some European countries; (4) consumers in 1980 in the USA paid more than $8000 million for prescriptions containing active substances obtained from plants.

In the recent past, a combination of data obtained empirically with the most technically advanced experimental laboratory and clinical procedures has provided several important contributions to medicine. Some well known examples include: *Atropa belladonna* L. (atropine; anticholinergic); *Digitalis purpurea* L. (digoxin; cardiotonic); *Colchicum autumnale* L. (colchicine; anti-gout); and *Cinchona officinalis* L. (quinine; antimalarial).

Conclusions

The aim of updating the work of Plenck is to help to preserve the knowledge of the plants that have been traditionally used in renal therapy. These plants represent a useful source for screening, chemical analyses and clinical trials of new diuretic drugs. Except in the above mentioned cases, however, ethnopharmacobotany has been effectively ignored in these days of great biotechnologic advances in medicine and plant biology.

It is hoped that physicians, laboratory scientists and botanists can now join forces in a united search for more effective diuretics.

References

1 Holubar K, Frankl J: Joseph Plenck (1735–1807). A forerunner of modern European dermatology. J Am Acad Dermatol 1983;326–332.
2 Holubar K: Early Dermatology in Central Europe: Joseph Plenck in Tyrnau, Budapest and Vienna. Koroth, 1984, 414–420.
3 Puschmann TH: Die Medizin in Wien während der letzen 100 Jahre. Vienna, Verlag von Mortiz Perles, 1884.
4 Zimmerman FJ: Rede zur Gedächtnis des verstobenen KK Rathes und Professors Herrn Joseph Jacob von Plenck. Vienna, P.H. Bauer, 1808.
5 Endre H: Tudomany egyete Orvosi Karanak Multjarol Es Jelenerol. Budapest, Az Atheneum, 1896.
6 Michaud M: Plenck Joseph-Jacques; in Biographie Universelle. Akademische Druck- und Verlagsanstalt, Graz, 1970, pp 514, 515.
7 Tibor G: Magyarorszag Orvosi Bibliographija 1472–1899. Budapest, Az Atheneum, 1,900.
8 British Library General Catalogue of Printed Books to 1975, p 405.

Am J Nephrol 1994;14:383

Alberto Tizianello

Department of Internal Medicine,
Division of Nephrology,
Genoa, Italy

Introduction

In Venice in 1562, F. Sansovino printed a textbook of therapy, *Secreti Medicinali*, by Pietro Bairo, physician at the court of Charles II, Duke of Savoy (1486–1553), in Turin (fig. 1). Calculi are by far the major topic in the section dealing with diseases of the kidney and urinary tract. The titles of the chapters are: renal abscess; prevention of stone formation; treatment of stones in the urinary tract; bladder stones and their complications; bladder stones in children; and bladder ulcerations.

Diabetes is also mentioned, and the balance between urine excretion and water intake is stressed. At that time, the sweet taste of urine was an important aid in the diagnosis of diabetes. This diagnostic test was commonly the task of an assistant. The birth of modern nephrology was still very far off, and the position of assistants often very uncomfortable!

In 1844 Liebig reported the results of various experiments in man [1]. His conclusions were the following:

> 'I have ascertained that the salt content of the urine, passed shortly after a copious drink of water, always exceeds that of the water, whereas in the later samples its content of salts, including phosphates, becomes vanishingly small. It follows that all salts present in the urine must be regarded as transient blood constituents which are excreted precisely because they are no longer appropriate to the normal blood constitution.'

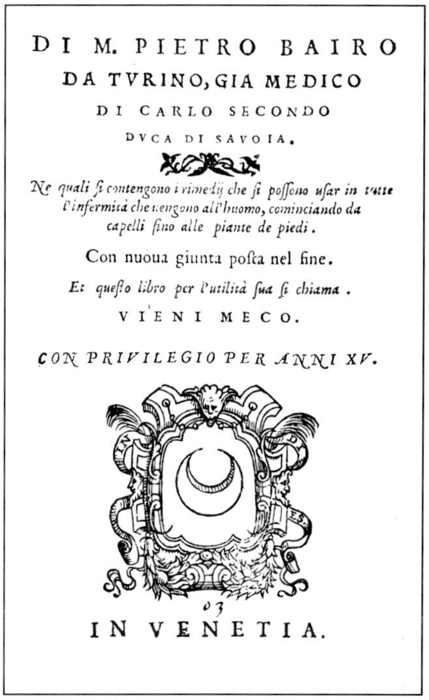
DI M. PIETRO BAIRO
DA TVRINO, GIA MEDICO
DI CARLO SECONDO
DVCA DI SAVOIA.
Ne quali si contengono i rimedij che si possono usar in tutte l'infermità che vengono all'huomo, cominciando da capelli fino alle piante de piedi.
Con nuoua giunta posta nel fine.
Et questo libro per l'utilità sua si chiama.
VIENI MECO.
CON PRIVILEGIO PER ANNI XV.
IN VENETIA.

Fig. 1. Title page of *Secreti Medicinali* by Pietro Bairo.

Liebig was a pioneer in providing information on the role of the kidney in maintaining the physicochemical stability of the animal organism. The concept of homeostasis was clearly outlined by Claude Bernard about 30 years after the publication of Liebig's paper.

In the early years of the 20th century practical medicine was still largely empiric. Diagnosis was derived almost completely from a patient's history and physical examination, while support from laboratories was very poor. Moreover, treatment was mainly symptomatic, and few specific drugs were available. English empiricism, developed by Locke, Berkeley and Hume in the 17th and 18th centuries, according to which knowledge derives only from experience and observation, was the philosophy followed by physicians. Soon, however, medical science with the support of other sciences, mainly chemistry and physics, was able to rapidly develop. Modern medicine was born.

Reference

1 Liebig J: Uber die Constitution des Harns der Menschen und der fleischfressenden Thiere. Am Chem Pharm 1844;50:161, cited in Gorman A Hills: Acid-Base Balance. Baltimore, Williams and Wilkins, 1973, p 85.

Alberto Tizianello, MD
Department of Internal Medicine
Division of Nephrology
Viale Benedetto XV, 6
I-16132 Genoa (Italy)

0250–8095/94/0146–0383
$8.00/0

Am J Nephrol 1994;14:384–390

Francesco Rossi
Mario Mangrella
Anna Loffreda
Enrico Lampa

Institute of Pharmacology and Toxicology,
Faculty of Medicine and Surgery, Second
University of Naples, Naples, Italy

Wizards and Scientists: The Pharmacologic Experience in the Middle Ages

Key Words

Pharmacology
Pharmacy
Middle Ages
Formularia
Magic ritual

Abstract

During the Dark ages, Greco-Roman science survived in the eastern Roman Empire and the most important advances in pharmacology and pharmacy were made in Byzantium. As the Arab empires spread in the 7th and 8th centuries, they incorporated earlier learning, and the most important contribution of Arabic medical writers was probably the introduction of formularies to aid in the preparation of medicines. In turn, the later spread of Arabic knowledge to the West introduced little-known plants and fostered an interest in collecting and cultivating them, and also introduced the palatable dose forms preferred by the Arabic doctors. In the West, however, the Christian Church taught a doctrine of unquestioning faith, and despite the centers of learning, e.g. at Salerno, most ordinary people depended on the healing power of faith, religious relics and traditional folk medicine. Hydrology was also well developed in the Middle Ages. The *formularia* that survive describe many indigenous plants, but with few illustrations. Their gathering and preparation is generally guided by magic ceremonies and ritual, and plants often took their properties from their habitat, e.g. the wayside plantain was thought good for tired or wounded feet. Concepts of therapeutic plants were also influenced by alchemy and were linked to related metals and planets.

Introduction

Social, economic and ideologic causes have been invoked to explain the severe decline of the sciences in the Catholic West between 500 AD and 1,000 AD. The collapse of the western Roman Empire in 476 AD led to a disintegration of political authority and concomitantly to a cultural decline in western Europe. These cultural changes resulted from the conflict of Roman and Germanic outlooks, and from the contemporary expansion of the Christian faith. Moreover, in the preceding centuries, the work of philosophers of the stoic, epicurean and neo-platonic schools and the expansion of mysticism among the common people increased scepticism about naturalistic studies. The wide diffusion of mysticism, primarily originating in the Alexandrian schools of philosophy and promoted by some Eastern religious cults and doctrines, including gnosticism, theologism and magianism, to some extent supported the spread of Christianity, which shared some of the principles of those doctrines, e.g. the search for everlasting happiness through the separation from earthly matters and the devotion to spiritual life [1].

Francesco Rossi, MD
Institute of Pharmacology and Toxicology, Faculty of
Medicine and Surgery, Second University of Naples
Via Costantinopoli 16 – Via S. Andrea delle Dame 8
I–80138 Naples (Italy)

It was against this background that the Greco-Roman heritage survived in the eastern Roman Empire, and it was in Byzantium that the most important advances in pharmacology and pharmacy occurred during the Middle Ages [2].

Arabic Medicine and the Classical Tradition

While many non-rational elements of Alexandrian culture were absorbed into Byzantine practices, medicine and pharmacy generally followed the Greek and Roman patterns. The most important tenet of Byzantine practitioners was the perfection and adaptation of Galen's teaching in the tradition of Oribasius [2]. Oribasius, who is properly considered among the best of Byzantine physicians, lived from 325 AD to 403 AD. He shared Galen's ideas on urine, based on developments of the uroscopic methods of Hippocrates. The Hippocratic school already placed considerable importance on evaluation of the quantity and quality of urine, how it was excreted, and the stage of a disease indicated by a relative lack or excess of urine [2]. Hippocrates described urine *tenuis,* i.e. light; urine *crassa,* i.e. thick; and other types of urine, called *albicans, biliosa, rubiconda* (or *rubra*), *cruenta, nigricans, aeruginosa* and *varia.* He also distinguished different types of urinary sediment.

The schools of medicine that followed (the Galenic school, and even more so, the Arabic school) extended examination of the urine by increasing the types described and the characteristics of the sediment, including the position and structure of the sediment within the liquid part. Numerous treatises on the diagnostic usefulness of urine examination were compiled in the Middle Ages, particularly by the pupils of the Salerno School of Medicine.

Oribasius based his knowledge of uroscopy on these theories. His works included *Synopsis,* which was a travel edition of *Singaghe, Europista,* which became a popular book of therapeutics, and a Galenic summary dedicated to Julius, the Byzantine Emperor. Like Oribasius, other Byzantine medical writers also had knowledge of ancient texts about the necessity of experience with pharmaceuticals. Chief among these writers were Aetius of Amida, Alexander of Tralles and Paul of Aegina [2].

In the 7th and 8th centuries, great Arab empires spread across North Africa to Spain and across the Middle East and Persia to India. Arab civilization gained its initial impetus from the religious doctrine of Islam, but the extraordinary culture that subsequently developed in literature, architecture, philosophy and science, including

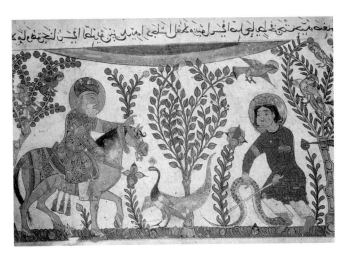

Fig. 1. Miniature from an Arabic manuscript of the 13th century, showing two physicians gathering ingredients for medicines.

medicine and pharmacy, was derived from the cultures of the many nations incorporated into the Arab Empire.

The most important contribution of Arabic writers to medical literature was probably the introduction of a new genre of professional sources of information, the formularies, intended for the use of pharmacists and other who prepared medicines (fig. 1). These books consisted of compilations of formulas and recipes for medications arranged in orderly (usually alphabetic) fashion and included instructions for compounding and suggestions for use [2]. The prototype of these formularies was *Al Aqrabadhin al Kabir,* a book compiled by Sabur ibn Sahl in the mid-9th century. A very important formulary was *Al Dukkan, (The Apothecary Shop)* by Ibn'Abd Rabbih. This formulary was distinguished by its descriptions of the dose forms preferred by Arab doctors, including syrups, conserves and confections, some of them incorporating spices and perfumes [2].

In the 11th century appeared a formulary compiled by Al Biruni, entitled *Kitab al Saydanah fi al Tibb, (Book of Pharmacy in the Healing Art).* This work, in addition to being enchanting for its description of more than 1,000 simple remedies, represents a quantum leap towards the identification of the complementary roles of pharmacist and physician, and documents the high profile of pharmacy in the Arabic world. The author of this book wrote that pharmacy is: 'the art of knowing ... simple ingredients in their various species, types and shapes. From these a pharmacist prepares compounded medications as prescribed by and ordered by the prescribing physician'. The formulary compiled in Spain by Ibn al Baytar in the 13th

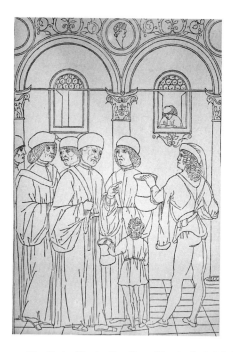

Fig. 2. An illustration from *Fasciculo de Medicina,* an illuminated manuscript published in Venice in the 14th century, depicting a consultation on urine. In the foreground, 4 long-robed doctors are standing round an older one, the professor, to whom a young man and a child stretch out their *matulae* to receive an opinion on their urine.

century was even more extensive, including 800 botanic drugs, 145 mineral drugs, and 130 animal drugs [2].

After the spread of Arabic medical knowledge to the West, urine testing became more and more important. It acquired a 'uromantic' character, because it was thought that the inspection of urine could give complete information about the diagnosis and prognosis of diseases. Urine examination was performed by studying the liquid in a broad-necked, pot-bellied glass vase, called a *matula,* carried by the physician in a straw basket. This vessel, also described by Avicenna, was often seen as the symbol of a physician [2]. Figure 2, taken from *Fasciculo de Medicina,* an illuminated manuscript published in Venice in the 14th century, shows a consultation on urine. In the foreground, 4 long-robed doctors stand round an older one, the professor, to whom a young man and a child stretch out their *matulae* to receive an opinion on their urine.

The wide diffusion of Arabic medical knowledge had several consequences. First, the prescription of plants that were not well known fostered an interest in the search for and cultivation of such primary ingredients. It is known that, even before Arabic medical writings were translated into Latin, monks of European monasteries were copying

prescriptions calling for drugs that could have originated only in the Middle East, the Far East, or Africa. Some of them, e.g. ambergris (from the Arabic ambar) and camphor (from the Arabic kafour), were unknown in the *materia medica* of the ancient and classical worlds. Secondly, the introduction of dose forms new to the West represented a very important contribution to the development of medicine and must be considered a precious heritage from the Arabic apothecaries, who had advanced knowledge of grinding, mixing and dissolving.

The blending of traditional Western knowledge of drugs and the Arabic apothecary's art introduced new materials and advanced dose forms, including syrups, conserves, confections, juleps and electuraries, all of which made use of sugar or honey and confounded the old notion that only bitter medicines were efficacious. In addition flavoring extracts, e.g. rosewater, orange and lemon peel and tragacanth, enhanced the preparation and administration of drugs.

The use of earths as therapeutic agents was widespread. Clay and alkaline earths, formerly recommended by the Greeks, became trading commodities under the Arabs. Packets of earth were marked with a seal, from which the name *terrae sigillatae* originated; the seal attested the country of origin, e.g. *terra samia, terra cimolia, terra lemnia.* In the Middle Ages, white clay from the Milk Grotto in Bethlehem was highly prized. Women who were having difficulty in breast-feeding used the miraculous drug, called 'Mary's milk', in the hope that it would increase the flow of milk [3]. Drinking vessels were also made from these earths, and it was said that anyone drinking from these would be immune to any kind of poisoning. Water kept in these vessels was used as a remedy for snake-bites.

Medicine and Pharmacy in the Western World

The Germanic tribes that dominated western Europe after the collapse of the western Roman Empire added little to the medicine and pharmacy that the classical and Arabic worlds had developed. Christianized Europe fell back on the healing power of faith, religious relics and traditional folk medicine [2].

The learning of Rome and Byzantium, however, was not completely without heirs. Under the domination of unquestioning faith, there were small signs indicating encouragement to the development of sciences. For example, in the monasteries the monks worked to acquire and preserve ancient knowledge. A central figure in the development of medicine in this period was Aurelius Cassiodorus (485–585 AD), chancellor to Theodoric the Great. After retiring into private life, he founded a monastery at Vivarium (Calabria, Italy) in about 540 AD, in which a community was devoted to study, contemplation and the care of sick patients and pilgrims [1]. The major text compiled by Cassiodorus was *Institutiones,* in which the author directed the monks to acquaint themselves with the works of Dioscorides and to read the works of Hippocrates, Galen and others, collected by himself in the library of the monastery. Cassiodorus advised them to: 'learn the characteristics of the herbs and the compounding of medicines', and admonished them to: 'place all your hopes on the Lord'. The work of Cassiodorus began the outline of the monastic medicine that in the Christianized West would be organized in the schemes of the Benedictine doctrine.

Following the example of the Eastern monasteries, from which Western monasticism took birth, charitable institutions called *xenodochia* were founded. The monks, whose approach to healing was based on Christian charity, with scientific observation taking second place, were familiar with a good deal of ancient learning, but their medicine and pharmacy was based largely on empiricism (fig. 3). The medical training of the monks was promoted by the intense activity of copying, collecting and preserving codex versions of the classical writers and the scientific writings of contemporary authors. These activities took place in the *scriptoria.*

The main credit for bringing Roman horticultural techniques from Italy to the rest of Europe must lie with the Benedictine monks. In the monasteries founded by St. Benedict of Nursia in Italy and in Europe (Cluny, San Gallo, Cologne, Lorsch, Canterbury, York), sickrooms operated and pharmacies were organized. At Reichenau, Walafrid Strabo (809–849 AD) wrote didactic poems in hexameter verse containing information about the rearing, cultivation and use of medical herbs known at that time [3].

The tradition of the monastic schools was carried on by university scholars who combined ancient doctrines with Arabic learning. Some important advances, however, were made by independent scholars, e.g. Albertus Magnus, Arnold of Villanova and Raimond Lull. The insights derived from the works of independent or scholastic researchers were collected in the Benedictine *scriptoria* and used by physicians and apothecaries in their practices. The concepts introduced by men like Arnold of Villanova and Albertus Magnus were an indication of the complete change in scientific outlook that would later characterize the Renaissance. Following the work of the

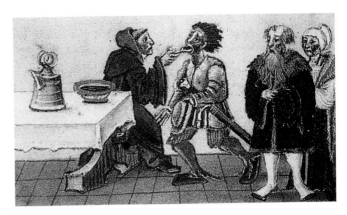

Fig. 3. An illuminated page from a 16th century manuscript, in which is depicted a Benedictine monk about to administer holy wine to a sick man.

independent scholars of the Middle Ages, the men of the modern age would embark on the unification of scientific knowledge and provide the basis for the development of the modern science.

Early Medieval Pharmacy

At the start of the Middle Ages the most consulted books of medicine were the *Herbarium Vires et Curationes* by Pseudo Apuleius, and *Medicina ex Animalibus* by Sestus Placitus. This latter was undoubtedly the most widely used textbook of remedies obtained from animals [1]. One of the treatises of the Abbess Hildegarde of Bingen (1098–1179 AD) was a textbook of *materia medica* which, though influenced by ancient writings, also contains a great deal of information about folk medicine. Among the indigenous medicinal herbs she mentioned are marshmallow, valerian, absinth, lovage, thyme, dandelion, St. John's wort, coltsfoot, lavender and poppy [3].

A vernacular literature of recipes also developed. Old English, Irish, French and German works appeared, with Roman, Celtic and Teutonic folk medicine much in evidence.

A major change in Western attitudes towards pharmacy and drug therapy took place through transmission of the Arabic and Greek compilations, in their entirety, to western Europe [2]. Two centers of learning arose: one at Toledo in Spain, where a school of translators was founded by Archbishop Raymond in the 11th century, and another, the more important, at Salerno, where the medical center attracted both patients and students in the 10th century.

The Salerno School of Medicine (fig. 4), which could be viewed as Europe's first university, was responsible for

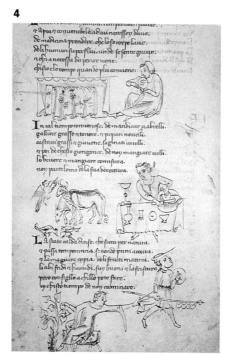

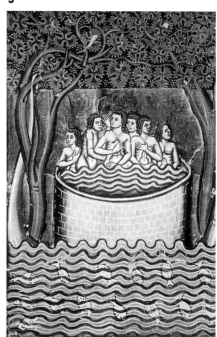

Fig. 4. An illuminated page from *Regimen Sanitatis Salernitanum,* kept in the National Library of Naples.

Fig. 5. A miniature showing the *Cantarelli* bath from Peter of Eboli's *De Balneis Puteolanis.*

major contributions to medicine and pharmacy, not simply for translations of medical texts. Even before Constantinus Africanus (said to be a merchant turned monk) went to Salerno, the *Passionarius Galeni* was compiled, probably by the Italian physician Gariopontus [2]. The Salerno School of Medicine made significant contributions to the diagnostic evaluation of urine. Uroscopy, a science that had arisen from Hippocratic observations on the characteristics of urine (color, appearance, quantity), was developed by the medical schools of Byzantium and the Arabic scientific works. The Salerno School of Medicine added the Arabic knowledge of uroscopy to the Hippocratic ideas, and introduced esoteric elements from the Alexandrian writers.

Among the many treatises of the Middle Ages, e.g. the books of Gilles de Corbeil, Isaac Judaeus and Magister Maurus, the most interesting is *Regulae Urinarium,* compiled by Ursone Salernitano and comprehensive of all the most widely diffused knowledge about this matter. Magister Maurus, in his book *De Urinis,* discriminates 4 related regions in urine as in the human body as a whole. The regions of the body were: brain and living limbs; heart and spiritual limbs; liver and nourishing limbs; kidney, testicles and lower organs. The related regions of urine were: circulation; surface (or aerial matter); substance; and grounds. In the Middle Ages, the works of the Arabic doctors and the writings of the Salerno School of Medicine

aided in developing a novel specialty – urology – into a field that until then had been dominated by empiric concepts and surgical measures.

Hydrology

Hydrology was well developed in the Middle Ages. According to the *Regimen Sanitatis* of the Salerno School of Medicine, many thermal baths were noteworthy for their therapeutic properties against many diseases. A very important source of information about these practices is the illuminated manuscript *De Balneis Puteolanis,* a collection of epigrams written by Peter of Eboli, a pupil of the Salerno School of Medicine [4]. This work, which has been known since the 13th century, described the thermal baths of two Neapolitan centers, Baia and Pozzuoli. The name of the bath *De Petra* may derive from the surrounding volcanic stone, but the author of the book declares that the name is due to the litholytic action of the water of this bath. In particular, the water of the bath *De Petra* was considered diuretic and efficacious for the elimination of small renal calculi. Peter of Eboli writes:

'Many people, suffering from nephrolithiasis, gave out rapidly a urine full of calculous residues' [4].

Another thermal bath praised in *De Balneis Puteolanis* for its therapeutic properties against urinary calculi is the bath *Sancti Georgi,* the water of which was known to be

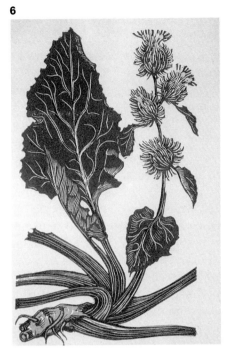
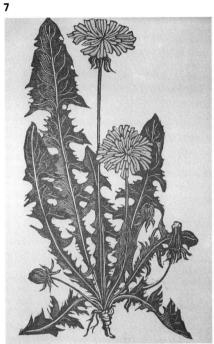

Fig. 6. *Arctium lappa* (great burdock).
Fig. 7. *Taraxacum officinale* Weber (dandelion).

diuretic. In the bath Cantarelli (fig. 5) boiling water spouted directly from the sea and was restrained and collected by clay constructions. Peter of Eboli named the bath *Sudatorium* as being useful in cases of salt/water imbalance [4].

None of the baths described by Peter of Eboli still exists. The unstable volcanic ground of the areas in which they were sited meant that the distribution and sources of thermal water changed rapidly with time. Today the significance of thermal remedies in the Middle Ages can only be deduced from the marvelous pictures by Peter. The existence of a vernacular translation of Peter's work into an ancient Neapolitan dialect testifies to the high regard in which hydrology was held [4].

Herbal Remedies and Magic

Jorimann classifies formularies of the early Middle Ages into *antidotaria* and *formularia* [3]. In *antidotaria* a list of indications revealing the antitoxic character of the antidote can be found; preparation was complicated and costly. Precious drugs, including pulverized pearls, gold and silver, figured prominently in the preparations of antidotes. The use of metals like gold was a link with alchemy, and drinkable gold was a principle related to the 'Great Elixir', the magistery. The horn of the mythical unicorn was an important component of many antidotes. The powder obtained from this horn was considered very

efficacious against poisoning and as prophylaxis against many diseases [1].

In contrast, the *formularia* included many indigenous drugs which were easy to procure; their remedies were also based on religious and magical concepts [3]. In addition to preparations based on metals and folk imagination, the most important items in the paraphernalia of the physician and apothecary were herbs. The herbaria were widely used, primarily because the herbal drugs were certainly more available than the animal ones [1]. Any pharmacologic substance unmixed with others was called a simple. At first, minerals and animal parts were called simples, but later this term was reserved for plants, their parts and their derivatives.

For the most part, herbaria have survived without illustrations, and where these are available they are always inaccurate and vague. It is possible that the information necessary for recognizing the different plants was almost all orally transmitted and acquired by experience [1].

Among the herbs commonly used were the following. *Arctium lappa* (great burdock) (fig. 6), belonging to the *Astaraceae* family had choleretic and diuretic effects by virtue of its content of α-hydroxymethylacrylic acid [5]. Celandine was recommended in icterus, gravel and hydropsy. *Taraxacum officinale* Weber (dandelion) (fig. 7), the leaves of which were depurative and diuretic, was also used prophylactically in patients with lithiasis. *Equisetum* sp., or horsetail, had a particular diuretic action because of the abundance of potassium salts that it contained. Butcher's-broom, in association with fennel, parsley, celery and asparagus (the five root mixture) was recommended by Dioscorides, Pliny, Matthioli and Leclerc for urinary diseases. Dog-rose had diuretic properties and preventive actions against renal calculi. The leaves of bearberry were an excellent remedy in diseases of the genital and urinary tracts, and the leaves and young branches of mistletoe had hypotensive and diuretic effects [5].

Of the most ancient known illuminated Western herbarium, only 2 illustrations survive in the so-called Johnson's papyrus (400 AD) [1]. In the 7th–10th centuries, however, many copies of the 6th century codex of Dioscorides and of Pseudo Apuleius' *Herbarium* (4th century) were made. The *Herbarium* of Pseudo Apuleius, also called *De Medicaminibus Herbarium,* is a compilation of medical recipes taken from, among others, Dioscorides, *Medicina Plinii* (3rd century) and Pliny's *Naturalis Historia.* Pseudo Apuleius' *Herbarium* contained lists of plants, including their synonyms, and lists of the diseases cured. The recipes collected in this textbook were copied for many centuries, often badly.

References to magic and astrology were numerous. For example, plantain, which grows by the roadside and is crushed underfoot by man and animals, takes from this the magical property of healing disorders that arise from the road, e.g. wounds of the feet and tiredness. Moreover, the properties of herbs were linked to the position of the stars at the time of their harvesting or their medical use. For example, 7 twigs of a herb, without roots, had to be boiled when the moon was waning. The water was used to sprinkle the sick man, but the remedy was efficacious only in the first part of the night [1]. In some illustrations, the part of the plant is surrounded by snakes or insects to remind the physician that those herbs were effective against the bites and stings of the animals shown. The symbolic substitution of the simple roots with animals or parts of the human body became more and more common in the following centuries and was found throughout the herbaria of the Middle Ages [1].

Herb harvesting was often guided by magic ceremonies, which were described in many herbaria. The herba-list often a woman, had not only to study the position of the planets and stars (lunar phase, dawn and sunset, dominant constellation, etc.), but also to observe precepts about his/her own person, including ritual purification, sexual abstinence, nakedness, or the use of clothes without a belt [1]. Some plants also required particular procedures in order to neutralize harmful influences; for example, magic circles were traced out around mandrakes and magic formulas or prayers, like *praecatio terrae,* were often said [1]. Plants were not to be harvested by means of iron tools, but only by using wooden, precious metal, or other special instruments. For example, the ground around a mandrake was removed with an ivory tool. When harvesting by hand, only certain fingers could be used, usually the middle ones, called 'medicinal fingers'.

The concepts about therapeutic plants were influenced by alchemy, which introduced the relationship between a metal and a star or planet (gold–Sun, silver–Moon, lead–Saturn, iron–Mars, copper–Venus, tin–Jupiter, mercury–Mercury). Thus, a plant influenced by the Sun was thought to be related to gold, and a plant of the Moon to silver. Accordingly, alchemists used herbs to produce the so-called 'powders of projection', in order to try to transform metals into gold or silver.

The magianic view of the world, however, did not only lead to superstition. The people of the Middle Ages experienced a strong linkage between universal order and human life. The substances used as therapeutic agents also acquired spiritual significance and power, because the combination of spirit and matter itself represented the order of Nature.

References

1 Zanca A: Il Farmaco nei Tempi. Dalle Origini ai Laboratori; Parma, Astrea Coop, 1987.
2 Crown DL, Helfand WH: Pharmacy. An Illustrated History. New York, Harry N Abrams, 1980.
3 Mez Mangold L: A History of Drugs. Basel, Hoffmann-La Roche, 1989.
4 Mangrella M: Magister Petrus de Ebulo. Eboli, Giordano, 1981.
5 Borsatti G, Leboroni ME: La Via dei Semplici. Perugia, Guidi, 1988.

Am J Nephrol 1994;14:391–398

Sandra Sabatini

Departments of Physiology and Internal
Medicine, Texas Tech University Health
Sciences Center, Lubbock, Tex., USA

Women, Medicine and Life in the Middle Ages (500–1500 AD)

Key Words

Women's status
Middle Ages
Hildegarde von Bingen
History of pharmacology
Pharmacy and magic

Abstract

The status of women in the Middle Ages was ambiguous, because although they had great responsibility and expertise in practical affairs they were viewed as chattel and inferior to men. They were skilled in cookery, often of highly spiced dishes using a variety of ingredients and flavorings, and they were taught the use of medicinal herbs. They were often skilled in simple first aid, though they were not allowed to practise outside the home. An important exception to this was Hildegarde von Bingen, whose *Physica* brought her great renown. In it she became the first woman to discuss plants in relation to their medicinal properties. For most people in the Middle Ages, treatment revolved around herbs and diet, together with faith and holy relics and the use of (forbidden) pagan incantation and ritual. Astrology was often a necessary adjunct to treatment. In Salerno, however, medicine had been practised from classical times, and medical training could last for 7 years or more. One of the greatest medieval medical texts is the *Tacuinum Sanitatis,* which describes in detail the 6 essentials for the preservation of man's health. Several vegetables and herbs are mentioned in connection with the kidneys, the picking and preparation of which are imbued with magic.

Introduction

'There are waste places in the earth which fill one with terror ...' [1]. So wrote Sir William Osler in 1913 of the land we call 'Europe'. When desolation takes over the flourishing of man's mind and hand, a chill runs to the heart and one trembles with a sense of human instability. This is the way the Middle Ages began:

'Following the glory that was Greece and the grand era that was Rome, a frigid chill came upon the civilized world, in which the light of learning burned low, flickering almost to extinction' [1].

How did the gifts of these two great civilizations virtually vanish, and what was life and medicine like in this black and evil period from 500 AD to 1500 AD?

To address the first question, scholars believe that these civilizations were decimated primarily for 3 reasons [2]. First, virtually all the important cities were destroyed in the 400s when the 'barbarians' invaded southern Europe (table 1). As people fell, so did the writings and pictures of the times. Secondly, Christianity preached death, judgment, heaven and hell, and it was thought that only a few could 'save' the many. Thirdly, illness and the plague of the 6th century destroyed much of the Roman world. The Mausoleum of Hadrian shows an angel with a drawn

Sandra Sabatini, PhD, MD
Department of Physiology
Texas Tech University
Health Sciences Center
Lubbock, TX 79430 (USA)

Table 1. A few events of the Middle Ages (500–1500 AD)

Year (AD)	Military and political	Scientific and medical	Other
476	The fall of Rome		
581	Monte Cassino destroyed	Death of Anthimus, Theodoric's Greek physician (526)	Lombards invade Italy
768–814	Charlemagne	Rhazes, Persian physician (850)	Romanesque architecture
1020–1053	Normans conquer southern Italy	Hildegarde von Bingen (1098)	Normans conquer England (1066)
1095–1099	1st Crusade	Paper made in Spain (1150)	Gothic architecture
1204	4th Crusade (Constantinople captured)	Gold coins minted in Italy (1252)	Thomas Becket murdered (1170) Magna Carta (1215) Dante born (1265) Marco Polo in China (1271–1292)
1323–1328	Flanders social revolt	Black Death (1348)	Chaucer (about 1340–1400) The 100 Years War (1337–1453)
1400	Erasmus (1465–1536)	Henry the Navigator Printing from metal reaches Italy (1465)	Turks capture Constantinople (1453) The Italian language The Medici in Florence
1500	The Renaissance		

Data from Ref. 4, pp. 214–221.

sword unsheathed as victory over the plague. Catastrophic illness continued intermittently throughout the Middle Ages, culminating with the Black Death in 1348 (table 1).

Life and medicine in the Middle Ages, the subject of this paper, will examine the everyday life of women and doctors and shall show how the two were inextricably linked to the health and well-being of the populace. Some of the 'therapies' that affected the kidneys are also discussed before briefly reviewing the role of magic in medicine, because even though it was illegal, it pervaded the practice of medicine.

Women in the Middle Ages

Women in the Middle Ages found themselves perpetually oscillating between a 'pit and a pedestal'. The Church's view, as broadcast by monks, clergy and friars, was that women were instruments of the devil (the supreme temptresses) and as such, must necessarily both be evil and inferior to man. Women's actual condition varied not only from century to century, but also from class to class. The well-born woman's lot differed from that of the rich merchant's wife, and even more from that of the serf's wife. Regardless, most men agreed that all women were inferior beings. This gave men the right to inflict corporal punishment on 'their women' [2, 3]. A Dominican declared in the 13th century:

'A man may chastise his wife and beat her for correction, for she is of his household, therefore the lord may chastise his own' [4].

Canon law stated:

'It is plain that wives should be subject to their husbands and should be servants' [4].

Even the kindly and affectionate Goodman of Paris in the 14th century, told his wife:

'... to watch the behavior of a dog who always has his heart and his eye upon his master, because even were his master to beat him, the dog follows wagging his tail' [4].

One statute states:

'All inhabitants of Villefranche have the right to beat their wives, provided they do not kill them' [4].

Perhaps it was in the sphere of marriage that women's lot was the hardest, and it was worse for those in the lowest positions [3]. Marriages were not a matter of choice, but were arranged by parents, guardians, overlords – even the Church. The overriding consideration was financial gain or territorial aggrandizement. The Church's attitude towards divorce did not make a woman's lot enviable. According to Canon law, a marriage once made was unbreakable. The furthest the Church would go was to declare a marriage 'null and void'. A satirical poem from the time of Edward II tells us [4]:

'If a man have a wife,
And he love her not,
Bring her to the consistory court.
There truth should be wrought.
Bring two false witnesses with him,
And himself the third,
And he shall be separated,
As far as he would bide from his wife;
He shall be backed up full well
To lead a disreputable life.'

Some men, after spending their wives fortunes, deserted them, delighting in the game of searching for a 'handsomer and wealthier' mate.

Despite the sombre plight of women in the Middle Ages, however, there were happy marriages. Writings and romantic poems are documented in the late Middle Ages, the most famous of which was *The Romance of the Rose* [2, 3]. An idealistic view of women began to grow in the 12th century because of the adoration given to the Virgin Mary. Aristocratic women poets began to appear as troubadours in southern France. All wrote in praise of their lovers or on the escapades of King Arthur and Charlemagne.

Most women, however, even of the aristocratic class, were occupied with very practical affairs. An outstanding characteristic of medieval wives, regardless of status, was their capacity to deal not only with the management of their households – a matter complicated enough in itself – but also with the running of the estate during their husbands' absences on Crusades, at wars, or in courts. A woman was hostess in the lord's absence, meeting guests as they arrived onto the property. The woman of the castle trained her young children as well as those older girls sent from neighboring castles and great houses. These children were expected to behave demurely, be courteous, be silent, be modest, and when walking, not to 'trot or run'. When sitting a young woman must have her hands folded with her eyes modestly turned down [3, 4]. How times change, but how they still remain the same!

Spinning, weaving and the making of clothes were skills possessed by almost all women in the Middle Ages.

In matters of household management, women excelled. As women supervised the servants they needed a knowledge of every household task. As cooks they were experts. Records show that food was extraordinarily spicy and it was cooked in tremendous quantities [3, 4]. Medieval dishes were strongly seasoned with pepper, cloves, garlic, cinnamon, vinegar and wine, virtually all medicinal in some fashion. Ale was often used for cooking fish, and saffron was favored for coloring. One ancient recipe shows that: 'One hundred eggs are to be beaten into eight pints of milk', to which was added mint, sage, marjoram, fennel, parsley, beets, spinach, lettuce and powdered ginger [4]. Such a mixture of flavors must have been overpowering in smell and cholesterol, the latter earning the wrath of the American Heart Association today. Many birds not usually eaten today were often served in banquets – swans, cranes, herons and peacocks. Meat, poultry and fish were eaten in quantity, all heavily salted for preservation.

Women were also taught the use of medicinal herbs and became skilled in simple first aid, though they were not allowed to practise outside the home as doctors or surgeons. An exception to this was Hildegarde von Bingen, who is discussed later.

Doctors in the Middle Ages

The great schools of medicine were virtually decimated by the year 500 AD. A few monks kept medical and other knowledge alive during the centuries of barbarism. This care for the ailing was at first directed mainly towards the monks themselves, and then towards the lay brethren working within the monasteries. Nobles and kings had their own physicians, but almost all were clerics. The masses, by and large, had to depend on their womenfolk or on 'quacks and women pretenders'. This was particularly true in Europe, except in southern Italy where the Salerno School of Medicine flourished [4, 5].

Most treatments revolved around the use of herbs and adherence to diets, but numerous stories of miraculous cures by the Virgin Mother are found. Alongside this widespread belief in the healing power of the Christian faith was the use of pagan incantation and practices, highly tinged with sorcery. These were strictly forbidden by the Church, but under the sign of the cross or diluted by an admixture of Christian names and phrases, pagan practices persisted. Herb gatherers, busily plucking flowers or digging roots, under the influence of an appropriate planet, would be heard to mutter:

'Holy Goddess, Earth, Parent of Nature, the Great Mother ... come to me with thy healing powers and grant favorable issues to whatever I shall make from these herbs and plants. I beseech thee that thy gifts shall make those who take them, whole' [6].

Astrology was regarded as a necessary adjunct to the practice of medicine throughout the Middle Ages, even by the most scientifically minded. For example, there were lucky and unlucky days for blood-letting. One of the first inquiries a doctor made was to ask the patient his star sign, as certain remedies were associated with certain planets. Even then, it was essential to drink the medicine only when the moon was in a favorable position [6].

Urinalysis was a favored method for the diagnosis of disease. In the 9th century Notker, a monk from St. Gall, performed unbelievable wonders of healing by this method [4]. When the Duke of Bavaria became his patient, the Duke substituted the urine of a pregnant woman for his own, in order to test Notker. After the doctor's analysis of the *matula,* the monk turned to the Duke and said: 'God is about to perform a miracle. Within 30 days the Duke will give birth to a child'! Needless to say, Notker was appointed as ducal physician. Many tables and graphs were drawn up during the Middle Ages showing the significance of the color of urine for the diagnosis of disease. A fairly common sight was a servant carrying a urine flask through the street to be examined by a physician.

Not all medicine, however, was practised in this way. In Italy, trained laymen continued to practise medicine from classical times. Salerno, on its beautiful and sheltered bay, had long been a health resort, and by the 9th century was a flourishing medical center [4]. By the 11th century the Salerno School of Medicine had developed into one of the earliest and most important foundations of scientific and technical knowledge of the Middle Ages in Europe. There, 3 years of study in the liberal arts was followed by 4 years of medical study before a student could qualify as a physician. If the student intended to practise surgery, an additional 1 year of anatomy was compulsory.

One of the most famous teachers in Salerno was Constantinus Africanus, who was born in Carthage early in the 11th century [7, 8]. Africanus knew Arabic but not Greek, and thus he took to Salerno Arabic books and a thorough knowledge of Arabic medicine [4]. Duke Robert of Salerno invited Africanus to become his physician, and he spent most of his time translating medical works from Arabic into Latin. The works included those of Hippocrates, Galen and Celsus as well as the writings of the Arabic physician, Avicenna. A popular book containing certain maxims for health was composed at Salerno and the following has been translated [3]:

'If you would health and vigor keep,
Shun care and anger ere you sleep.
All heavy fare and wine disdain,
From noon-day slumber, too, refrain,
Each day to walk awhile you should
For this will work you naught but good.
The urgent calls of Nature heed.
These rules obey and you will find,
Long life is yours and tranquil mind.'

One of the most widely used Salernitan rules for health remains applicable today [4]:

'Use three physicians still – first Dr. Quiet
Next Dr. Merryman and third Dr. Diet.'

A vivid picture of the 11th century doctor can be gained from reading the *Instructions for the Physician Himself* from Salerno [4]. The physician is described on his way with a messenger who has summoned him to visit a patient. The physician is told to question the servant closely as to the exact nature and circumstances of his master's illness:

'Then, if not able to make a positive diagnosis after examining the patient's pulse and urine, he will at least excite astonishment for his accurate knowledge of the symptoms of the disease, and so win his confidence. The fingers should also be kept on the pulse, until at least the hundredth beat, to judge its character. Those standing around will be all the more impressed by the delay. On entering the house, the physician should not appear too haughty, but greet with kindly demeanor those present. Then, after seating himself by the sick man, he should accept the drink offered and proceed to put the patient at his ease before examining him.'

The *Instructions* also advised that the physician should have well-shaped nails, and that his hands should be: 'cleansed from all blackness and filth'. The doctor was further advised to learn proverbs pertaining to his craft in comforting patients, for if a doctor could tell good tales which made his patient laugh, he would: '... induce a light heart to the sick man' [4]. These insights speak of the importance of the medical history and of having a 'good bedside manner'. It is also clearly one of the first revelations of the importance of cleanliness in the practice of medicine.

Tacuinum Sanitatis
Perhaps one of the greatest medical texts in the Middle Ages is the *Tacuinum Sanitatis*. This collection was first discovered in 1875, though it appears that much had been written by the end of the 12th century. The term *tacuinum*

Table 2. Food and herbs beneficial to the kidney

From the garden	Use in the Middle Ages[1]	Composition[2] (g/100 g or % (water))					
		water	sodium	potassium	calcium	phosphorus	fiber
Watermelons, cucumbers	Stimulate urine output Cause 'pain in the loins'	96	2	410	29	21	1.7
Onions, leeks	Enhance urine output Stimulate sex and libido	89	1	130	32	44	0.8
Pignola (pine nuts)	Stimulate the kidneys and the bladder Enhance libido	3	0.3	420	74	324	2.2
Beans *(fava)*	Stimulate urine output	12	1	1,300	163	437	4.9
Fennel	Stimulates urine output Enhances vision						
Sugar	'Good' for the kidneys and bladder Stimulates thirst	0	0	0	0	0	0
Figs	'Clean the kidneys'	21	34	780	162	116	1.4
Turnips	Decrease swelling Increase sperm	91	37	230	40	34	1.1

[1] From *The Medieval Health Handbook (Tacuinum Sanitatis)* [9].
[2] From *Geigy Scientific Tables* [10].

is derived from the Arabic *taqwim,* meaning tables, and is a series of beautifully colored drawings complemented with a text on medicine and health. The manuscript was originally in Arabic, but precisely when it was translated into Latin has not been established with certainty [9]. Much of the information concerning this work revolves around the Arabian physician, Ibn Botlan, who lived in Egypt in 1047. Botlan occupied himself with theologic questions and wrote many works on medicine and health. It appears that a Latin translation must have been available by the year 1266, as an inscription in the Marciano Library in Venice reads [9]:

'Here begins the book of the *Tacuinum,* translated from Arabic into Latin at the court of the illustrious King Manfred, lover of science.'

This inscription indicates both when and where the translation was done. Manfred was King of Sicily from 1254 to 1266 AD and his court was in Palermo. While it is not known whether this represents the first translation, the text was widely distributed throughout Europe by the 14th and 15th centuries. The work was a summary of everything needed to live a healthy life. The following is taken from the preface [9]:

'The *Tacuinum Sanitatis* is about the six things that are necessary for every man in the preservation of his health, about their correct uses and effects. The first is the treatment of air which concerns the heart. The second is the right use of foods and drinks. The third is the correct use of movement and rest. The fourth is the problem of prohibition of the body from sleep, or excessive wakefulness. The fifth is the correct use of elimination and retention of humors. The sixth is regulating of the person by moderating joy, anger, fear and distress. The secret of the preservation of health, in fact, will be in the proper balance of all these elements, since it is the disturbance of this balance that causes illnesses which the glorious and most exalted God permits. Listed under these six classifications are many useful varieties whose nature, God willing, we shall explain. We shall speak, furthermore, about the choices suitable to each person owing to his constitution and age, and shall include all these elements in the simple form of tables because the discussion of the sages and the discordances in many different books may bore the reader. Men, in fact, desire from science nothing else but the benefits, not the arguments but the definitions. Accordingly, our intention in this book is to shorten long-winded discourses and synthesize the various ideas. Our intention also, however, is not to neglect the advice of the ancients.'

Table 2 lists some of the vegetables and herbs considered in the *Tacuinum* to be beneficial to the kidneys. Watermelons and cucumbers were thought to be particularly important in that they: 'cool hot fevers and purify the urine'. Also of value were turnips, particularly long and

Table 3. Food and herbs harmful to the kidney

	Adverse effects[1]	Composition[2] (g/100 g or % (water))				
		water	sodium	potassium	calcium	phosphorus
'Old' cheeses	Cause kidney stones	38	400	100	440	570
Sweet pomegranates	Cause swelling (Stimulates libido)					
Sorghum (melega)	Causes swelling (Good for peasants and swine)	24	43	1,238	273	16
Capers	Decrease urine output Decrease sperm					
Dill	'Harmful' to the kidney Causes nausea					

1 From *The Medieval Health Handbook (Tacuinum Sanitatis)* [9].
2 From *Geigy Scientific Tables* [10].

dark ones, as they: 'increase sperm and make the body less subject to swelling'. Pine nuts *(pignola):* 'stimulate the bladder, the kidneys, and the libido'. Onions and leeks: 'stimulate urination, influence coitus, and mixed with honey clear up catarrh of the chest'. Leeks were thought to be of particular value for individuals in cold climates during the winter. Listed with these foods are their mineral and fiber contents [10]. No clear pattern emerges, but most have high water and potassium contents and a low sodium content. These foods also contain substantial fiber, and today are recommended by the National Cancer Institute to: 'aid digestion and decrease cancer'! The 'beneficial' foods also have strikingly parallel effects on urine and sexual intercourse!

Table 3 lists some food and herbs cited in the *Tacuinum* as harmful to the kidney. 'Old' cheese causes kidney stones, and an analysis of the mineral content of cheese reveals a high calcium and phosphorus content. Except for its high potassium content, most people would agree that it should be restricted to 'swine'!

In the midst of this compendium, the issue of 'magic' is encountered. Most of the information does not reflect explicitly on the relationship between medicine and magic, nor does it indicate which of the cures are 'occult' as opposed to 'pharmacologic' [6]. Doubtless, most experts of the day would have argued that the curative power of their remedies was born out by the 'scientific' experience.

Magic is encountered in several different areas. First, the preparation of drugs and herbs often involved the observance of taboos. This was thought important for maintaining the 'purity' of the healing substance or for enhancing the power of the healer. For example, ashes from burnt ravens were effective against gout and epilepsy, but only if the birds were taken live from their nest, carried without touching the ground, and burned in a new pot! Also, herbs and foods had to be picked both barefoot and in silence, and the gatherer should abstain from sexual contact before collecting these herbs or foods. A herb should be dug from the ground without using an iron implement.

Secondly, the choice of healing ingredients was sometimes dictated by the symbolic considerations of perceived magic. Thus, animals known for their strength, speed or ferocity were preferred over gentler beasts. A bull or ram was considered more important as regards healing powers than was the female counterpart of the species.

Thirdly, even apart from the rise of a systematic form of astrology, medical procedures often involved explicit or implicit attention to the effects of heavenly bodies. Certain plants and herbs were thought to cure lunacy if they were wrapped in a red cloth and tied around the patient's head, particularly if the: 'appropriate astrologic sign was present and the moon was waxing'.

Finally, a specialized language rapidly developed which only the healers understood. Many new words appeared, often garbled and uninterpretable – not unlike the medical jargon that has developed in the 20th century. Thus, while the use of herbs and potions was both magic and medicine, the medieval practitioner and his patient could not separate one from the other.

Sabatini

Therapy in the Middle Ages

Hildegarde von Bingen

As discussed earlier, women were taught the use of medicinal herbs and became skilled in simple first aid, but they were not allowed to practise outside the home as doctors or surgeons. The medieval illustration of Tobit, lying blind and ill on his couch, while his wife Anna prepared medicine for him, mirrors many contemporary scenes [4]. Anna is seen reading her book of medical recipes and numerous copies still remaining testify to their popularity.

One particularly important woman of the Middle Ages was Hildegarde von Bingen [11]. Hildegarde was born in 1098 in the little German town of Böckelheim near Mainz. She was the daughter of a knight and for reasons of economy, protection, or recognition of exceptional talent was placed in a Benedictine convent at the age of 8 years. From early childhood, Hildegarde was subject to visions which became more frequent, intense and vivid as she attained maturity. At the age of 42 years she began to write about her visions, and some members of the 2nd Crusade believed she was a true prophetess of God. In 1148 Hildegarde took 18 of her nuns from Bingen and established a new convent, where she remained until her death in 1179.

In addition to her gifts as a mystic, she was said to have a reputation for learning. During her tenure at the new convent, she wrote the *Physica (Natural Science),* which brought her renown. This is the first book in which a woman discusses plants, trees and herbs in relation to their medicinal properties [11]. It is the earliest book on natural history written in German and, in essence, is the foundation of botanic studies in northern Europe. Hildegarde's *Physica* influenced the later 16th century works of Brunfels, Fuchs and Bock, the so-called 'German Fathers of Botany'.

At first glance this may seem a strange vocation for a cloistered nun, but it was an outgrowth of her duties in the convent. Almost all medicine in the Middle Ages had profound religious overtones. In the 12th century, particularly north of the Alps and far from Salerno, the practice of medicine was largely in the hands of the clergy. These clergy treated not only monks and nuns but also those laymen who worked their land; this later extended to the villagers and nearby parishes; it finally encompassed wayfarers whom the Christian faith exhorted its faithful to treat with charity and mercy. It is thus easy to understand how Hildegarde absorbed so much medical knowledge.

Hildegarde's *Physica,* in addition to displaying a complete knowledge of what was then known about the natural world, gives us a reliable picture of how medicine was practised by the clergy. She included recipes handed down by generations of her predecessors. She wrote her own observations on diseases and cures and of the various folk remedies of the day. In the course of gathering such information, she came on plant names that were not easily translated into Latin, a language that she knew intimately. Faced with this difficulty, the very practical and teutonic Hildegarde simply kept the original name. In her work are the first recorded uses of such names as *hymelsluszel* (heaven's keys, for the primrose) and *storkschnaubel* (a species of geranium).

Hildegarde wrote clearly that peas were considered inferior to beans as food (beans were thought useful as a diuretic (table 2). They are very high in potassium, low in sodium, rich in phosphorus, and very high in fiber. For whatever reason, she knew that beans were an almost complete food source. She also documented in elaborate detail (perhaps during one of her 'visions') that cannabis relieved headache, nutmeg purified the senses and lessened the evil humors, and that rose leaves would clarify sight. Such things had been said for more than 1000 years before and would continue to be said until the 19th century. It is not their efficacy that is in question, nor should Hildegarde be censured for plagiarism. What is important is that she has given us an unretouched view into the beliefs and practices of medieval man.

Hildegarde also provided some drawings in the *Physica.* In one, a physician is seen holding the famous 'urine cup' *(matula)* in order to determine whether the patient should be bled or not and from which site. Later, other artists sketched interpretations of her writings. This remarkable woman was also a composer. In 1981, hyperíon (England) recorded a series of her works entitled 'A feather on the breath of God: Sequences and Hymns by Abbess Hildegarde of Bingen '(Gothic Voices directed by Christopher Page). In his notes, Maestro Page describes her as '... one of the most remarkable creative personalites of the Middle Ages ...'. Does he know about her contributions to medicine, too?

Conclusions

While medicine in the Middle Ages was very primitive by modern standards, it was quite complex as regards rituals and taboos. The *Tacuinam Sanitatis* provides insight as to those foods and herbs deemed important for all aspects of life, concentrating on many aspects of therapy for the kidneys. Yet it is a limited treatise, considering the restrictions imposed by the Church and the undercurrents of magic and astrology. The hopelessness and despair of the populace, particularly women, that pervaded this era can be clearly sensed. Were it not for the survival of the Salerno School of Medicine and the 'common sense' that survived in southern Italy, what might have resulted and how much longer the world might have waited for the Renaissance are matters for speculation.

Acknowledgements

This work was supported in part by grants from the National Institutes of Health, numbers R01-DK-36119 and R01-DK-36199. The author would like to thank Ms. Liz Lund for typographic assistance.

References

1 Osler W: The Evolution of Modern Medicine. A Series of Lectures Delivered at Yale University on the Silliman Foundation in April, 1913. Birmingham, The Classics of Medicine Library, 1982.
2 Crump CG, Jacobs EF (eds): The Legacy of the Middle Ages. Oxford, Clarendon, 1926.
3 Wright T: Womankind in Western Europe. Groombridge, 1869. (citation from Ref. 4, p. 224).
4 Rowling M: Everyday Life in Medieval Times. New York, Dorset Press, 1968.
5 Haskins CH: Studies in the History of Medieval Science. New York, Frederick Ungar, 1967.
6 Kieckhefer R: Magic in the Middle Ages. Cambridge, Cambridge University Press, 1990.
7 Inglis B: History of Medicine. London, Weidenfeld and Nicolson, 1965.
8 McKinney LC: Early Medieval Medicine. Baltimore, John Hopkins University Press, 1937.
9 Arano LC: The Medieval Health Handbook, *Tacuinum Sanitatis*. New York, George Braziller, 1976.
10 Lentner C: Geigy Scientific Tables. West Caldwell, Ciba-Geigy Corporation, vol 1, 1981.
11 Anderson FJ: An Illustrated History of the Herbals. New York, Columbia University Press, 1977.

Am J Nephrol 1994;14:399–411

Giovanni Aliotta
Antonino Pollio

Department of Plant Biology, University of Naples Federico II, Naples, Italy

Useful Plants in Renal Therapy according to Pliny the Elder

Key Words
Pliny the Elder
Medicinal plants
Renal disease
History of pharmacology

Abstract
The *Naturalis Historia* of Pliny the Elder consists of 37 books, of which 16 are devoted to botany. About 900 plants are named, but many names are synonyms and identification is often impossible. Where identification is possible it is achieved by comparison of the actual names with the vernacular names in related languages or by indirect evidence from their medical use. In this way 130 plants used in renal therapy during Roman times can be identified. Many were eaten as part of the diet, and the distinction between medicinal and edible plants was not clearcut. Pliny was also the first author to comment that wild species are more active than cultivated ones. Most of the plants reported by Pliny are also mentioned by Dioscorides, and more than 30 of them were also listed by Plenck. Several are still quoted in modern pharmacopeias.

Introduction

In their search for food, early men gained a close acquaintance with the properties of many plants by trial and error. The process of discovering food plants revealed that some species could affect the functioning of the human body and mind. Moreover, they learned that a few plants could be dangerous or even fatally poisonous [1, 2]. Although ancient civilizations rose by virtue of the material achievements of agriculture, evidence suggests that man's first scientific approach to plants was awakened by their medicinal properties. There seem to be no agricultural reports as early as the earliest documentary evidence on medicinal plants, e.g. the Ebers papyrus (1500 BC).

The *Naturalis Historia* of Pliny the Elder (23–79 AD) represents the most important encyclopedic account of the scientific knowledge of plants in ancient times. This monumental work is composed of 37 books, it quotes more than 2,000 manuscripts and discusses about 33,000 facts, concerning cosmology and geography (books I–VI); anthropology and zoology (VII–XI); botany (XII–XXVII); medicine and pharmacology (XXVIII–XXXII) and mineralogy and art (XXXIII–XXXVII). Fortunately the *Naturalis Historia* has been preserved through the centuries (table 1).

Writing the *Naturalis Historia* was the main task of many years of Pliny's life. Pliny was not only a serious scholar interested in understanding natural phenomena, but he was also actively engaged in politics. He served the Roman Empire first as a captain of cavalry in Germany, then as procurator in Spain, and finally as Commander of the Fleet at Misenum, a bay in the gulf of Naples. Pliny was still holding this rank when he died of asphyxia while trying with some ships to help people escaping from Pompeii, Stabiae, Oplontis and Herculaneum, during the eruption of Vesuvius in August 79 AD.

Professor Giovanni Aliotta
Dipartimento di Biologia Vegetale
Università di Napoli Federico II
Via Foria 223
I-80139 Naples (Italy)

The influence of Pliny's work was enormous for more than 1000 years, but from the Renaissance until the present his fame suffered an eclipse. Pliny is accused of being uncritical and without originality. Indeed, it is still difficult to establish the defects and merits of Pliny [4, 5]. However inadequate, *Naturalis Historia* remained for centuries the only reflection of the theoretic synthesis achieved in Greek science by philosophers. Pliny pointed out that the knowledge of herbs played a major role in Greek and Roman medicine, and in turn botany was chiefly the study of medicinal plants, with the exception of the work of Theophrastus, (370–285 BC; Aristotle's successor in the Lyceum) who considered botany in a broader sense [6].

The number of plants named by Pliny is about 900, but many names are synonyms and identification is often impossible, as descriptions are fragmentary or lacking and there are no illustrations. This paper presents an attempt to produce a checklist of the scientific names of plants mentioned in the *Naturalis Historia* as useful in renal therapy. A brief comparison of these plants with those reported in the *De Materia Medica* of Dioscorides and in more recent herbals is also presented.

Table 1. Bibliography of *Naturalis Historia* [3]

Manuscript copies	A palimpsest copy, the *Nonantulus* of the 5th or 6th century AD, from the Benedictine monastery at Nonantula, near Modena In Rome (at unnamed location) in 1956
Earliest manuscripts	*Codex Bamburgensis,* 10th century AD *Leidensis Vossianus,* 11th century AD or earlier *Codex Parisinus Latinus* 6795, 10th or 11th century AD
Early editions	1st edition by Johann Spira, Venice, 1469 1st illustrated edition by Melchiorr Sessa, Venice, 1513 1st commentary and correction of manuscript texts: Hermolaus Barbarus, *Castigationes Plinianae,* Rome, 1492
English translations	Philemon Holland, London, 1601; selections available Bostock and Riley, London, 1855–1957; reprint available Loeb Classical Library, London and Cambridge, Mass., 1938–1962

Plants Named by Pliny the Elder

The naming of a specific plant referred to in older literature often presents grave difficulties, due to doubts about its identity and to the absence of any systematic nomenclature that was commonly accepted before the Linnaean classification [6]. Plants must usually be identified principally by philologic comparison of the actual names with the vernacular names in related languages or by indirect evidence from their medical use. The reference work used here is the edition of *Naturalis Historia* published in Italy in 1982–1987 by Elinaudi Press [7], which is based on that of Mayoff published in Stuttgart (1967–1970). Invaluable help has come from Andre's book *Les Noms des Plantes dans la Rome Antique* [8].

Table 2. Index of useful plants in renal therapy mentioned by Pliny in *Naturalis Historia*

Scientific and vernacular name	Name in Pliny Plant processing Location in *Naturalis Historia*	Therapeutic purposes		
		diuretic	stones	urinary affections
Achillea ageratum L. Sweet yarrow	Ageraton Plant smoke XXVII, 13	X		
Achillea millefolim L. Yarrow or *Myriophylium spicatum* L. Spiked milofoil	Milifolium Plant steeped in water XXVI, 78		X	
Acorus calamus L. Sweet flag	(H)arundo Root decoction XXIV, 85	X		

Table 2 (continued)

Scientific and vernacular name	Name in Pliny Plant processing Location in *Naturalis Historia*	Therapeutic purposes		
		diuretic	stones	urinary affections
Adiantum capillus-veneris L. Southern maidenhair, Venus' hair	Adiantum Plant steeped in wine XXII, 62	X		
Ajuga spp. Bugle	Chamaepitys Plant decoction XXIV, 29	X		
Allium ampeloprasum L. Wild leek	Ampeloprason Cooking of the plant XXIV, 136	X		
Anagallis arvensis L. Scarlet pimpernel	Anagallis Unspecified processing XXVI, 80	X		
Apium sp. Celery	Silaus Cooking of the plant XXVI, 88			X
Apium graveolens L. Celery	Apium Seed decoction XX, 112	X	X	
Aristolochia rotunda L. Birthwort	Malum erraticum Root decoction XXVI, 88		X	
Artemisia abrotanum L. Southernwood	Habrotanum Seed and leaf decoction XXI, 160			X
Artemisia sp. Sagebrush	Artemisia Plant in sweet wine decoction XXVI, 81		X	X
Asarum europaeum L. Wild ginger	Asarum Plant steeped in wine XXI, 134	X		
Asparagus officinalis L. Asparagus	Asparagus Root and seeds steeped in wine XX, 108	X	X	X
Asphodelus sp. Asphodel	Asphodelus Root steeped in wine XXII, 67	X	X	
Asplenium sp. Spleenwort	Callithrix Plant steeped in wine XXVI, 87		X	
Aster linosyris Bernh. Aster	Chrysocomes Root as food XXI, 148	X		
Atractylis gummifera L. Distaff thistle	Chamaleon Root decoction XXII, 45	X		X

Table 2 (continued)

Scientific and vernacular name	Name in Pliny Plant processing Location in *Naturalis Historia*	Therapeutic purposes		
		diuretic	stones	urinary affections
Berula erecta (Hudson) Coville Stalky berula	Sium Plant as food or in decoction XXII, 84	X	X	X
Beta vulgaris L. subsp. *maritima* (L.) Arcan Sea beet	Beta Plant as food XX, 69	X		
Brassica oleracea L. Wild cabbage	Brassica Cooking of leaves XX, 86			X
Bunium aromaticum L. Hawk nut, or *Pimpinella cretica* Pimpinella	Pseudobunium Potion of shoots XXIV, 153			X
Bunium ferulaceum Sibth et Smith Hawk nut	Napus Flower decoction XX, 21	X		X
Bupleurum fruticosum L. Shrub thoroughwax	Bupleurum Root steeped in wine XXII, 77	X		
Capparis spinosa L. Capers	Capparis Root chopped with barley meal steeped in water XX, 165		X	
Carum copticum B. et H. Ajowan caraway	Ami Seeds; unspecified processing XX, 163	X		
Celsia sp. Celsia	Arction Root decoction XXVII, 33			X
Centaurea spinosa L. Centaurea	Hippophaes Plant juice XXII, 29	X		
Ceratonia siliqua L. Carob, St John's bread	Siliqua Fruit as food XXIII, 151	X		
Cicer arietinum L. Chick-pea	Cicer Seeds as food XXII, 149	X	X	
Cichorium intybus L. Chicory	Cichorium Plant juice XX, 74			X
Citrullus colocynthis (L.) Schrader Colocynth, bitter apple	Colocynthis Fruit infusion XX, 14			X

Table 2 (continued)

Scientific and vernacular name	Name in Pliny Plant processing Location in *Naturalis Historia*	Therapeutic purposes		
		diuretic	stones	urinary affections
Clinopodium vulgare L. Cushion calamint	Clinopodium Plant steeped in water XXIV, 137			X
Cressa cretica L. Unknown	Anthyllium Plant steeped in water XXI, 175		X	X
Crithmum maritimum L. Samphire	Crethmos Plant steeped in wine XXVI, 82			X
Crocus sativus L. Saffron crocus	Crocus Flowers; processing not clear XXI, 138–139	X		X
Cucumis sativus L. Cucumber	Cucumis Seed steeped in wine XX, 10	X	X	X
Cupressus sempervirens L. Italian cypress	Italian Cypress Roots and leaves steeped in water XXIV, 15			X
Cymbopogon schoenanthus Spreng. Unknown	Juncus odoratus Plant; unspecified processing XXI, 120	X		X
Cynodon dactylon (L.) Pers. Bermuda grass	Gramien Root and seed decoction in wine XXIV, 180	X	X	X
Cyperus esculentus L. Chufa flat sedge or *Cyperus rotundus* L. Nut grass	Cyperus Root steeped in water XXI, 118	X	X	
Danaë racemosa (L.) Moench. Alexandrian laurel	Chamaedaphne Plant juice XXIV, 132	X		
Daucus carota L. Wild carrot	Staphylinus Seeds minced, steeped in wine XX, 30	X		
Dracunculus vulgaris Schott. Stink dragon	Aron Plant steeped in water XXIV, 142	X		
Equisetum arvense L. Field horsetail	Equisaetum Plant juice in wine XXVI, 134	X		
Eryngium campestre L. Snakeroot eryngo	Erynge sive Eryngion Plant in water and honey XXII, 18			X

Table 2 (continued)

Scientific and vernacular name	Name in Pliny Plant processing Location in *Naturalis Historia*	Therapeutic purposes		
		diuretic	stones	urinary affections
Erysimum cheiri (L.) Crantz Wallflower	Viola lutea Plant dried; unspecified processing XXI, 130	X		
Euphorbia lathyrus L. Caper euphorbia	Lathyris Seeds steeped in water XXVII, 95	X		
Evernia sp. Evernia	Sphagnos sive sphaco sive bryo Plant steeped in wine XXIV, 27	X		
Ficus carica L. Fig	Ficus Fruit as food XXIII, 120	X		
Foeniculum vulgare Miller var. *dulce* (Miller) Thell. Florence fennel	Feniculum Root added with barley infusion XX, 257	X	X	
Frankenia hirsuta L. Frankenia, sea heath	Empetros Plant decoction XXVII, 75		X	
Gladiolus segetum Gawler Corn flag gladiolus	Xifio Root steeped in water XXVI, 79	X		
Glycyrrhiza glabra L. Licorice	Glycyrrhiza Root; unspecified processing XXII, 24		X	
Hedera helix L. English ivy	Hedera Plant steeped in water XXIV, 75	X		
Helichrysum spp. Everlasting flower	Heliochrysos Plant steeped in wine XXI, 168	X		
Hypericum olympicum L. or *Polemonium caeruleum* L. Greek valerian, Jacob's ladder	Polemonia Plant steeped in wine XXVI, 78		X	X
Hypericum spp. St. John's wort	Hypericon Seeds steeped in wine XXVI, 85	X		X
Juniperus spp. Juniper	Iunipirus Seeds steeped in wine XXIV, 54	X		
Laurus nobilis L. Grecian laurel	Laurus Root steeped in wine XXIII, 153		X	
Lithospermum officinale L. Gromwell	Lithospermum Fruits steeped in wine XXVII, 98		X	X

Table 2 (continued)

Scientific and vernacular name	Name in Pliny Plant processing Location in *Naturalis Historia*	Therapeutic purposes		
		diuretic	stones	urinary affections
Lonicera sp. Honeysuckle	Peryclymenon Leaf decoction XXVII, 120	X		
Lupinus albus L. White lupin	Lupinus Root decoction XXII, 154	X		
Marrubium vulgare L. White horehound	Marrubium Plant; unspecified processing XX, 241	X		
Matthiola incana (L.) R. Br. Stock	Viola alba Plant; unspecified processing XXI, 130	X		
Mentha pulegium L. Pennyroyal	Puleium Plant decoction in wine XX, 153	X	X	
Meum athamanticum Jacq. Baldmoney	Meum Minced root steeped in water or in decoction XX, 253	X		X
Myriophyllum spicatum L. Spiked milfoil	Milifolio sive myriophyllon Plant; unspecified processing XXIV, 152	X		X
Myrtus communis L. True myrtle	Myrtus sativa candida Fruit juice XXIII, 159	X		
Nasturtium officinale L. Water cress	Sysymbrium sylvestre Plant steeped in wine XX, 247	X	X	
Nigella sativa L. Black cumin	Git Plant juice XX, 182	X		
Ocimum basilicum L. Basil	Ocimum Plant used as a compress XX, 121	X		
Olea europaea L. Olive	Olea Fruit as food XXIII, 73		X	
Onobrychis caput-gali (L). Lam. and *Onobrychis viciaefolia* Scop. Sainfoin	Oenobreches Dried powdered plant steeped in water XXIV, 155			X
Ononis antiquorum L. Restharrow	Anonis Plant steeped in water with honey XXVII (29)		X	

Table 2 (continued)

Scientific and vernacular name	Name in Pliny Plant processing Location in *Naturalis Historia*	Therapeutic purposes		
		diuretic	stones	urinary affections
Onopordum acanthium L. Scotch cotton thistle	Onopradon Plant; unspecified processing XXVII, 110	X		
Origanum dictamnus L. Dittany of Crete	Dictamnum Plant; unspecified processing XXVI, 78			X
Origanum majorana L. Sweet marjoram	Amaracum o Sampsuchum Plant decoction XXI, 163	X		
Origanum heracleoticum Rchb. Oregano	Origanum heraclium Plant as food XX, 177	X		
Orlaya grandiflora (L.) Hoffm. False carrot	Caucalis Plant juice XXII, 83	X	X	X
Paeonia officinalis L. Peony	Glycisides Roots steeped in wine XXVII, 84			X
Paliurus spina-christi Miller Christ's thorn	Paliurus Leaves steeped in water XXIV, 115	X	X	
Pancratium maritimum L. Pancratium	Pancratium Plant juice with honey XXVII, 118	X		
Pastinaca sativa L. Garden parsnip	Siser Plant as food XX, 34	X		
Phillyrea sp. Mock privet	Tilia Leaves; unspecified processing XXIV, 50	X		
Physalis alkekengi L. Chinese lantern	Vesicaria Plant; unspecified processing XXI, 177		X	X
Picea excelsa (Lam.) Link Norway spruce	Picea Bark's ash steeped in water XXIV, 28	X		
Pimpinella anisum L. Anise	Anesum Plant juice and minced seeds XX, 189	X		
Pinus pinea L. Italian stone pine	Nucibus pineis Bark in wine decoction XXIII, 142		X	X

Table 2 (continued)

Scientific and vernacular name	Name in Pliny Plant processing Location in *Naturalis Historia*	Therapeutic purposes		
		diuretic	stones	urinary affections
Pistacia lentiscus L. Lentisk pistache	Lentiscum Fruits, bark and sap; unspecified processing XXIV, 36	X		
Plantago major L. Ripple-seed plantain	Plantago Plant steeped in wine XXVI, 78		X	X
Polygonum aviculare L. Knotgrass	Polygonum Seeds steeped in water XXVII, 114	X		
Portulaca oleracea L. Purslane	Porcillaca Plant juice XX, 214	X		X
Potentilla reptans L. Creeping cinquefoil	Quinquefolium Plant in wine decoction XXVI, 79			X
Prunus amygdalus Stokes Almond	Amygdalis Fruits as food XXIII, 144	X		
Prunus avium L. Sweet cherry, or *Prunus cerasus* L. Sour cherry	Cerasium Fruits as food XXIII, 141	X		
Psoralea bituminosa L. Scurf pea	Trifolium Root steeped in water XXVI, 89			X
Raphanus sativus L. Radish	Raphanus sativus Plant as food and root decoction XX, 23	X	X	
Rosa gallica L. French rose	Rosa Seeds; unspecified processing XXI, 124	X		
Rubus fruticosus L. European blackberry	Rubus Fruit as food XXIV, 117	X		
Rumex sp. Dock	Lapathum Root juice XX, 234	X		
Ruscus aculeatus L. Butcher's broom	Oxymyrsine sive chamaemyrsine sive ruscum – Myrtus silvestris Root in wine decoction XXIII, 165	X		X
Ruta graveolens L. Rue	Ruta Plant decoction XX, 139	X		

Table 2 (continued)

Scientific and vernacular name	Name in Pliny Plant processing Location in *Naturalis Historia*	Therapeutic purposes		
		diuretic	stones	urinary affections
Salvia officinalis L. Sage	Elelisphacos, sphaco, (lens sativa) Plant as food XXII, 146	X		
Sambucus ebulus L. Danewort	Sabucus Fruits steeped in water XXIV, 51	X	X	
Santolina chamaecyparissus L. Cypress cotton lavender	Habrotanum montanum Leaf and seed decoction XXI, 160	X		
Satureja hortensis L. Summer savory	Cunila Plant; unspecified processing XX, 173	X		
Scandix pecten-veneris L. Shepherd's needle	Scandix Plant decoction XXII, 80	X		
Scolymus maculatus L. or *Scolymus hispanicus* L. Spanish oyster plant	Scolymos Plant as food XXII, 86	X		
Sedum cepaea L. Stonecrop	Cepaea Plant steeped in wine XXVI, 84		X	
Sempervivum arboreum Houseleek	Holochrysos Plant as food XXI, 148	X		X
Smyrnium olusatrum L. Alexanders	(H)olusatrum Root decoction and seeds steeped in wine XX, 117		X	X
Sonchus oleraceus L. Sow thistle	Soncos Plant; unspecified processing XXII, 88		X	
Spartium junceum L. Weaver's broom	Genista Crushed seeds steeped in water XXIV, 65			X
Spiraea filipendula L. Dropwort	Oenanthe herba Root; unspecified processing XXI, 167			X
Stachys officinalis L. Betony	Vettonica Plant infusion XXVI, 78		X	X
Symphytum tuberosum L. Tuberous comfrey	Alum Root; unspecified processing XXVII, 41			X

Table 2 (continued)

Scientific and vernacular name	Name in Pliny Plant processing Location in *Naturalis Historia*	Therapeutic purposes		
		diuretic	stones	urinary affections
Teucrium chamaedrys L. Wall germander, and *Teucrium lucidum* L. Sage-leaved germander	Chamaedrys Plant steeped in water XXIV, 130	X		
Teucrium scordium L. Water germander	Scordion Root decoction XXVI, 89	X		
Thymus serpyllum L. Mother-of-thyme	Serpyllum Plant steeped in water XX, 245			X
Umbilicus pendulinus DC. Navelwort	Cotyledon Plant; unspecified processing XXVI, 80		X	
Uriginea maritima (L.) Baker Sea onion	Scilla Roasted bulb decoction XX, 100	X		
Urospermum picroides Schm. Sheep's beard	Laetuca Plant juice XX, 63	X		
Urtica dioica L. Stinging nettle	Urtica Plant juice XXII, 36	X		
Vaccinium uliginosum L. Bog bilberry	Hyacinthus Root steeped in wine XXI, 170	X		X
Valeriana celtica L. Valerian	Nardus gallicum Plant decoction XXI, 135	X		
Verbena officinalis L. European verbena	Verbenaca Plant steeped in water XXVI, 78		X	
Vicia ervilia (L). Willd. Bitter vetch	Ervum Seed roasted and minced with honey XXII, 151			X
Vitex agnus-castus L. Lilac chaste tree	Vitex Plant; unspecified processing XXIV, 59	X		
Vitis vinifera L. Grape	Uva passa sive Astaphida Dried fruit as food XXIII, 15			X

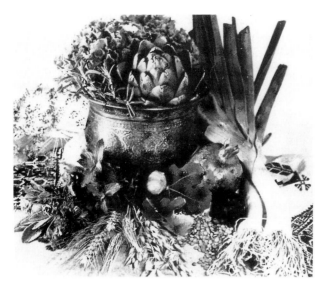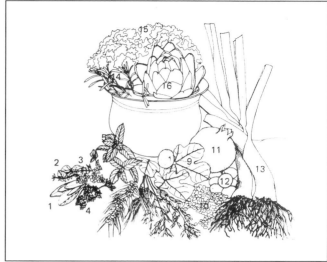

Fig. 1. Plants of Mediterranean or Middle Eastern origin. 1 = sage; 2 = thyme; 3 = oregano; 4 = parsley; 5 = mint; 6 = wheat; 7 = barley; 8 = oats; 9 = fig; 10 = lentils; 11 = pomegranate; 12 = olives; 13 = leeks; 14 = rosemary; 15 = lettuce; 16 = artichoke [11].

Naturalis Historia reports 130 plants used in renal therapy during Roman times (table 2). Some plants, e.g. *Asparagus officinalis, Berula erecta, Cucumis sativus* and *Cynodon dactylon,* were considered effective as diuretics as well as useful against stones and urinary infections. Many plants were processed mainly in boiling water or in wine, while 13 plants were eaten directly without undergoing processing. Diet thus constituted a fundamental aspect of traditional medicine, and the distinction between edible and medicinal plants was not clearcut in the ancient medicine of Western countries (table 3, fig. 1), as in many other societies [11]. It is difficult to establish whether Pliny knew the doctrine of signature, which originated in China and which suggested that for every ailment there is a specific plant remedy, the clue existing in the plant's shape. Whether or not he did know of it, the use against renal stones of fruits of *Lithospermum officinale* represents one of the best examples of this doctrine.

Even though the toxicity of wild plants was well known in Greek medicine [12], Pliny was the first author to point out that weeds are more active as medicine than cultivated species. A close relationship between cultivation and the biologic activity of plants has been ascertained; in fact, the levels of secondary products of plant metabolism, i.e. alkaloids, phenolic compounds and glycosides, responsible for the pharmaceutic effects are significantly reduced in cultivated species [13].

Table 3. Common edible and medicinal plants cultivated by the Romans [11]

Cereals	Barley, wheat
Vegetables	Asparagus, beans, beet, broad beans, carrots, chick peas, chicory, garlic, lettuce, leeks
Fruits	Apples, apricots, cherries, figs, grapes, peaches, pears
Condiments	Basil, celery, dill, fennel, marjoram, mint, parsley, pepper, rue, thyme

The distinction between wild and cultivated species is also shown in the organization of *Naturalis Historia.* Cultivated plants are described in 2 separate books (book XX, vegetables; and book XXIII, fruit trees), while the medicinal action of weeds of the Mediterranean region is the subject of books XXI and XXV–XXVII.

Most of plants and their therapeutic purposes reported by Pliny are also mentioned by the famous Greek physician Dioscorides (1st century AD) in his *De Materia Medica* [14]. Nowhere, however, did Pliny mention Dioscorides. Probably Pliny and Dioscorides wrote simultaneously and did not know of each other's work. They often made very similar statements about medicinal plants, because they consulted a common source, perhaps Diocles of Carystos, a contemporary of Theophrastus in

Athens, and Crataeus, a herbalist who was a court doctor of King Mithradates VI of Pontus (120–60 BC).

Pliny obviously had a genuine interest in plants and an enthusiasm that finds frequent expression. There is evidence that both Pliny and Dioscorides were able to recognize the plants mentioned in their respective treatises. Pliny emphasized that:

'Experience, the most efficient teacher of all things especially in medicine, gradually degenerated into mere words and verbiage. For it was pleasanter to sit diligently listening in lecture-rooms than to go out into the fields and look for different plants at the different seasons of the year.' *Naturalis Historia* XXVI, 11

This was also the opinion of Dioscorides and Galen, who recommended that every doctor should learn to recognize medicinal plants by seeking practical training from an expert. Unfortunately, their suggestion was not accepted for many centuries.

It should be noted that more than 30 plants considered by Pliny as useful in renal therapy were quoted by the Austrian physician Plenck (1735–1807) in his outstanding work *Icones Plantarum Medicinalium* [15]. Moreover, many species reported by Pliny are still mentioned in several pharmacopeias throughout the world [16]. Finally, 8 species *(Achillea millefolium, Ceratonia siliqua, Crocus sativus, Cyperus esculentus, Glycyrrhiza glabra, Pimpinella anisum, Plantago major, Uriginea maritima)* have been included in a list of very useful plants compiled by the World Health Organization [17].

Naturalis Historia, as other outstanding herbals, e.g. *De Materia Medica* of Dioscorides, brings into perspective the massive knowledge acquired in the classical period to maintain health by using common plants. In this respect, biomedical scientists of today could find important data in the neglected botanic work of Pliny [18].

It can be concluded that a study of the botanic portion of the *Naturalis Historia* reveals that Pliny is an invaluable source for tracing the development of early botany, and that he made important contributions of his own. The present authors agree with Stannard [5], who affirmed that there are good reasons for asserting that if Theophrastus was the father of botany, to Pliny belongs the honorary title of 'father of the history of botany'.

References

1 Lewis WH, Elvin-Lewis PF: Medical Botany. New York, Wiley Interscience, 1977.
2 Aliotta G: Edible wild plants of Italy. Inform Bot Ital 1987;19:17–30.
3 Anderson FJ: An Illustrated History of the Herbals. New York, Columbia University Press, 1977.
4 André J: Pline l'Ancien botaniste. Rev Etudes Latines 1955;33:297–318.
5 Stannard J: Pliny and Roman botany. Isis 1965;56:420–425.
6 Morton AG: History of Botanical Science. London, Academic Press, 1971.
7 Plinio: Storia Naturale. Turin, Einaudi, 6 vols, 1982–1987.
8 André J: Les Noms des Plantes dans la Rome Antique. Paris, Les Belles Lettres, 1985.

9 Saccardo PA: Cronologia della Flora Italiana. Bologna, Edagricole, 1971.
10 Tannahill R: Food in History. Bungay, The Chaucer Press, 1973.
11 Simpson BB, Conner-Ogorzaly M: Economic Botany. New York, McGraw-Hill, 1986.
12 Hippocrates: Hippocratic Writings, translated by Chadwick J, Mann WN. New York, Ronald Press, 1978.
13 Johns T: With Bitter Herbs They Shall Eat It. Tucson, University of Arizona Press, 1990.
14 Dioscorides: De Materia Medica. London, New York, Hafner, 1933.

15 Plenck JJ: Icones Plantarum Medicinalium, Secundum Sistema Linnaei Digestarum cum Enumeratione Virium et Usus Medici, Chirurgici atquae Diaetetici. Vienna, Apud Rudolphum Graeffer et Soc, 8 vols, 1788–1812. (Volumes 7 and 8 were edited by JL Kerndl after the death of the author).
16 Penso G: Index Plantarum Medicinalium Totius Mundi Eorumque Synonymorum. Milan, Organizzazione Editoriale Medico Farmaceutica, 1983.
17 Penso G: Le Piante Medicinali nell'Arte e nella Storia. Basel, Ciba-Geigy, 1986.
18 De Santo NG, Capasso G, Ranieri Giordano D, Aulisio M, Anastasio P, Annunziata S, Armini B, Coppola S, Musacchio R: Nephrology in the *Naturalis History* of Pliny the Elder (23–79 AD). Am J Nephrol 1989;9:252–260.

Am J Nephrol 1994;14:412–417

Manuela De Matteis Tortora

Orto Botanico, University of Naples
Federico II, Naples, Italy

Some Plants Described by Pliny for the Treatment of Renal Diseases

Key Words
Pliny the Elder
Medicinal plants
Renal diseases
History of nephrology

Abstract
Pliny the Elder described medicinal plants in books XX–XXVII of *Naturalis Historia,* reporting the therapeutic properties and preparations of the plants for use in different parts of the body. An exhibition of 20 plants chosen from those indicated for renal diseases is described.

In books XII–XXVII of *Naturalis Historia,* Pliny the Elder deals with botany, describing exotic, local, wild and cultivated plants. He passes from an essentially botanic treatment, concerning above all trees (books XII–XVI), to a strictly agricultural one (books XVII–XIX).

Books XX–XXVII deal with medicinal plants, and particularly with the healing properties of 'vegetables', 'flowers', 'food plants and foodstuffs', 'vine, olive and fruit trees', 'officinal wild plants' and 'officinal volunteer herbs'. In these books the author reports the therapeutic properties and preparations of the plants for use in different parts of the body and enriches the text with historical news.

The last paragraphs of book XXV and book XXVI are particularly interesting because Pliny inverts the order of describing the subject matter and lists remedies according to the plants that give them.

On the occasion of the 1st International Conference on the History of Nephrology, the Orto Botanico of Naples exhibited 20 plants chosen from those indicated by Pliny for the treatment of renal diseases. Table 1 lists the species (sometimes only the genus), the family name, the uses and the properties of each one. Photographs of the specimens, as displayed at the conference, are shown in figs. 1–21.

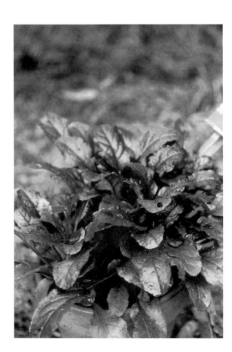

Fig. 1. *Ajuga* spp.

Dr. Manuela De Matteis Tortora
Orto Botanico
Università di Napoli Federico II
Via Foria 223
I-80139 Napoli (Italy)

Table 1. Some species named by Pliny as being useful in renal diseases

Species	Name according to Pliny	Uses and properties according to Pliny
Ajuga spp. *(Lamiaceae)*	Chamaepitys	Decoction with barley flour is good for kidneys and bladder. Potion in water cures dysuria
Crithmum maritimum L. *(Apiaceae)*	Crethmos	Decoction is diuretic; in potion with wine cures strangury
Cupressus sempervirens L. *(Cupressaceae)*	Cupressus	Root potion minced with leaves cures bladder diseases and strangury
Cynodon dactylon (L.) Pers. *(Poaceae)*	Gramen	Root decoction in wine cures dysuria and bladder ulcers and breaks stones. Seed is a very strong diuretic
Juniperus communis L. *(Cupressaceae)*	Iuniperus	Seeds are diuretic
Marrubium vulgare L. *(Lamiaceae)*	Marrubium	Diuretic, but is dangerous with bladder ulcers and if renal diseases are present
Myrtus communis L. *(Myrtaceae)*	Myrtus	Berries in wine are of use against bladder diseases. Berry juice is diuretic
Ocimum basilicum L. *(Lamiaceae)*	Holochrysus	With wine it cures stragury
Origanum majorana L. *(Lamiaceae)*	Amaracum	Good for patients with urinary troubles
Origanum spp. *(Lamiaceae)*	Origanum	Diuretic
Phillyrea sp. *(Oleaceae)*	Tilia	Leaves are diuretic
Pinus pinea L. *(Pinaceae)*	Pinus	Pine nuts are good for kidneys and bladder
Pistacia lentiscus L. *(Anacardiaceae)*	Lentiscus	Fruits, bark and sap are diuretic
Prunus avium L. *(Rosaceae)*	Cerasus	Dried cherries are diuretic
Rumex sp. *(Polygonaceae)*	Lapathum	Root potion in wine cures stones. Root juice is diuretic
Ruscus aculeatus L. *(Liliaceae)*	Ruscus	Root potion drunk on alternate days cures stones and is good for strangury and when there is bloody urine
Ruta graveolens L. *(Rutaceae)*	Ruta	Potion in wine is of use against renal diseases. Diuretic also when there is bloody urine
Salvia officinalis L. *(Lamiaceae)*	Salvia	Diuretic
Thymus serpyllum L. *(Lamiaceae)*	Serpyllum	Potion in water cures urinary troubles
Vitex agnus-castus L. *(Verbenaceae)*	Vitex	Diuretic

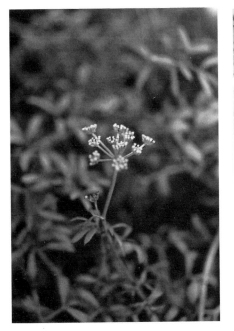

Fig. 2. *Crithmum maritimum.*

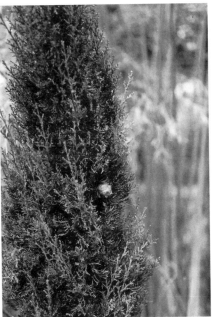

Fig. 3. *Cupressus sempervirens.*

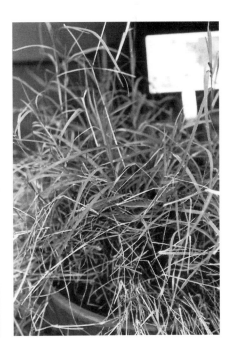

Fig. 4. *Cynodon dactylon.*

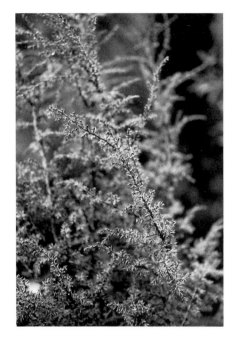

Fig. 5. *Juniperus communis.*

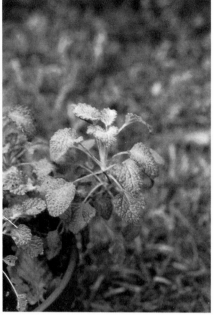

Fig. 6. *Marrubium vulgare.*

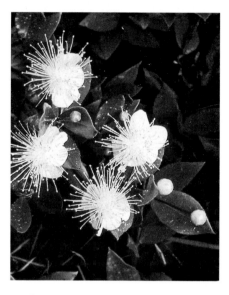

Fig. 7. *Myrtus communis.*

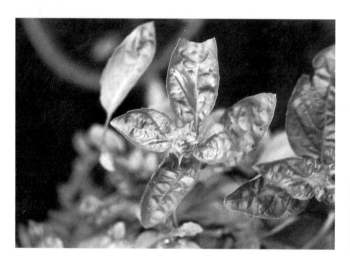

Fig. 8. *Ocimum basilicum..*

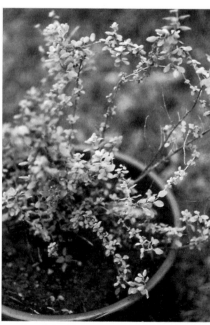

Fig. 9. *Origanum majorana.*

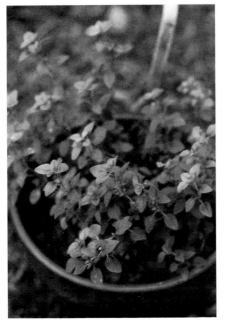

Fig. 10. *Origanum* spp.

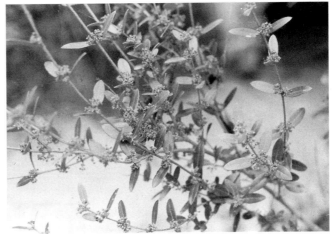

Fig. 11. *Phillyrea* sp.

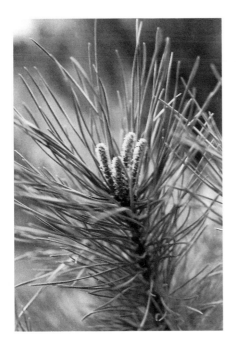

Fig. 12. *Pinus pinea.*

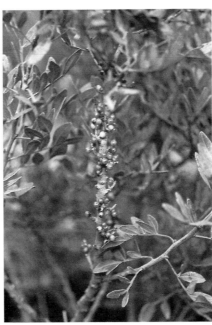

Fig. 13. *Pistacia lentiscus.*

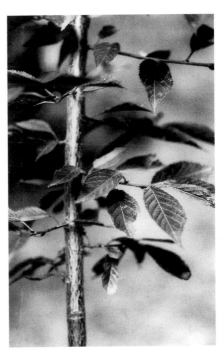

Fig. 14. *Prunus avium.*

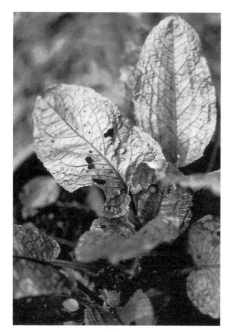

Fig. 15. *Rumex* sp.

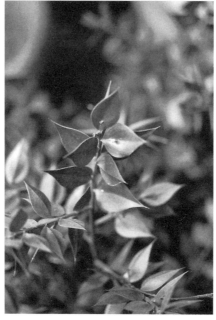

Fig. 16. *Ruscus aculeatus.*

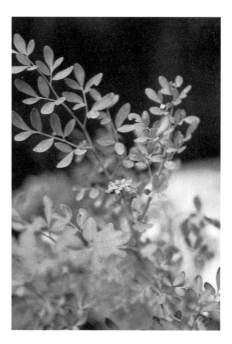

Fig. 17. *Ruta graveolens.*

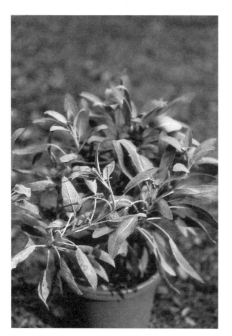

Fig. 18. *Salvia officinalis.*

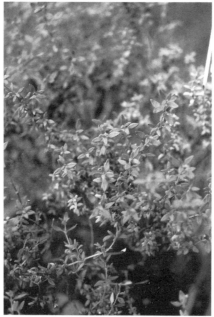

Fig. 19. *Thymus serpyllum.*

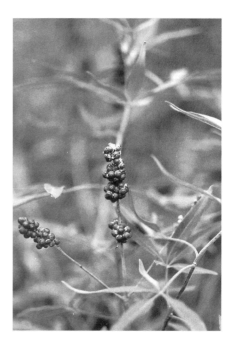

Fig. 20. *Vitex agnus-castus.*

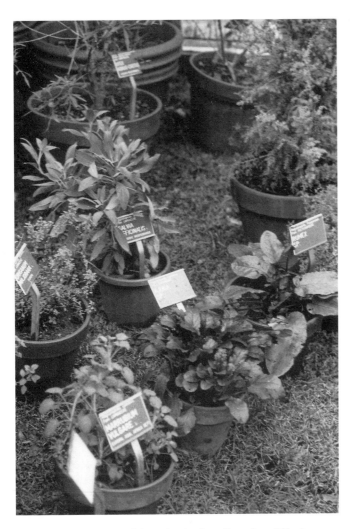

Fig. 21. Exhibition of plants by the Orto Botanico of Naples.

Further Reading

Pignatti S: Flora d'Italia. Bologna, Edagricole, vols 1–3, 1982.

Plinio: Storia Naturale. Turin, Einaudi, 1982–1988.

Tutin TG, Heywood VH, Burges NA, Valentine DH, Walters SM, Webb DA: Flora Europaea. Cambridge, Cambridge University Press, vols 1–5, 1964–1980.

Am J Nephrol 1994;14:418–422

Manuela De Matteis Tortora

Orto Botanico, University of Naples
Federico II, Naples, Italy

Some Plants Described by Dioscorides for the Treatment of Renal Diseases

Key Words

Dioscorides
Medicinal plants
Renal diseases
History of nephrology

Abstract

The original *De Materia Medica* of Dioscorides has been lost, but several copies remain. Unlike the original, these contain an alphabetical listing of plants and color plates. The source for the plants described in this paper is a 16th century translation into vernacular Italian and the Codex Neapolitanus. In all, 12 plants listed by Dioscorides for treatment of renal diseases can be positively identified.

Pedanios Dioscorides from Anazarba in Sicily (1st century AD) was a great scholar of medicinal plants and described plants, animals and minerals with healing virtues in his treatise *De Materia Medica*. The text was arranged, as in a true pharmacopeia, according to the therapeutic properties; for example, the author reported 'habitat', morphology, properties, uses and preparations of each plant. The original work has been lost, but there are later manuscripts, some of which are supposed to be true copies and others only handbooks of the plants contained in *De Materia Medica*. The *Codex Neapolitanus*, also known as Dioscorides of Naples, is one of the latter; it is an ancient manuscript, kept in the National Library of Naples, whose origin and date are unknown. It is very similar to the *Dioscorides of Vienna*, that is the *Codex Vindobonensis* made in Constantinople about 512 AD. Historical and philologic studies suggest that the *Codex Neapolitanus* originated 1–2 centuries later than the *Codex Vindobonensis;* however, the information inferred from studies of both codices does not demonstrate conclusively either the existence of a common source or that *Codex Neapolitanus* is a copy from *Codex Vindobonensis.*

The main differences between the codices and the original work by Dioscorides are the alphabetic order of listing the plants and the presence of color plates, which were not in the original. The *Codex Neapolitanus* consists of 172 plates, each containing 2, sometimes 3, and very occasionally 4, plant drawings; plant name and text are under the figure.

The present paper concerns some plants indicated by Dioscorides for the treatment of renal diseases. To this end, a 'translation' of the text by Dioscorides, the treatise *I Discorsi ne i sei Libri della Materia Medicinale di Pedacio Dioscoride Anazarbeo,* was used. It was written in the *lingua volgare Italiana* (vernacular) by Doctor Pietro Andrea Matthioli in 1557 AD. The book, after a dedicatory epistle to Cardinal Christofano Madruccio and an introduction addressed to readers, opens with an index in which plants (and also animals and minerals) used by Dioscorides are arranged in alphabetic order. It continues with the *Tavola dei Rimedi di Tutti i Morbi del Corpo Umano (Table of the Remedies of All Diseases of the Human Body)* and the treatments illustrated plant by plant.

Dr. Manuela De Matteis Tortora
Orto Botanico
Università di Napoli Federico II
Via Foria 223
I–80139 Napoli (Italy)

Table 1. Plants named by Dioscorides as being of use in renal diseases. Only those that can be positively identified have been included

Species	Uses and properties from Matthioli
Acanthus sp. (Acanthaceae)	'Le radici, bevute, provocano l'orina' (Its roots, drunk, induce urine)
Adiantum capillus-veneris L. (Adiantaceae)	'Il decotto dell'erba, bevuto, giova all'orina ritenuta e rompe le pietre' (The decoction of the herb, drunk, is of use for the retention of urine and breaks stones)
Anagallis sp. (Primulaceae)	'Il succo, bevuto con vino, giova contro i difetti delle reni' (Its juice, drunk with wine, is of use against defects of the kidneys)
Capparis spinosa L. (Capparaceae)	'Il frutto, bevuto quaranta giorni continui, fa orinare i trombi del sangue' (Its fruit, drunk for 40 continuous days, causes blood thrombi to pass in the urine)
Foeniculum vulgare Miller (Apiaceae)	'Il decotto delle fronde, bevuto, perchè provoca l'orina, 'côferisce' ai dolori delle reni ed ai mali della vescica' (The decoction of leaves, because it induces urine, is of use for renal aches and bladder diseases)
Glycyrrhiza glabra L. (Fabaceae)	'Il succo delle radici, bevuto con vino passo, sana la rogna della vescica e i dolori delle reni. Vale a tutte queste cose il decotto della radice fresca' (The juice of its roots, drunk with raisin wine, cures bladder itch and kidney aches. The decoction of fresh root is of use for all these things)
Juniperus communis L. (Cupressaceae)	'I frutti provocano l'orina' (Its fruits induce urine)
Paeonia officinalis L. (Paeoniaceae)	'Giova ai dolori delle reni e della vescica' (It is good for bladder and renal aches)
Plantago sp. (Plantaginaceae)	'Si mangiano fronde e radici con vino passo nelle ulcere delle reni e della vescica' (Leaves and roots are eaten with raisin wine for renal and bladder ulcers)
Ruscus aculeatus L. (Liliaceae)	'Le fronde e parimente i frutti, bevuti nel vino, fanno orinare, rompono le pietre della vescica e giovano alle distillazioni dell'orina. Fa i medesimi effetti il decotto della radice bevuto nel vino' (Its leaves and likewise its fruits, drunk in wine, induce urine, break bladder stones and are good for the distillation of urine. The decoction of its root, drunk in wine, produces the same effect)
Ruta graveolens L. (Rutaceae)	'Provoca l'orina' (It induces urine)
Salvia officinalis L. (Lamiaceae)	'Il decotto delle sue fronde e parimente dei rami, bevuto, fa orinare' (The decoction of its leaves and likewise of its branches, drunk, induces urine)

In the epistle, Matthioli told of his diligent and scrupulous translation of the treatise by Dioscorides. He did not clearly disclose his source, however, but he specified that he added: 'natural and live figures of all plants and animals about which Dioscorides wrote and told' with the help of the painter Giorgio Liberale from Udene, who drew them: 'with art, talent and inestimable patience'. In his work, Matthioli also adds personal notes and plant descriptions from Pliny, Galen and other important scholars of botany.

Table 1 lists 12 different plants indicated by Dioscorides for the treatment of renal diseases; these are the

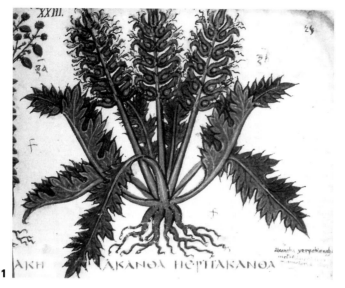

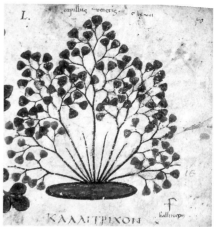

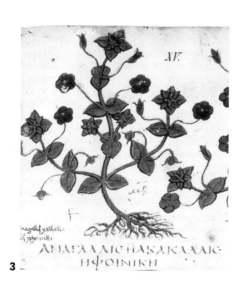

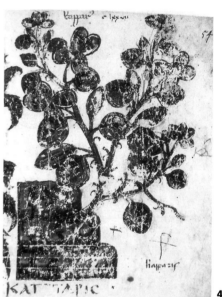

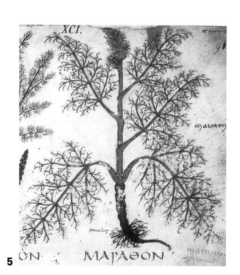

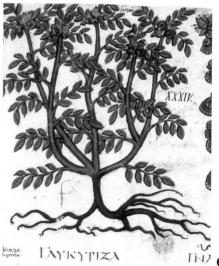

7

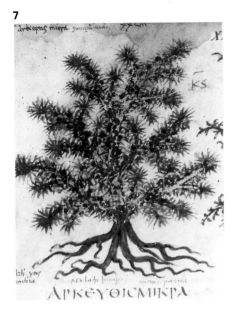

ΑΡΚΕΥΘΙΟΜΙΚΡΑ

8

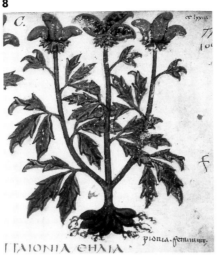

ΠΑΙΟΝΙΑ ΘΗΛΙΑ

9

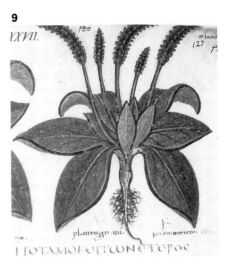

ΠΟΤΑΜΟΓΟΙΤΩΝΕΤΕΡΟΟ

10

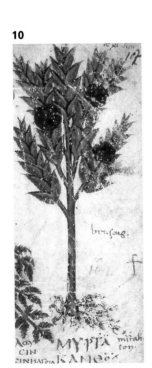

ΜΥΡΤΑ ΚΑΝΘΟΟ

11

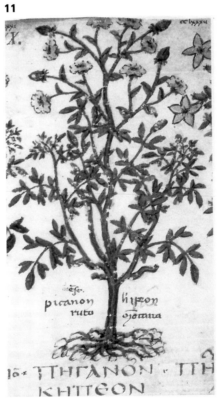

ΠΗΓΑΝΟΝ ΠΗ ΚΗΠΕΟΝ

12

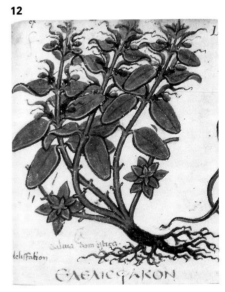

ϹΑΕΛΙϹϤΑΚΟΝ

Fig. 1. *Acanthus* sp.
Fig. 2. *Adiantum capillus-veneris.*
Fig. 3. *Anagallis* sp.
Fig. 4. *Capparis spinosa.*

Fig. 5. *Foeniculum vulgare.*
Fig. 6. *Glycyrrhiza glabra.*
Fig. 7. *Juniperus communis.*
Fig. 8. *Paeonia officinalis.*

Fig. 9. *Plantago* sp.
Fig. 10. *Ruscus aculeatus.*
Fig. 11. *Ruta graveolens.*
Fig. 12. *Salvia officinalis.*

plants contained in the *Codex Neapolitanus* whose species or genus identification is certain. To achieve this, it was necessary to combine careful observation of the figures in the *Codex Neapolitanus* and diligent reading of the text with consultation of different floras. The table reports the species (or the genus), the family, the uses and the properties of each plant. The figures relating to these plants in the *Codex Neapolitanus* are shown in figs. 1–12.

Acknowledgements

The author is grateful to Dr. Bruno Menale, Dr. Paolo Caputo and Mrs. Maria Gabriella Tinè for their assistance during this work.

Further Reading

Fiori A: Nuova Flora Analitica d'Italia. Florence, Ricci, vols 1–2, 1923–1929.

Matthioli PA: I Discorsi di M Pietro Andrea Matthioli Medico Sanese, ne i sei Libri della Materia Medicinale di Pedacio Dioscoride Anazarbeo. In Vinegia, nella Bottega d'Erasmo, Appresso Vincenzo Valgrifi, e Baldassar Costantini. Bologna, Arnaldo Forni Editore, 1984.

Pignatti S: Flora d'Italia. Bologna, Edagricole, vols 1–3, 1982.

Tutin TG, Heywood VH, Burges NA, Valentine DH, Walters SM, Webb DA: Flora Europaea. Cambridge, Cambridge University Press, 1964–1980.

Zangheri P: Flora Italica. Padua, Cedam, vols 1–2, 1976.

Am J Nephrol 1994;14:423–425

Luigia Melillo

Cattedra di Storia della Medicina, Facoltà di Medicina, II Università degli Studi di Napoli, Naples, Italy

Diuretic Plants in the Paintings of Pompeii

Key Words

Pompeii
Mosaics
Medicinal plants
Edible plants

Abstract

The plants that appear in the paintings and mosaics of Pompeii are chiefly edible and medicinal, though flowers with purely esthetic appeal are also shown. An important example is one of the floor mosaics from the House of the Faun, in which it is possible to identify lemon, cherry, strawberry, pomegranate, grape and olive, leaves of grape, fig, apple and olive, and flowers of corn cockle. The diuretic properties of some of these plants are mentioned in the *Naturalis Historia* of Pliny the Elder. A silver cup from the House of Menandro, one of the most refined examples of plant decoration in antiquity, shows olive branches and fruits. The presence of plants in such artefacts confirms that people of classical times were conscious that plants were important producers of food, oils, fibers, woods and medicines.

Introduction

The pictorial and written records of ancient civilizations are a witness to the fact that men had begun to be consciously aware of plants and to consider them in a way that marks a first step towards scientific study. Symptomatic of this change is the appearance of artistic representations of plants in wall paintings and sculptures [1]. About 1800 BC craftsmen of the Minoan civilization in Crete painted frescoes in the great king's palace at Knossos and introduced the images of a number of plants that interested them. In Egyptian paintings plants also appeared, e.g. the representation of fruit trees and the reaping of wheat found in a grave in Thebes (fig. 1) [2].

Paintings and Mosaics in Pompeii

As reported in the last century by Comes [3], the plants that appear in the paintings and mosaics of Pompeii, recovered many centuries after the destruction of the city by an eruption of Vesuvius in 79 AD, are chiefly edible and medicinal, though flowers whose appeal was purely esthetic are also shown. An important example is one of the floor mosaics of the House of the Faun (fig. 2). The house, which was discovered in 1830, was a very large upper-class residence, with two atria and two peristyles (fig. 3). It was named after the discovery of a bronze statue of a faun. Its rich floor decoration was compromised by the removal and transfer of its mosaics to the Naples Museum.

The mosaics were composed of very small *tesserae,* clearly of Alexandrian inspiration, dated to about 120 BC. In the mosaic shown in fig. 2 it is possible to identify lemon, cherry, strawberry, pomegranate, grape and olive, leaves of grape, fig, apple and olive, and flowers of corn cockle. The diuretic properties of some of these plants are mentioned in the *Naturalis Historia* of Pliny the Elder (23–79 AD).

The sweet cherry (*Prunus avium* L.) is a deciduous tree that grows up to 20 m tall and is a native of Eurasia; it was imported into Italy by Lucullus. According to Pliny: *Ce-*

Professor Luigia Melillo, MD
Cattedra di Storia della Medicina, Facoltà di Medicina
II Università degli Studi di Napoli
Via Puccini 19
I–80127 Naples (Italy)

© 1994 S. Karger AG, Basel
0250–8095/94/0146–0423
$8.00/0

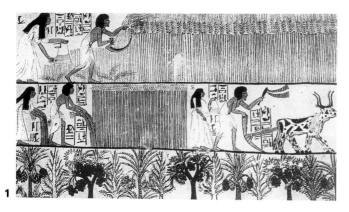

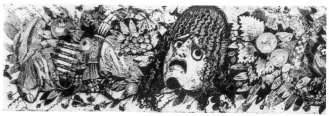

Fig. 1. Paintings from a grave at Thebes, Egypt, 1400 BC.
Fig. 2. Floor mosaic in the House of the Faun in Pompeii.

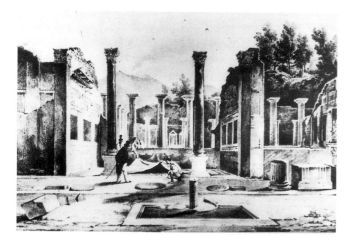

Fig. 3. The House of the Faun in Pompeii.

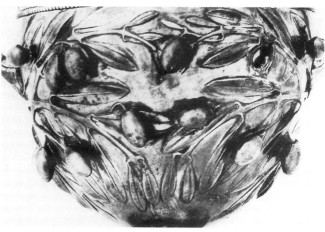

Fig. 4. A silver cup decorated with olive branches and trees, found in the House of Menandro in Pompeii (Archaeologic Museum of Naples).

rasi ante victoriam mithridaticam Luculli non fuere in Italia. In fact, the sweet cherry is not mentioned in *De Agricultura* written by Cato the Elder (234–149 BC). It should be noted that the famous Villa of Lucullus (*Castrum Lucullianum*) where he planted many species from Eastern countries, was located in Naples, on the hill called Pizzofalcone. Pliny also reports that the edible dried drupes of sweet cherry are diuretic (*Naturalis Historia* XXIII, 141). The fruits and fruit stalks are currently mentioned in 6 pharmacopeias as astringents and diuretics [4].

Corn cockle (*Agrostemma githago* L.) is an annual herb with a slender stem which is native to Eurasia. It is a common weed of cereal fields. Once used in medicine as a diuretic and an emmenagogue, seeds of corn cockle have also been used to treat dropsy.

The grapevine (*Vitis vinifera* L.), a native of western Asia, is one of the oldest of cultivated plants; it was known to the ancient Egyptians about 6000 years ago. Even Noah planted the grape after the flood and made wine therefrom: *Noè plantavit vineam bibensque vinum inbriatus est* (*Genesis* 9, verse 20). Wine grape cultivation spread from the eastern Mediterranean region to France and later to Spain, Portugal, Italy and Algeria. The Greeks developed viniculture to a high degree. They stored their wine in vessels smeared with pine pitch to prevent leakage, a practice that accounts for the Greek fondness for a resinous flavor in wine. The Romans did not use pitch on their wine vessels, which is one reason why Italian wines surpassed Greek wines in popularity under the Roman Empire [5]. Pliny reports that dried grapes used as food were considered diuretic (*Naturalis Historia* XXIII, 15).

Ivy (*Hedera helix* L.) is an ornamental evergreen vine. In olden days, the leaves formed the poet's crown as well as the wreath of Bacchus, to whom the plant was dedicated. A garland of ivy was hung outside wayside inns to indicate that wine was sold therein. Greek priests presented a wreath of ivy to newly married coupless, symbolizing fidelity [6]. Pliny reports that ivy steeped in water is diuretic (*Naturalis Historia* XXIV, 75).

Olive (*Olea europaea* L.) is a native of the Mediterranean region, and there are many references to it in the Bible and in classical writings. Figure 4 shows a silver cup *(cantharos)* found in the House of Menandro in Pompeii and transferred to the Archaeologic Museum of Naples. This cup is one of the most refined examples of plant decoration in antiquity. The cup is surrounded by a decoration representing olive branches and fruits. The olive is a small, slowly growing tree which often lives to a great age. The fruit of this plant has been valued since ancient times, not only as food but also as a source of oil. This oil was not only edible, but could also be used for lamps. In some religions it is prepared for burning in sanctuary lamps and for anointing. The oil also has medicinal and cosmetic uses. The fruits as food were considered useful in renal therapy as diuretics and against stones.

Fig (*Ficus carica* L.) is a native of western Asia and has been grown for its fruit since very early times. It was often represented in Roman frescoes as evidenced by paintings from Pompeii and the floor mosaic described earlier (fig. 2). The fig is a small deciduous tree with flowers borne inside the fruit. Pollination is achieved by the female fig wasp. Figs are eaten fresh, dried, or preserved. They have many medicinal uses, and syrup of figs is a well-known medicinal preparation, included in several pharmacopeias. In addition, figs have mild diuretic and laxative properties: in fact, niter (potassium nitrate) pomade with figs was rubbed on the bellies of dropsical patients [7]. Furthermore, codex 97 kept in the Abbey of Montecassino reports: *cum ficu sicca iydropicos curat* [8].

Although the representation of plants in ancient paintings and mosaics tends in general to be less accurate than that of people and animals, it should be emphasized that probably all decorative plants were also, and indeed primarily, used either as food or as medicine. The presence of plants in such paintings confirms that people of classical times were conscious that plants were important producers of food, oils, fibers, woods and medicines.

References

1 Morton AG: History of Botanical Science. London, Academic Press, 1971.
2 Penso G: Les Plantes Médicinales dans l'Art et l'Histoire. Paris, R. Dacosta, 1986.
3 Comes O: Pflanzen in den Malereien von Pompeji. Stuttgart, Nagele Verlag, 1895.
4 Penso G: Le Piante Medicinali nella Terapia Medica. Milan, Org Ed Med Farm, 1987.
5 Simpson BB, Conner-Ogorzaly M: Economic Botany. New York, McGraw-Hill, 1986.
6 Duke JA: Medicinal Plants of the Bible. Owerry, New York, London, Tado-Medic Books, 1983.
7 De Santo NG, Capasso G, Ranieri Giordano D, Aulisio M, Anastasio P, Annunziata S, Armini B, Coppola S, Musacchio R: Nephrology in the *Naturalis Historia* of Pliny the Elder (23–79 AD). Am J Nephrol 1989;9:252–260.
8 Codicum Casinensium Manuscriptorum Catalogus. Monti Casini, 1915, p 96.

Am J Nephrol 1994;14:426–431

Massimo Cirillo
Giovambattista Capasso
Vito Andrea Di Leo
Natale Gaspare De Santo

Chair of Nephrology, Department of
Pediatrics, 2nd University of Naples,
Naples, Italy

A History of Salt

Key Words
Salt
Salt taxes
Salt monopolies
Symbolism of salt
Human evolution
Dietary salt
Medical use of salt

Abstract
The medical history of salt begins in ancient times and is closely related to different aspects of human history. Salt may be extracted from sea water, mineral deposits, surface encrustations, saline lakes and brine springs. In many inland areas, wood was used as a fuel source for evaporation of brine and this practice led to major deafforestation in central Europe. Salt played a central role in the economies of many regions, and is often reflected in place names. Salt was also used as a basis for population censuses and taxation, and salt monopolies were practised in many states. Salt was sometimes implicated in the outbreak of conflict, e.g. the French Revolution and the Indian War of Independence. Salt has also been invested with many cultural and religious meanings, from the ancient Egyptians to the Middle Ages. Man's innate appetite for salt may be related to his evolution from predominantly vegetarian anthropoids, and it is noteworthy that those people who live mainly on protein and milk or who drink salty water do not generally salt their food, whereas those who live mainly on vegetables, rice and cereals use much more salt. Medicinal use tended to emphasize the positive aspects of salt, e.g. prevention of putrefaction, reduction of tissue swelling, treatment of diarrhea. Evidence was also available to ancient peoples of its relationship to fertility, particularly in domestic animals. The history of salt thus represents a unique example for studying the impact of a widely used dietary substance on different important aspects of man's life, including medical philosophy.

Introduction

The dietary intake of salt, i.e. sodium chloride, is believed to play a role in the pathogenesis of many disorders, e.g. hypertension, nephrolithiasis, asthma, gastric cancer and osteoporosis [1–5]. Humphry Davy discovered the element sodium, the cation of salt, in 1807, and since that time several studies have shown that sodium is the principal cation in human blood and tissue fluids. The medical history of salt begins in ancient times, however, and is closely related to different aspects of human history. Only the first era – the era of cooking salt – will be addressed in the present review, as the era of chemical salt (artificial soda) mainly developed in industrial times [6].

Massimo Cirillo, MD
Nefrologia – Padiglione 17
Nuovo Policlinico
Via Sergio Pansini 5
I–80131 Naples (Italy)

Salt Production

An extensive analysis of the problems of salt production has been carried out by Multhauf [6]. The technologies used for salt production vary in different geographic areas depending on the sources used. Salt may be extracted from sea water, mineral deposits (rock salt), surface encrustations, saline lakes and brine springs. There are good and bad salts, i.e. salts with low and high contents of other minerals.

Sea Salt

The sea is a saline solution containing about 3.5% of salts, 2.5% of which is sodium chloride, which can be precipitated by reducing the solution to a small fraction of its original volume. In northern Europe, owing to the generally dull climate and the low salt concentration of the sea, sea water was artificially warmed or boiled in many ways, a very ancient one involving the use of clay dishes (briquetage). The technique of burning peat deposits impregnated with salt was also widely used. In warm areas salt was produced by the natural evaporation of sea water, advantage being taken of lagoons close to the sea which seasonally dried up. In other areas, evaporation of sea water was accelerated by channel and pool systems hardened by the hot ground [7]. In such warm regions the salt harvest took place at the end of the hot season, thereby becoming an auxiliary occupation of farmers.

Brine Salt

This source was important in inland areas of northern Europe owing to the high costs of transporting salt overland from sea sources. Brine was warmed using many techniques: forest timber in central northern Europe (Hall, Tyrol; Reichenhall, Bavaria; Hallein, Salzburg) was used as fuel for these procedures. Salt production thus initiated many environmental problems in Europe, because entire forests were completely burned as a result of this activity.

Rock Salt

In ancient times salt deposits were mined mostly where they reached the surface, as in Transylvania. Salt bricks were used for construction in Gerra, Arabia, according to Pliny [8]:

'Gerris Arabiae oppido muros domosque massis salis faciunt aqua feruminantes.'

Both houses and the mosque were made of salt bricks extracted from a mine 1 m below the surface in Teghaza,
the so-called 'city of salt' in the Sahara, a city which has played a central role in African history since the 11th century [9]. The Chinese had already discovered vast underground salt deposits by drilling deep over 1000 years earlier than the Europeans.

In the 18th century the western Carpathian regions (Wieliczka, Poland and Soovar, Hungary) and Transylvania (Siebenbürgen) became the most renowned for their salt mines. In Poland, the salt mine of Wieliczka was a major source of wealth and the underground workings extended for more than 30 km^2 and included a sumptuous chapel and a vast ballroom for festivities [6].

Socioeconomic Aspects

Salt played a central role in the economies of many regions [6]. The very first roads were made for salt transportation and some of the earliest cities were established as centres of the salt trade [10]. Salt production is often expressed in the name of the site, as for example in Salzburg (Austria), Salzkotten (Prussia), Saltcoats (Scotland) and Lavanapura (India). Salt production was a major source of income in these sites; for example, in Reichenhall the entire population was dependent on the salt industry and its related activities and occupations (woodsmen, traders, workmen, etc). Salt production was also related to the problem of bad working conditions in industry, with women and children working up to 16–18 h/day.

Religious centers and monasteries were founded close to important salt sources [11]. Proprietorship and production rights involved not only the Church, but also the local nobility and those who actually produced the salt. The appearance of coal as the dominant fuel in the 16th century replaced the use of wood as fuel, thereby limiting the importance of the nobility as main fuel suppliers and linking the salt industry directly to the coal industry.

Salt has been mentioned as a main item of Venetian commerce since the 6th century [12]. It was produced in Chioggia, Cervia (south of Ravenna), Alexandria, Cyprus, and the Balearic Islands (Ibiza). Later, Pisa and Genoa entered the trade, controlling salt exportation from Sardinia and Provence. The 'invention' of salted herring (14th century) caused an increase in the northern European salt trade and led to a development of the concentration of sea salines around the harbours of northern Europe. The nearest available sources, e.g. Luneburg (England) and the Low Countries increased their salt production, which was then replaced by the so-called 'bay salt' produced along the French Atlantic coast. This salt was dark in color but cheap. The Dutch managed to improve the color and quality of bay salt, thus regaining a central role as importers/exporters of salt by the end of the 16th century. Thereafter (17th century), the Iberian peninsula became a very important center, with salt produced both in Spain and Portugal. In the course of the 17th and 18th centuries Britain once more became the largest producer and trader in the salt industry, which was favored by an already well-developed shipping industry, including the mastery of channel technology, the discoveries of coal and rock salt, and the ventures of the East India and British America companies involved in supplying the colonies with salt.

Taxation and Monopoly

Salt consumption for culinary use is related to population size and has been used as a basis for population censuses and taxation purposes. Salt monopoly has been practised in many ancient and modern states and represents an important source of revenue or a mean for maintaining low retail prices.

Despotic governments of antiquity, e.g. in ancient Egypt or ancient Israel, imposed a salt tax, while Athens and early republican Rome did not [13]. In ancient Egypt the salt tax, which was paid in addition to the cost of the commodity, was smaller for women than men and children were exempt. In medieval Europe, the introduction of salt monopolies paralleled the formation of nation states and the cost of military ventures. For example, in the 13th century Charles of Anjou, son of Louis VIII of France, introduced a salt tax in Provence to finance the conquest of the Kingdom of Naples [6]. *Gabelle,* a word that is used in many countries to refer to taxes, was introduced in France to refer solely to the salt tax. The word comes from the Latin *gablum,* deriving in turn from the Hebrew *gab* meaning tribute. In the last years before the French Revolution more than 3,500 people were condemned for offences against the salt laws. The salt tax was indeed considered a cause of the French Revolution, and the salt tax was soon repealed by the Revolutionary Government, only to be restored in 1805 to raise funds for the war [14].

Salt was also a factor in the Indian War of Independence. In India, the supply of salt was monopolized by the British, with foreign salt accounting for one-third of the total consumption despite inexhaustible Indian supplies of it. The low sodium content of cereals and green foods in India exacerbated the salt problem, as Indians are predominantly vegetarians and rice-eaters, and therefore depend on adding sodium to their food to avoid sodium deficiency [15].

Cultural, Symbolic and Religious Aspects

Salt has been invested with many meanings, and conversely, words such as salacious or salary (coming from Via Salaria, the Roman road for exporting salt) derive from salt. Its main characteristics – purity, whiteness, incorruptibility, obtainable from sun and sea – contributed to salt becoming an emblem in many cultures. In ancient Egypt, salt was placed over a dead person's body to express the wish for prolonging life; similarly in Scotland, salt was used as a symbol of the immortal spirit in contrast to earth, which was the emblem of the corruptibility of the body [16]. Salt was regarded as the essence of living things and life, and as the very soul itself. Nothing could be eaten without salt and to be without salt was to lack an essential element [17]. A civilized life was believed to be impossible without salt, and its name was also used to refer to mental pleasures:

'Sales appellantur omnisque vitae lepos et summa hilaritas laborumque requies non alio magis vocabulo constat' [8].

As indicated by the word salary, salt was used as money in many regions, and even recently salt money has been found in Africa, Borneo and China [18].

Salt has long been considered a divine gift and sacred object: a religious procession was performed to seek a new spring after a disaster had diluted the spring at the Grande Saunerie of Burgundy [6]. Salt was important in many rites related to hospitality, oaths and betrothals [19]. It was included in religious oblations:

'And every oblation of thy meat offering shalt thou season with salt.'
(Leviticus 2, 13)

A similar use was practised by the Greeks, salt being appreciated by their Divinities [20], and salt is still given during Roman Catholic baptism. The use of salt in so many rituals can be related to the concept of salt as a bond, in which it is viewed as having the capacity to transfer its properties to another substance, thus preserving it from decay. For these characteristics and for its natural affinity with water, magical powers were attributed to salt.

In the Bible salt carries various connotations, including perpetuity (*Numbers* 18, 19: 'a covenant of salt before the Lord for ever'), wealth (*Ezra* 4, 14: 'those who eat the salt of the royal palace'), purity and strength (*Ezekiel* 16, 4: 'in the day thou was born... thou was not salted at all'). Similarly, in the new Testament it is equated with knowledge (Paul to the *Colossians* 4, 6: 'let your speech be always with grace, seasoned with salt', and *Matthew* 5, 36; *Luke* 14, 34–35; *Mark* 9, 50: the Disciples had to be for men what salt is for food) and strength (*Mark* 9, 49: 'For everyone shall be salted with fire').

Man's Evolution and Salt Intake

The importance of finding salt is underlined by the fact that an appetite for salt is innate and salt is a primary taste function in vertebrates. According to Manley [19]: '... the universal existence of an appetite for salt indicates that the substance serves more important functions than that of merely gratifying the palate ...', an adequate amount of additional sodium being needed for fetal growth in utero and for lactation.

The sodium-deficient environment of inland areas far from the coast can affect herbivores, vegetarians and omnivores, which may experience conditions close to sodium deficiency brought about by sodium losses due to infectious diseases (diarrhea and vomiting) or hot weather (sweating). This risk is not shared by carnivores, which ingest enough sodium from their prey and do not depend on the sodium content in the environment. Anthropoids are vegetarians, and man is similar to vegetarians both in dentitian and in the gastrointestinal tract [21]. Hominid evolution, initiated 30 million years ago mainly in tropical warm regions, was associated with a substantially vegetarian diet, and some evidence supports the thesis that the diet of feral man even in relatively recent times was mainly vegetarian and characterized by a very low sodium intake [16]. The development of salt-saving mechanisms would thus have been favored by selection pressure and also because of the assumption of the upright posture, as reflected by the known effect of posture on plasma aldosterone concentration [16].

The hypothesis has been put forward that the practice of adding salt to food is typical of agricultural-vegetarian lifestyles, as there is no need to add salt when food contains a sufficiency of it [22]. In recent times, ethnic differences in the habit of taking salt have supported this interpretation. Individuals consuming milk and meat almost exclusively (nomads of northern Russia and Siberia, the Kirghiz of Turkestan, the Numidians) or drinking heavily salted waters (the Bedouins of Arabia) do not salt their foods, whereas vegetarians do [19].

Some rather intriguing speculation proposes that endo-cannibalism is also related to the need for an adequate sodium intake [16]. This might represent the ritualization of an ancient method of recycling important minerals, including sodium. This ritual, begun under conditions of mineral deficiency, would have continued for the induced sense of well-being in men living in warm regions on a low mineral (sodium, calcium and phosphate) intake.

Medical Views of Dietary Salt Intake and Medical Uses of Salt

One of the most ancient notions on the medical aspects of salt comes from China, where even more than 4,500 years ago it was already known that an elevated dietary intake of salt hardens the pulse [23], an observation which is perfectly in keeping with the current view of the relationship between salt intake and blood pressure level [1].

From the chemical point of view, the main characteristics of salt, according to Galen, were those of being warm and having an earthy structure [24]. The use of salted bread was recommended by Aristotle [25], Averroes [26] and Avicenna [27]. Galen [28] advised an adequate intake of salt through the use of salted bread for everyone except athletes and children. The introduction of salted bread into the Papacy was supported in a book [24] of the 16th century as a particularly useful habit for elderly and obese individuals. This proposal is in sharp contrast with the present view of the cardiovascular effects of a high salt intake, but was based on the idea that salt could favor the humoral excretion of noxious substances, which naturally occurs in athletes due to their sweating. It is to be noted that the same book [24] also reports that non-saline water, rather than salt, is indicated in urinary stone disease:

'Adhaec Tyberis aqua ad calculos gignendos in renibus et vesica et generandas obstruciones in visceribus aptissima est.'

The reasons for this idea are not described, but this same concept may still be valid today [2]. The advice regarding salt in bread, however, was not accepted; in fact, bread is still not salted in most of central Italy, unlike northern and southern Italy.

Since ancient times salt has been known to counteract putrefaction, an effect due to the high osmolarity of saline solutions which arrests bacterial growth, as had been described by Plutarch [20] and Pliny [8]. An extensive

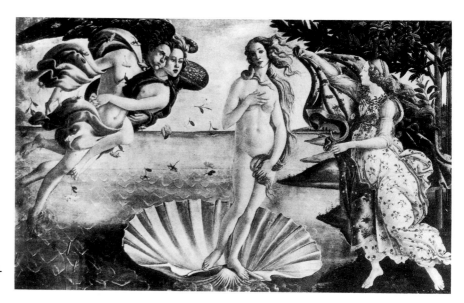

Fig. 1. Venus Saligena by Botticelli (Uffizi Gallery, Florence).

description of the ancient medical uses of salt and saline solutions is provided by Pliny the Elder [8] in book XXXI book of his *Naturalis Historia.* Pliny reported the use of sea water for bruises and osteoarthropathies:

'Medendi modus idem et in marinis erit, quae calefiunt ad nervorum dolores, feruminanda a fracturis ossa, contusa, item corpora siccanda, qua de causa et frigido mari utuntur.'

This use was probably based on the capacity of saline solutions to reduce tissue swelling through osmotic pressure. Pliny also recommends the use of sea water as a purge, and describes a preparation called *thalassomeli,* which consisted of sea water, honey and rain water:

'Inveteratur et quod vacant thalassomeli aequis portionibus maris, mellis, imbris.'

For therapeutic purposes, Pliny also gives instructions for the preparation of a solution similar to sea water, starting from water and salt:

'Verum et hoc cura providit inventa ratione, qua sibi quisque aquam maris faceret.'

Saline solutions were advised in many conditions and also in cases of diarrhea, a piece of advice which may still be valid today. Finally, Pliny describes the medical use in burns of *garum,* a well-known ancient food prepared by allowing fish intestines to ferment in the presence of salt, as an antiseptic substance: '... et garo ambusta recentia sanatur ...'.

The role of salt in reproduction and fertility is reflected in the ancient myth of Venus Saligena, who rises from the sea (fig. 1). Aristotle observed that in many species, litter size and milk production are increased by a diet with a high salt content:

'... sheep are much improved in condition by drinking, and accordingly the flocks are given salt every 5 days ...', and '... salt in the food tends to increase the quantity of milk in ewes ...' [29].

Similar concepts were expressed by Plutarch [30] and Pliny [8]:

'Quin et pecudes armentaque et iumenta sale maxime sollicitantur ad pastus, multo tum largiore lacte multoque gratiore etiam in caseo doet.'

Accordingly, reproduction of vegetarian animals appears to be affected by the salt level in the environment under both free-living and experimental conditions [16]. The relationship between adequate salt intake and fertility could have been relevant to man, particularly considering that salt intake was quite low in regions where hominids developed.

Adequate salt intake is also important in warm tropical areas to enable acclimatization to intense sweating. In such regions, the risk of experiencing sodium depletion can be increased by infectious diseases causing post-fever sweating, diarrhea and vomiting. This notion was already known as early as the 15th century according to the reports of Cadamosto [31], a Venetian traveller who described the importance of salt and its trade in central Africa (Timbuktu). In the equatorial climate, a common remedy was to take a small piece of salt, mix it in a jar with some water and drink it every day. As late as the end of the 19th century, agricultural populations living around the Niger were particularly avid for salt and their children commonly sucked a stick of salt [32].

Conclusions

The history of the medicinal use of salt in Western culture shows that greater consideration was given to the positive aspects of its use. Different explanations may be proposed in this regard. First, evidence was available to support the role played by salt in reproduction. Secondly, the positive religious and symbolic meanings ascribed to salt favored the medical use of this substance, in that medical science had long been guided by philosophic beliefs rather than by truly scientific observations. Finally, observations in early antiquity indicated that salt was able to counteract putrefaction [8, 20].

In the 19th century the idea arose that, although an adequate amount of salt is indispensable for life, too high a salt intake could be unhealthy. As for many other dietary items that are harmless when taken in moderation:

'... it is possible to eat salt in such quantities as to produce very injurious results' [19].

This opinion is close to the present medical view of salt, which considers overuse of this commodity to be related to the development of many disorders. The history of salt, therefore, represents a unique example for studying the impact of a widely used dietary substance on different important aspects of man's life, including medical philosophy. It also shows how changes in dietary habits experienced by man throughout his history may relate to different pathologies, which represent opposite states according to the deficiency or excess of a particular dietary item.

References

1 Stamler J: Dietary salt and blood pressure. Ann N Y Acad Sci 1993;6:122–156.
2 Cirillo M, Laurenzi M, Panarelli W, Stamler J: Urinary sodium to potassium ratio and urinary stone disease. Kidney Int 1994, in press.
3 Burney PG, Britton JR, Chinn, S, Tattersfield AE, Platt HS, Papacosta AO, Kelson MC: Response to inhaled histamine and 24-hour sodium excretion. BMJ 1986;292:1483–1486.
4 Correa P: Is gastric carcinoma an infectious disease? N Engl J Med 1991;325:1170–1172.
5 Goulding A, Campbell DR: Effects of oral loads of sodium chloride on bone composition in growing rats consuming ample dietary calcium. Miner Electrolyte Metab 1984;10:58–62.
6 Multhauf RB: Neptune's Gift: a History of Common Salt. Baltimore, Johns Hopkins University Press, 1978.
7 Rutilius Numantius: De Reditu, caput 416, page 14. Florence, Sansoni, 1967.
8 Pliny: Naturalis Historia, book XXXI, 54–98.
9 Caillié R: Travels through Central Africa to Timbuctu. London, vol 2, 1830, 119–128.

10 Bloch MR: The Social Influence of Salt. SA 1963;209:89–98.
11 Krunitz JG: Salz, in Oeconomisch-technische Encyclopädie. Berlin, 1823, 133–135, 1773–1858.
12 Cassiodorus: Variae, caput 537.
13 Schleiden MJ: Das Salz. Leipzig, 1875.
14 Trébuchet A: Sel, in Baudrimont A et al. (eds): Dictionnaire de l'Industrie, Paris, vol 10, 1841.
15 Gandhi M: Monograph on Common Salt. Calcutta, Federation of Indian Chambers of Commerce and Industry, 1929.
16 Denton D: The Hunger for Salt: an Anthropological, Physiological and Medical Analysis. New York, Springer-Verlag, 1982.
17 Plutarch: Moralia VIII: Table Talk IV, Symmachus Discourses.
18 Parsons JA: Sodium Chloride: the Salt of Life. Discovery 1951, pp 360–385.
19 Manley JJ: Salt and other condiments. London, Clowes, 1884.
20 Plutarch: Quaestiones Conviviales, 684f.

21 Oakley KP: Skill as human possession, in Singer C (ed): History of Technology. London, Oxford University Press, vol 1, 1954.
22 Lapique L: Documents ethnographiques sur l'alimentation minérale. L Anthropologie 1896;7:35.
23 Ruskin A: Classics in Arterial Hypertension. Springfield, Illinois, Charles C. Thomas, 1956.
24 Vicinanza M: De Salis Natura ac Sale cum Panibus Commiscendo Commentarius – 1585–1590? Salerno, Centro Studi e Documentazione della Scuola Medica Salernitana, 1992.
25 Aristotle: Book XXI, problem 5.
26 Averroes: Colliget, book V, caput 31.
27 Avicenna: Book II, 2, caput 573.
28 Galen: Book I, caput 4.
29 Aristotle: Historia Animalium, book VIII, problem 10.
30 Plutarch: Natural Causes, caput 3.
31 Jarcho S: A note on the medical use of salt in 15th century Africa. Med Hist 1958;2:226–228.
32 Dastre A: Le sel. Revue des Deux Mondes 1901;1:1.

Am J Nephrol 1994;14:432–435

Arturo Borsatti[a]
M. Rippa-Bonati[b]
August Antonello[a]

[a] Department of Internal Medicine,
Division of Nephrology;
[b] Institute of History of Medicine,
University of Padua, Padua, Italy

Familial Hypertension in Morgagni's *De Sedibus et Causis Morborum per Anatomen Indagatis*

Key Words

Familial hypertension
History of hypertension
Bladder stones
Edema
Stroke

Abstract

Morgagni was a contemporary of Malpighi, but unlike the latter he concentrated on macroscopic clinical and anatomic observations. His *De Sedibus et Causis Morborum per Anatomen Indagatis* consists of 5 books, written as letters to other scientists and members of foreign academies. He dealt with diseases of the head, the chest and the abdomen and with surgically treatable diseases. The final book contains corrections to the previous 4 in the light of new studies and extended clinical experience. One case history presented, of a patient of Valsalva's who died with edema and a bladder stone, can probably be considered as the first description of familial hypertension. From his clinical and autopsy investigations, Morgagni concluded that the patient died of hereditary bladder stone disease and apoplexy.

Introduction

The concepts of Morgagni (fig. 1) cannot be fully appreciated unless it is realized that he was a contemporary of Malpighi, from whom he derived his mechanistic concept of the human body. According to Morgagni, the human body is constructed like a machine, which consists of a huge number of subunits called *glandules*. Life is thus the result of the harmonious working of the many subunits of this machine. The rupture of this *harmonius vitale* brings about progressive functional deterioration, which finally results in a disease whose clinical manifestations and severity depend on the focal point of the malfunction and the magnitude of the damage [1].

What distinguished Morgagni from Malpighi was his technical approach. The basis for the mechanistic approach of Malpighi was the microscope, an instrument which, considering the technology of the time, Morgagni did not know very well and distrusted. Being gifted with a more powerful clinical analytic ability, Morgagni preferred macroscopic rather than microscopic anatomy [2]. This is implicit in the title of his book, *De Sedibus et Causis Morborum per Anatomen Indagatis (The Seats and Causes of Diseases Investigated by Anatomy)* (fig. 2), published in Venice in 1761 [3] when Morgagni was almost 80 years old.

The *De Sedibus* of Morgagni

The way in which Morgagni wrote this book undoubtedly qualifies him more as a European than as a purely Italian scientist and as a forerunner of European literature. The form used by Morgagni in *De Sedibus* was

Professor August Antonello, MD
Department of Internal Medicine
Division of Nephrology
University of Padua
I–35100 Padua (Italy)

© 1994 S. Karger AG, Basel
0250–8095/94/0146–0432
$8.00/0

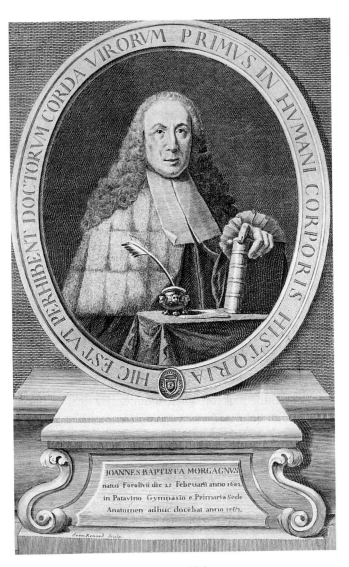

Fig. 1. Engraving of Morgagni by Volpe.

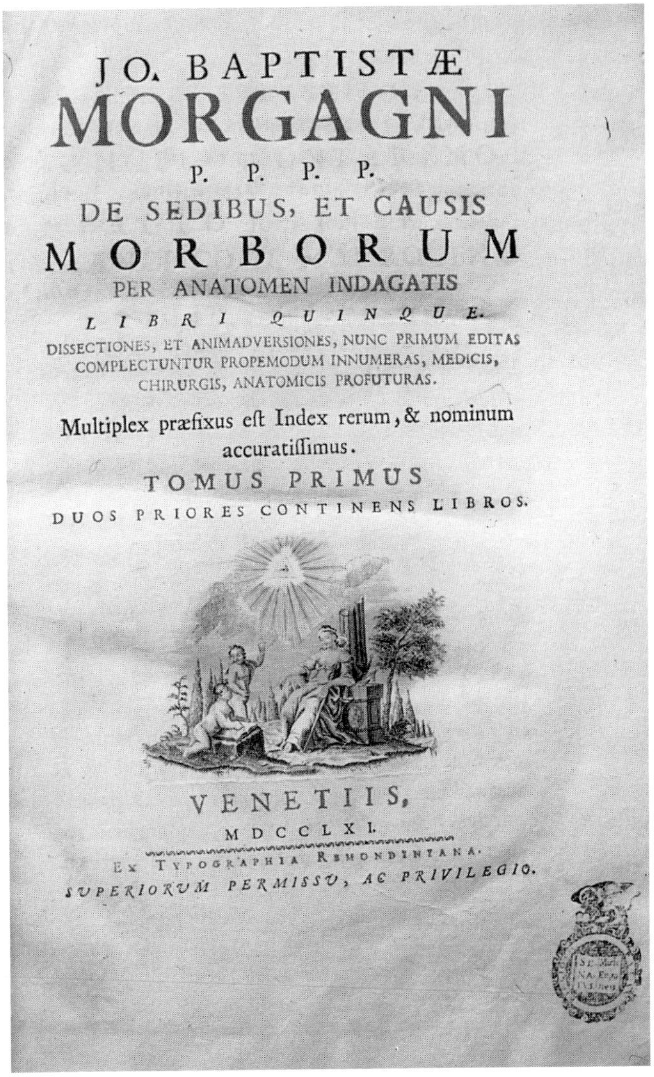

Fig. 2. Title page of the first edition of Morgagni's *De Sedibus et Causis Morborum per Anatomen Indagatis,* published in Venice in 1761. Translated, it reads: 'The Seats and Causes of Diseases Investigated by Anatomy in five books containing a great variety of dissections, with remarks. To which are added very accurate and copious indexes of the principal things and names therein contained'.

that of letters written to other scientists and members of foreign academies, using knowledge and developing hypotheses which were no longer the patrimony of a single scientist but pertained to other scholars, thus establishing a common link between scientists of the whole European continent [1]. Furthermore, *De Sedibus* consists of 5 books or *libri,* each of which is dedicated to a foreign academy of which Morgagni was a member. The 1st book, which deals with diseases of the head, was dedicated to the German Cesarea Academia Nature Curiosorum and

is dated 1708; the 2nd book is concerned with diseases of the chest and was dedicated in 1724 to the Royal Academy of London; the 3rd has as its topic diseases of the abdomen and was dedicated to the Académie Royale des Sciences de France in 1731; the 4th considers surgically treatable diseases and was dedicated to the Russian Academia Imperialis Petropolitana in 1735; and the 5th is a kind of *errata corrige,* in which Morgagni reconsidered previous studies making corrections and adding new considerations in the light of new studies and his improved clinical experience. This final book was dedicated to the Regia Academia Berolinensis in 1754 [2].

De Sedibus is essentially a collection of anatomoclinical records, in which Morgagni developed correlations between the signs and symptoms presented by patients and the anatomic lesions found at autopsy. Such an approach was not original, having been attempted earlier by Bonnet, though not with the same logical consistency as Morgagni. This was properly placed in perspective by Laennec, who characterized Bonnet's book as a 'compilation indigeste et incohérent' [1]. The anatomoclinical records reported by Morgagni in *De Sedibus* are not simply the result of his own observations, but refer also to what he inherited from his teachers, particularly from Valsalva, with whom Morgagni had been a fellow in Bologna [2].

A Case History Concerning Hypertension
In the first book of *De Sedibus,* in the *Lettera Anatomo Clinica IV,* a case history is reported of a friend of Valsalva:

'The father of Zani died of apoplexy and his grandfather of bladder stone, when he was more than 70. He [Zani] was corpulent, flabby, with a very large short neck, a very red face and lead a sedentary life devoted to literary studies and generous meals, as it is convenient for a noble person, was already 40 when he first started making stones which he passed with the urine.'

At age 63 years, the patient started complaining of painful micturition, passing large quantities of watery urine alternating with periods of oliguria. Together with such symptoms Zani also complained of: 'tormenting headaches, owing to which his senses became dull and the movements of the right side of his body feeble'. Immediately afterwards: 'during the Autumn his feet became edematous and from the right foot a large quantity of limpid liquid came out, since the skin had corroded, the liquid, heat coagulated, was similar to egg albumen'. The patient did not improve and started feeling sleepy: '... afterwards, during the Winter when the austral winds blew, he was found without the use of speech, and with the right side of his body almost unmovable'. The patient died 5 days later.

At autopsy the kidneys were normal, as was the bladder, which contained a stone the size of an egg, with an oval shape, but depressed, with a rough surface, and with a color which was not white as his grandfather's stone had been, but reddish. The lungs were red and the heart was large. Inside the skull the dura mater was wrinkled and beneath the pia mater among the sulci of the brain had collected a clear liquid, like a shiny glass. Finally, both carotid and vertebral arteries showed inside the wall small and scattered bodies, white and fixed, most of which had a cartilaginous consistency which in some was bony. Morgagni concluded:

'... therefore Zani was affected by a twofold disease, which was hereditary: bladder stone disease and apoplexy.'

Zani almost certainly died of a stroke, like his father did. Equally certain was the fact that he was affected by atherosclerosis, as suggested by the anatomic finding of 'cartilaginous plaques' in both vertebral and carotid arteries. Considering the association between atherosclerosis and hypertension, it is always difficult to assess which comes first, the chicken or the egg. Obesity and a sedentary life-style, both of which afflicted Zani, favor both atherosclerosis and hypertension. In going through Morgagni's description, however, hypertension appears to be the primary problem. The edema presented by Zani was probably cardiac in origin, as the kidneys of the patient were normal. Furthermore, an enlarged heart and red lungs are in keeping with cardiac failure. The description of Zani's heart given by Morgagni is simply that of a 'big heart', and no information about the condition of the coronary vessels or the existence of myocardial scars is available. Considering that Morgagni had fixed his attention mainly on apoplexy, however, and taking into account his anatomic skills, it can safely be supposed that they were absent. These considerations support the idea that the cardiac enlargement presented by Zani was due to hypertension rather than to atherosclerotic heart disease. Concerning the bladder stone, it must be remembered that Zani's grandfather had also suffered a renal stone. This could represent a predisposition to hypertension, as a relationship between high blood pressure and nephrolithiasis is now recognized [4, 5].

If this interpretation is correct, it can be surmised that both Zani and his father were hypertensive and both died of the most common complication of high blood pressure – a cerebrovascular accident. In this sense, Morgagni's report might be considered as the first description of familial hypertension.

One final note has to be added. In 1965 in Padua, Avogaro and Crepaldi [6, 7] described a syndrome characterized by hyperlipidemia, obesity, mild diabetes without ketosis, and high blood pressure, which seems to portray patients like the one described by Morgagni. It is interesting to note that scholars from the same university have made similar observations after an interval of almost 2 centuries. A very long time indeed for a very short journey!

References

1 Giordano D: Morgagni. Turin, Unione Tipografica Torinese, 1941.
2 Belloni L: L'Opera di Giovanni Battista Morgagni. 25th Congresso della Società Italiana di Storia della Medicina. Forli, 1971, pp 239–246.
3 Morgagni GB: De Sedibus et Causis Morborum per Anatomen Indagatis. Venice, 1761.
4 Cirillo M, Laurenzi M: Elevated blood pressure and positive history of kidney stones: Results from a population-based study. J Hypertens 1988;6:485–486.
5 Cappuccio FP, Strazzullo P, Mancini M: Kidney stones and hypertension: Population based study of an independent clinical association. BMJ 1990;300:1234–1236.
6 Avogaro P, Crepaldi G: Essential hyperlipemia, obesity and diabetes. Abstract from the European Association for the Study of Diabetes. Montecatini Terme, 1965, p 58.
7 Avogaro P, Enzi G, Crepaldi G, Tiengo A: Associazione di iperlipemia, diabete millito e obesità di medio grado. Acta Diabetol Lat 1968;4:27–34.

Am J Nephrol 1994;14:436–442

Joachim Harlos
August Heidland

Department of Medicine, Division of
Nephrology, University of Würzburg,
Würzburg, Germany

Hypertension as Cause and Consequence of Renal Disease in the 19th Century

Key Words
History of nephrology
19th century
Bright's disease
Blood pressure measurement
Vascular pathology
Essential hypertension

Abstract

The pioneering work of Richard Bright, who introduced the concept of the renal origin of cardiovascular disease, initiated the continuous unfolding of knowledge on renal disease and its close interrelationship with arterial hypertension in the 19th century. Hypertension as a clinically and pathologically defined entity, however, was not established. The partial elucidation of the problem that the diseased kidney was sometimes the cause and sometimes the consequence of elevated blood pressure is not only fascinating but also remarkable, given the crude techniques available to physicians at that time. Subsequent workers came to regard 'Bright's disease' as consisting of several conditions differing in clinical manifestation and pathology. In particular, Johnson and Gull and Sutton drew attention to the small blood vessels in renal disease. Only the invention of a clinically applicable method of measuring blood pressure indirectly allowed Mahomed and Allbutt to show that hypertension may occur in the absence of renal disease. They paved the way for a clear separation of hypertensive renal disease from other forms of 'Bright's disease', culminating in the classification introduced by Fahr and Volhard.

Introduction

Although isolated observations had been made before, the continuous unfolding of knowledge and understanding of hypertension and its relation to kidney disease began with Richard Bright (1789–1858). His is the credit for having formulated a coherent concept of disease from a disparate body of knowledge, by linking clinical signs (dropsy, albuminuria, hard pulse) with the finding of anatomic lesions in the kidney and the heart. Educated in Edinburgh, he was appointed assistant physician to Guy's Hospital in London in 1820. Guy's Hospital was a center of modern medicine in England, which was inspired by the concepts and techniques of the Paris medical school. In 1827 he published his *Reports of Medical Cases Selected with a View to Illustrating the Symptoms and Cure of Disease by a Reference to Morbid Anatomy* [1]. He wrote:

'I have never yet examined the body of a patient dying of dropsy attended with coagulable urine in whom some obvious derangement was not discovered in the kidneys.'

Two further publications on kidney disease appeared in 1836. The 1st paper, a brilliant review of the natural course of nephritis, mentions the observation of a hard

Joachim Harlos, MD
University of Würzburg
Division of Nephrology
Josef-Schneider-Strasse 2
D–97080 Würzburg (Germany)

© 1994 S. Karger AG, Basel
0250–8095/94/0146–0436
$8.00/0

pulse and gives a detailed description of clinical signs (headache, loss of visual power, convulsions, dyspnea) following acute and chronic arterial hypertension, though Bright had no means of measuring blood pressure [2]. In the 2nd paper, dealing with systemic complications of renal disease, he noted that hypertrophy of the heart commonly accompanied contracted kidneys found at autopsy. Summarizing the results of his investigations in 100 patients with albuminuria, Bright wrote:

'The obvious structural changes in the heart have consisted chiefly of hypertrophy with or without valvular disease; and what is most striking, out of fifty-two cases of hypertrophy, no valvular disease whatsoever could be detected in thirty-four. This naturally leads us to look for some less local cause, for the unusual efforts to which the heart has been impelled' [3].

Bright suggested that the 'altered quality' of the blood in renal disease affected the peripheral vasculature, particularly capillaries, in such a way that an increased force was necessary for propelling the blood – an incredibly accurate prediction of the mechanisms involved in this process.

By considering renal disease to be primary and cardiac change secondary, Bright established the concept of the renal origin of cardiovascular disease. Subsequently, this principle of causality was taken for granted and it did not occur to contemporary physicians that elevated blood pressure might come first. It should be remarked, however, that Bright, in his usual cautious manner, acknowledged the possibility of a reversed causal connection.

Mechanism and Consequences of Hypertension in Renal Disease

The basis for further understanding the context of renal disease and cardiovascular disorders was provided by the growing knowledge of renal physiology and pathology. William Bowman (1816–1892) recognized in 1842 that glomeruli and tubules formed a functional unit [4]. He suggested that renal function was secretory, while 1 year later Carl Ludwig (1816–1890) developed the theory that urine excretion was based on mechanical filtration and osmosis [5]. Subsequently, in the mid-19th century, the pathoanatomic approach to medical research was extended by physiology, a process mainly initiated by the work of Carl Ludwig in his laboratory in Leipzig [6]. Particularly in Germany, research now went beyond anatomic description and tried to elucidate the pathologic processes underlying the organic changes found at autop-

sy, by combining study of the structure of an organ with knowledge of the physicochemical changes that occurred in its function.

Friedrich Theodor Frerichs (1819–1885), Professor in Kiel, Breslau and later in Berlin, postulated that the glomerulus was the initial site of injury in Bright's disease. He recognized that both hydrostatic pressure and pore size of the glomerular capillary wall were essential factors controlling the composition of the filtrate [7]. Frerichs reasoned further that:

'The disturbances of transudation [in Bright's disease] will be observed first in that part of the renal capillary system which under normal conditions has to withstand the highest pressure, i.e. the vascular Malpighian bodies.'

Frerich's observation could be interpreted as a forerunner of the concept of glomerular capillary hypertension [8]. Unfortunately, his theory concerning the origin of Bright's disease was based on investigation of a special case of albuminuria, the congested kidney, which is actually not albuminuric nephritis. Consequently, his further reflections on the interrelationship between renal and cardiovascular diseases went astray.

The most important German exponent of the new concept with a special interest in the relationship of renal and cardiac disorders was Ludwig Traube (1818–1876). Traube, an assistant of Schönlein in Berlin, was one of the first Jewish physicians to become a full professor in Germany. His work on the hemodynamics of the circulation was based on animal models, using the physiologic methods and concepts introduced by Ludwig and his coworkers. Independently of Bright (he was not aware of Bright's original papers), he noted the coincidental findings of shrunken kidneys and hypertrophy of the left ventricle. Traube recognized that albuminuric kidneys due to cardiac failure showed a totally different appearance at autopsy than kidneys with Bright's disease, and in contrast to Frerichs he clearly distinguished albuminuric nephritis from the congested kidney. In his monograph *Über den Zusammenhang zwischen Herz- und Nierenkrankheiten (The Connection between Cardiac and Renal Diseases)* published in 1856, Traube described the relationship between perfusion pressure in the kidney and urinary solute excretion, and demonstrated that elevated tension in the aortic system, i.e. hypertension, was the underlying pathophysiologic process of cardiac hypertrophy in Bright's disease. He further recognized the key role of hypervolemia in the pathogenesis of renal parenchymal hypertension [9]. Traube reasoned that a shrunken kidney would have two major consequences:

'It will act, first, by decreasing the blood volume which flows out in a given time from the arterial system into the venous system. It will secondly act by decreasing the amount of liquid which at the same time is removed from the arterial system as urinary secretion. As a result of both conditions, particularly because of the latter, the mean pressure of the arterial system [Aortenspannung] must increase. Consequently again, an increase in resistance is produced which opposes the emptying of the left ventricle. The left ventricle will dilate and this will be associated with an increase of the muscle fibers in the left ventricular wall.'

Less cautious than Bright in creating hypotheses to explain his observations, he attributed the raised pressure purely to the change in the kidney. Due to the rigidly mechanistic approach of his research concept, Traube misinterpreted the role of diminished renal perfusion in increasing peripheral vascular resistance. His lasting contribution, however, was to begin to elucidate the mechanism underlying renal parenchymal hypertension, thus making it evident that hypertension was the causal link between Bright's disease and the ensuing cardiovascular damage.

Experimental Renal Hypertension

Traube's work was based on the investigation of normal physiology. Two decades later the first experimental studies of hypertension were carried out in animal models. The earliest experimental approaches to hypertension were devoted primarily to determining the effect of nephrectomy and other manipulations of the kidney on the blood pressure and renal excretory function. In 1879 Grawitz and Israel induced hypertrophy of the heart by partial nephrectomy in rabbits, which they attributed to the development of hypertension [10]. Later, Pässler and Heineke demonstrated an increase in blood pressure by the same procedure in dogs [11]. In 1898 Bradford reported that in dogs, removal of renal tissue led to an increase in water and urea excretion, but not salt excretion [12]. In addition, a rise in arterial pressure could be observed and blood pressure remained elevated when the animals were moribund.

At the same time Tigerstedt and Bergman showed that a saline extract of rabbit kidney tissue produced a prolonged rise of arterial pressure when injected into other rabbits [13]. They named the active principle 'renin'. Their demonstration of a pressor substance was the forerunner of a vast number of experiments to determine whether various procedures on the kidney could release renin.

Clinical Tools for Detection of High Blood Pressure

Richard Bright and his successors had to use simple tools to detect cardiac involvement in renal disease in living patients. For much of the 19th century no methods of measuring blood pressure indirectly were available. The only way to estimate arterial tension was by feeling the pulse and noting its degree of compressibility, a subjective and inexact diagnostic tool. With some skill, cardiomegaly could be detected by percussion. Because of their limited comprehension of Bright's findings, most practitioners directed attention to the pulse only after the urine had been found to be abnormal. This point is of some importance, as it hampered the recognition that high blood pressure could occur without any sign of renal damage.

In the middle of the 19th century, diagnostic techniques were enlarged by the adoption of an instrument initially used for physiologic investigation. The ophthalmoscope was invented by Hermann von Helmholtz (1821–1894) in 1851 and rapidly came into clinical use [14]. Five years later, the German ophthalmologists Friedrich Heymann (1828–1870) and Albrecht von Graefe (1828–1870) described a characteristic alteration of the ocular fundus in Bright's disease [15, 16]. Further investigations were carried out by Liebreich [17], who named the finding *retinitis albuminurica*, i.e. retinitis angiospastica. Subsequently, ophthalmoscopy became a common method in the diagnosis of Bright's disease. A comprehensive list of signs by which left ventricular enlargement could be recognized during life was given by Traube. He pointed out that there was a close relationship between retinal change (retinitis albuminurica) found by fundoscopy and 'elevated arterial tension' in Bright's disease [18].

Contracted Granular (Arteriosclerotic) Kidney

One important question that arose from Bright's work was whether he had described a single disease or different conditions having in common only the finding of an altered kidney. Two major subdivisions could be found at autopsy: the large pale and the contracted granular kidney. In attempting to classify Bright's disease, most workers considered contracted granular kidneys to be a separate class [19]. Further clinical and pathologic observations led to the next landmark in the study of hypertension in renal disease: the recognition that renal damage could be the consequence of a generalized disease of the vasculature due to an (as yet) poorly understood pathologic process, i.e. essential hypertension.

Samuel Wilks (1824–1911), a physician at Guy's Hospital, reported in 1855 his observation that the natural history of these 2 types of Bright's disease differed considerably. He assumed that a slowly progressing form of contracted kidney could be caused by a disease of the arteries [20]. Similar observations were made by Carl Bartels (1822–1878), a clinician in Kiel. He separated acute and chronic forms of Bright's disease by clinical signs and suggested that shrunken kidneys can even appear without an antecedent acute stage. In his paper [21] published in 1871, he reported that such patients appeared healthy for a long time, then suffered from cephalalgia and vertigo, and some of them died from stroke or convulsions. If the disease lasted longer, then cardiac hypertrophy and retinitis albuminosa were common findings in these patients. Edema appeared only in the terminal stage of the disease and patients died with progressive uremia. Bartels' lucid description reflects the clinical course of what is today called arteriosclerotic renal shrinkage, or hypertensive nephrosclerosis.

Wilks' hypothesis was later pursued by Johnson, Gull and Sutton, who elaborated on Bright's findings with particular reference to the vascular pathology of contracted granular kidneys. Although microscopic examination of tissue slices had come into use in the middle of the 19th century, these studies were hampered by serious handicaps: methods of staining and fixation were primitive or non-existent and little was known about normal histologic appearances.

George Johnson, Professor of Physics at King's College Hospital, London, published extensively on renal disease with particular emphasis on microscopic anatomy [22]. In 1868 he described thickening of the muscular coat of arterial vessels not only in the diseased kidney but also in other tissues and organs [23]. He considered this to be a true hypertrophy, which was due to chemical alterations of the blood that caused obstruction in small arteries and consequently increased the work of the left ventricle. Like Bright he assumed that vascular and cardiac changes were secondary to renal damage. In contrast to Bright, however, he found that the site of vascular damage was small arteries rather than capillaries.

Four years later, in 1872, William Gull (1816–1890) and Henry Sutton (1836–1891) suggested that vascular disease could be responsible for the damage to the kidney. Gull, a physician at Guy's Hospital, and Sutton, a pathologist at the London Hospital, had found widespread 'hyaline-fibrinoid' material in the walls of arterioles and capillaries in patients suffering from contracted granular kidneys. They called this form of vascular sclerosis 'arteriocapillary fibrosis' [24]. They stated: '... that this change occurs chiefly outside the muscular layer, but also in the tunica intima of some arterioles'. Gull and Sutton regarded this as a generalized disease of blood vessels affecting many parts of the body, including the kidneys. In such cases, they postulated 'arteriocapillary fibrosis' to be the 'primary and essential change', i.e. the cause and not the consequence of diseased kidneys [25]. It must be assumed that Gull and Sutton described what we now call arteriosclerosis and arteriolosclerosis. Their paper [25] initiated a long-lasting controversy with Johnson, who vehemently attacked the concept of arteriocapillary fibrosis.

The main contribution of both research groups, however, was to draw attention to the small blood vessels in renal disease. Their observations were later confirmed, particularly by German workers. In 1877 Ernst Ziegler (1849–1905) published similar observations on the effects of arterial disease on the kidney and showed how atrophy of this organ could be caused by arteriosclerosis [26]. Carl Anton Ewald (1845–1915) examined the small vessels of the pia mater and found hypertrophy of the tunica media [27], while Leonhard Jores (1866–1835) laid emphasis on changes in the arterial intima, particularly a fatty hyaline thickening, which he found not only in the kidney but also in the organs generally [28].

It is somewhat surprising that neither Johnson nor Gull and Sutton understood the pathologic process underlying their findings. They found a full pulse in patients with contracted granular kidneys, and further described increased arterial pressure as resulting from increased peripheral resistance due to the decreased caliber of small peripheral vessels. For practical reasons, however, it did not occur to them that high blood pressure might cause vascular damage and precede renal disease. While in primarily renal disease alteration of the kidney (albuminuria, dropsy) as well as clinical signs of cardiovascular disease (full pulse, cardiomegaly) could be detected in living patients, renal deterioration due to vascular disease was a finding usually made at autopsy. When the problem of 'arteriocapillary fibrosis' was discussed at the Pathological Society in 1877, Gull and Sutton had to confess their inability to recognize the early stages of this disease during life [29]. Even if a full pulse or cardiomegaly were found in a patient, the early stages of deterioration of renal function could not be detected easily with the diagnostic tools (sediment, urinalysis) available at that time. To progress beyond simple observations during life and after death, actual measurement of arterial blood pressure was required.

Blood Pressure Measurement in the 19th Century

In 1828 Jean Léonard Marie Poiseuille (1799–1869) developed the mercury manometer, but for obvious reasons direct measurements of arterial pressure were carried out solely in experimental animals [30]. Although Faivre used Poiseuille's mercury manometer in 1856 to measure arterial pressure directly during limb amputation [31], determination of the behavior of blood pressure in man was based on indirect methods of measurement.

The first indirect instrument was that of Hérisson (1834). Its real purpose was to estimate the amplitude of the pulse, and measurement of arterial pressure was secondary and inaccurate [32]. In 1854 Karl Vierordt (1818–1884) designed an instrument specifically to measure arterial pressure. Weights were added to a scale pan placed on a lever which pressed on a button overlying the radial artery [33]. By adopting the principle of Ludwig's kymograph, Etienne-Jules Marey (1830–1904) in 1863 introduced a new instrument, the sphygmograph. Its purpose was to record amplitude, duration and compressibility of the pulse and to analyze its waveforms [34]. Frederick Akhbar Mahomed (1849–1884) later refined Marey's sphygmograph by adding a graduated wheel which allowed him to measure the force required to occlude the radial pulse [35]. Nevertheless, it was a very clumsy instrument. A more practical device for measuring blood pressure was developed by Samuel von Basch (1837–1905) in 1881, and he regarded pressures up to 150 mm Hg as normal [36]. All these instruments estimated blood pressure on the basis of the compressibility of the radial artery and/or the peripheral arterial pressure contour. Only the modern sphygmomanometric methods, attributable to Scipione Riva-Rocci (1863–1937), Heinrich von Recklinghausen (1867–1942) and Nikolai Korotkoff (1874–?) have focused attention on the numeric values of the systolic and diastolic pressure in the brachial artery [37–39].

Discovery of Essential Hypertension

The systematic study of arterial blood pressure in man began with Frederick Akhbar Mahomed (1849–1884). He combined for the first time measurement of arterial blood pressure with clinical and pathologic observations. In his first, classic, paper published in 1874, Mahomed described his observation that high arterial pressure was present before albumin appeared in the urine in patients developing Bright's disease following scarlet fever [40].

He called this finding the 'prealbuminuric stage of Bright's disease'. His further investigations advanced the view that high blood pressure could cause changes in small vessels and lead to contraction of the kidneys. Discussing the problem of 'arteriocapillary fibrosis', Mahomed suggested that:

'... it is very common to meet with people apparently in good health who have no albumin in the urine or any other sign of organic disease, who constantly present a condition of high arterial tension when examined by the aid of the sphygmograph' [41].

In 1879 Mahomed extended his observations by analyzing 100 cases of granular kidneys, relating the findings during life and after death. 'Ordinary signs of Bright's disease', i.e. dropsy and albuminuria, were prominent in only 26 patients, and these were found to have 'a yellow or mixed contracted kidney'. The remainder showed a 'red contracted kidney' and albuminuria was often absent. The predominant clinical manifestations were cerebral and cardiac in origin, and elevated blood pressure was a consistent finding. Mahomed drew the lucid conclusion that elevated arterial pressure was the cause and not the consequence of renal damage, preceding the latter by many years [42]. These clinical and pathologic findings provided strong support for the work of Gull and Sutton, and Mahomed stated that high arterial pressure was the clinical counterpart of 'arteriocapillary fibrosis'. His studies contain some accurate observations on the condition now commonly called essential hypertension: he noted the onset of hypertension even in young persons; the occurrence of a familial tendency; and the fact that it need not lead to renal disease at all [43].

Sadly, Mahomed died of typhoid fever at the age of 35 years, and his pioneering work was not fully appreciated by his contemporaries. The main reason for this was the continuing lack of a simple and accurate means of measuring blood pressure. The sphygmograph was a clumsy instrument, and its use too cumbersome for routine clinical application. Furthermore, Mahomed had adopted a rather extreme view of the causality between renal disease and arterial hypertension. He was convinced that hypertension always preceded renal damage in chronic Bright's disease. In this context his choice of the term 'prealbuminuric Bright's disease' was unfortunate and led to some misunderstanding. It could not appeal to physicians educated in the belief that albuminuria and Bright's disease were synonymous. Nevertheless, credit for the recognition of essential hypertension is rightly given to Mahomed. He perceived clearly what others later established more fully.

Harlos/Heidland

Hypertension in Renal Disease

Henry Huchard (1844–1910), Professor of Medicine in Paris, recognized in 1889 that hypertension might occur independently of nephritis. He stated that:

'Arterial hypertension is the cause of arteriosclerosis, preceding by a varying time interval the evolution of different diseases which are in turn secondary to vascular sclerosis' [44].

Huchard named this condition 'presclerosis'.

Similar observations were made by Clifford Allbutt (1836–1925), Regius Professor of Physics in Cambridge. His work paved the way for the acceptance of essential hypertension as a separate disease with its own natural history and consequences. Unlike others before, who based their conclusions on large series of autopsies, he pursued the fate of a small number of patients coming to his practice over long periods of time. In agreement with Mahomed, he reported in 1877 his observation that elevated arterial pressure can occur in the absence of albuminuria [45]. Nearly 20 years later he described 5 similar cases in elderly patients and called this condition 'senile plethora' [46, 47]. Later Allbutt introduced the term 'hyperpiesis' to describe a disease of middle-aged or elderly people who developed a rise in arterial pressure without general symptoms of renal disease, and in the early stages did not show evidence of damage in any organ at all [48]. Riva-Rocci's invention had enabled him to carry out accurate measurement of arterial blood pressure in his patients. Allbutt clearly recognized that 'hyperpiesis' (later called essential hypertension) was an entirely different class of disorder that was not caused by parenchymal renal disease and indeed did not necessarily lead to renal disease at all. By this he clearly differentiated hypertensive renal disease from the other forms of Bright's disease [49].

Conclusions

The rapid confirmation of Bright's findings by other workers led to a new eponym – Bright's disease – and throughout the last century the classification of renal lesions in Bright's disease dominated research. Simple observations during life and after death drew attention to the small vessels in renal disease but could not give a clear answer to the conundrum that renal disease was sometimes the cause and sometimes the consequence of cardiovascular disorders. Only the invention of instruments to measure blood pressure indirectly provided a modern view of the relationship between renal disease and high arterial pressure. Thus, by the turn of the century, it was appreciated that chronic parenchymal renal disease can lead to hypertension as a secondary phenomenon, but that hypertension and small vessel disease can also occur as a primary feature not necessarily secondary to a contracted state of the kidneys.

An early and surprisingly modern attempt to bring clinical findings and pathology into a coherent scheme according to these findings was that of Franz Volhard (1872–1950) and Theodor Fahr (1877–1945). Their monograph should be mentioned in this context, even though it was published in 1914 [50]. Summarizing the contemporary state of knowledge, their outstanding work did much to clarify concepts of renal and arterial disease. Volhard the physician and Fahr the pathologist divided Bright's disease into 3 major forms, namely the degenerative diseases or nephroses, the inflammatory diseases or nephritides, and the arteriosclerotic diseases or scleroses. This classification has been expanded and modified, but in essence remains acceptable today.

References

1 Bright R: Reports of Medical Cases, Selected with a View of Illustrating the Symptoms and Cure of Diseases by a Reference to Morbid Anatomy. London, Longman, Rees, Orme, Brown and Green, 1827.

2 Bright R: Cases and observations illustrative of renal disease accompanied with the secretion of albuminous urine. Guy's Hosp Rep 1836;1: 338–379.

3 Bright R: Tabular view of the morbid appearances in 100 cases connected with albuminous urine. Guy's Hosp Rep 1836;1:380–400.

4 Bowman W: On the structure and use of the Malpighian bodies of the kidney, with observations on the circulation through that gland. Philos Trans R Soc 1842;132:57.

5 Ludwig C: Beiträge zur Lehre vom Mechanismus der Harnsekretion. Marburg, Elwert, 1843.

6 Gerabek W: Der Leipziger Physiologe Carl Ludwig und die medizinische Instrumentation. Sudhoffs Arch 1991;75:171–179.

7 Frerichs FTH: Die Bright'sche Nierenkrankheit und deren Behandlung. Braunschweig, Vieweg, 1851.

8 Ritz E, Zeier M, Lundin P: French and German nephrologists in the mid-19th century. Am J Nephrol 1989;9:167–172.

9 Traube L: Über den Zusammenhang von Herz- und Nierenkrankheiten. Berlin, Verlag August Hirschwald, 1856.

10 Grawitz P, Israel O: Experimentelle Untersuchung über den Zusammenhang zwischen Nierenerkrankung und Herzhypertrophie. Arch Pathol Anat 1879;77:315.

11 Pässler H, Heinecke D: Versuche zur Pathologie des Morbus Brightii. Verh Dtsch Pathol Ges 1905;9:99.

12 Bradford JR: The results following partial nephrectomy and the influence of the kidney on metabolism. J Physiol 1898/1899;23:416–469.

13 Tigerstedt R, Bergman PG: Niere und Kreislauf. Skand Arch Physiol, 1898;8:223–271.

14 Helmholtz H: Beschreibung eines Augenspiegels zur Untersuchung der Netzhaut im lebenden Auge. Berlin, 1851.

15 Von Graefe A: Nachträgliche Bemerkung über Sclerotico-chorioideitis posterior. Graefes Arch Klin Exp Ophthalmol 1854/1855;1:307.

16 Heymann FM: Über Amaurose bei Bright'scher Krankheit und Fettdegeneration der Netzhaut. Graefes Arch Klin Exp Ophthalmol 1856;2. Cit. from: Vogel J, Virchow R (eds): Handbuch der speziellen Pathologie und Therapie. Erlangen, 1856–1865, vol 6/2:637.

17 Liebreich C: Ophthalmoskopischer Befund bei morbus Brightii. Graefes Arch Klin Exp Ophthalmol 1859;5:265.

18 Traube L: Nachträgliche Bemerkungen über den Zusammenhang von Herz- und Nierenkrankheiten, in Gesammelte Beiträge. vol 2, 1859, pp 421–437.

19 Johnson G: On the forms and stages of Bright's disease of the kidneys. Med Chir Trans 1859; 42:152–164.

20 Wilks S: Cases of Bright's disease, with remarks. Guy's Hosp Rep Ser 2 1853;8:232–315.

21 Bartels CHC: Klinische Studien über die verschiedenen Formen von chronischen diffusen Nierenentzündungen. Sammlung klinischer Vorträge von Volkmann 1871;25:160.

22 Johnson G: On the proximate cause of albuminuous urine and dropsy and on the pathology of the renal blood vessels in Bright's disease. Med Chir Trans 1850;33:107–120.

23 Johnson G: On certain points in the anatomy and pathology of Bright's disease of the kidney. Med Chir Trans 1868;51:57–76.

24 Gull WW: Chronic Bright's disease with contracted kidney (arterio-capillary fibrosis). BMJ 1872;2:673–674.

25 Gull WW, Sutton HG: On the pathology of the morbid state commonly called chronic Bright's disease with contracted kidney ('Arterio-capillary fibrosis'). Med Chir Trans 1872;55:273–326.

26 Ziegler E: Über die Ursachen der Nierenschrumpfung nebst Bemerkungen über die Unterscheidung verschiedener Formen der Nephritis. Dtsch Arch Klin Med 1880;25:585.

27 Ewald CA: Über die Veränderungen kleiner Gefäße bei Morbus Brightii und die darauf bezüglichen Theorien. Virchows Arch Pathol Anat Physiol 1877;71:453.

28 Jores L: Über die Arteriosklerose der kleinen Organarterien und ihre Beziehungen zur Nephritis. Virchows Arch Pathol Anat Physiol 1904;178:367.

29 Rault R: Enigma of contracted granular kidney: a chapter in the history of nephrology. Am J Nephrol 1991;11:402–408.

30 Poiseuille JLM: Recherches sur la force du cœur aortique. Paris, Didot, 1828.

31 Faivre J: Etudes expérimentales sur les lésions organiques du cœur. Gazette Méd 1856;11: 712.

32 Hérisson J: Le Sphygmomètre: Instrument qui Traduit à l'Œil Toute l'Action des Artères. Paris, Crochard, 1834.

33 Vierordt K: Die bildliche Darstellung des menschlichen Arterienpulses. Arch Physiol Heilk 1854;13:284.

34 Marey EJ: Physiologie Médicale de la Circulation du Sang. Paris, Delahaye, 1863.

35 Mahomed FA: The physiology and clinical use of the sphygmograph. Med Times Gazette 1872;1:62–64.

36 Von Basch SSR: Einige Ergebnisse der Blutdruckmessung an Gesunden und Kranken. Z Klin Med 1881;3:512.

37 Korotkoff NS: On methods of studying blood pressure. Izv Voennomed Akad 1905;11:365.

38 Von Recklinghausen H: Über Blutdruckmessung beim Menschen. Arch Exp Pathol Pharmakol 1901;46:78.

39 Riva-Rocci S: Un nuovo sfigmomanometro. Gazz Med Torino 1896;47:981.

40 Mahomed FA: The etiology of Bright's disease and the pre-albuminuric stage. Med Chir Trans 1874;57:197–228.

41 Mahomed FA: On the sphygmographic evidence of arterio-capillary fibrosis. Trans Pathol Soc 1877;28:394.

42 Mahomed FA: Some of the clinical aspects of chronic Bright's disease. Guy's Hosp Rep Ser 3 1879;39:363–436.

43 Mahomed FA: On chronic Bright's disease, and its essential symptoms. Lancet 1879;i:46.

44 Huchard H: Maladies du Cœur et des Vaisseaux. Paris, Doin, 1889.

45 Albutt TC: Pathology of granular kidney. Brit For Med Chir Rev 1877;60:279–298.

46 Allbutt TC: Senile plethora or high arterial pressure in elderly persons. Trans Hunterian Soc 1896;96:38–57.

47 Allbutt TC: Senile arterial plethora. Philadelphia Med J 1,900;5:859–914.

48 Allbutt TC: Rise of blood pressure in later life. Med Chir Trans 1904;86:323–343.

49 Allbutt TC: Arteriosclerosis and the kidneys. BMJ 1911;853–858, 922–927.

50 Volhard F, Fahr T: Die Bright'sche Nierenkrankheit. Klinik, Pathologie und Atlas. Berlin, Springer, 1914.

Am J Nephrol 1994;14:443–447

Eberhard Ritz
Sonja Küster
Martin Zeier

Department of Internal Medicine, Division
of Nephrology, Ruperto Carola University,
Heidelberg, Germany

Clinical Nephrology in 19th Century Germany

Key Words
Urinary sediment
Urinalysis
Bright's disease
Nephritis
19th century Germany

Abstract
Bright's work led to the recognition that coagulable protein in the urine indicated macroscopic kidney disease. After light microscopy was introduced, Simon, Nasse, Henle and Frerichs identified the major constituents of urinary sediment. By 1896, Senator had deduced that hyalin cylinders arise in the kidney tubules, and only the discovery of the Tamm-Horsfall protein in the next century separated him from the modern concept. Chemical analysis of urine also advanced greatly. Recognition of the pressure-volume relationship by Traube was probably the most brilliant achievement related to renal disease, and became the basis of the later pressure-natriuresis relationship. Traube also linked left ventricular hypertrophy with renal disease, recognizing that it maintained circulatory homeostasis at a higher level of pressure. The concept of nephritis changed considerably with technical progress, and Gluge was the first to see inflamed Malpighian bodies or glomeruli. The primary site of damage was disputed by many, including Henle, Pfeufer, Virchow, Reinhardt and Frerichs, but all these workers had to reconstruct the sequence of events leading to the autopsy findings. The term glomerulonephritis was first coined by Klebs, and the classification of nephritis adopted by Senator in 1896 led directly to the classic monograph of Volhard and Fahr (1914) on Bright's disease.

Introduction

It is certainly artificial, and somewhat dated, to view the development of science within narrow national boundaries. To quote Goethe: 'Der Geist kennt keine Grenzen' (the human mind does not respect frontiers). Nevertheless, linguistic and cultural barriers were certainly more marked in the 19th century and limited the exchange of ideas to a greater extent than today. It may therefore be useful to discuss separately the development of clinical nephrology in Germany during the last century. Limitations of space necessitate restriction of the discussion to a few particularly illustrative examples of the major contributions of German nephrologists (or rather internists with a special interest in renal disease).

Progress in Urinalysis – the Tools for Clinical Diagnosis

Richard Bright's breakthrough discovery led to the recognition that the presence of coagulable protein in the urine was linked to macroscopic disease of the kidney. Apart from proteinuria, he also noted erythrocytes ('the red particles in blood') in the urine of some patients.

Professor Eberhard Ritz, FRCP
Department of Internal Medicine
Bergheimer Strasse 58
D–69115 Heidelberg (Germany)

1

DIE ERKRANKUNGEN

DER

NIEREN.

VON

PROF. DR H. SENATOR

IN BERLIN.

WIEN 1896.

ALFRED HÖLDER

K. U. K. HOF- UND UNIVERSITÄTS-BUCHHÄNDLER

I. ROTHENTHURMSTRASSE 15.

2

II.

Die Fragmentation der rothen Blutkörperchen und ihre
Bedeutung für die Diagnose der Hämaturien.

Aus der medicinischen Klinik zu Jena.

Von

Dr. F. Gumprecht,

Assistenzarzt.

(Mit 7 Abbildungen im Text.)

Der morphologische Vorgang, welcher Gegenstand dieser Untersuchungen ist, verläuft folgendermaassen: Die rothen Blutkörperchen
strecken, nachdem ihr Protoplasma sich in zuweilen erkennbarer Weise
verändert hat, amöboide Fortsätze aus, so dass das gesammte Körperchen das Aussehen einer Keule, einer Flasche, eines Kreuzes, eines
Spirillum oder sonstiger Formen annimmt, die ausgestreckten Fortsätze ziehen sich zu hämoglobinhaltigen Kugeln zusammen, welche
entweder in Verbindung mit der Mutterzelle bleiben, nur durch eine
Scheidewand von ihr getrennt, durch einen Faden an ihr hängend,
oder sie reissen völlig von ihr ab und treiben als freie, gefärbte Kugeln
umher. Diese Kugeln erleiden schliesslich dasselbe Schicksal wie alle
rothen Blutzellen, sie entfärben sich, und die zurückbleibenden Schatten
lösen sich auf.

Die Einflüsse, welche solche Veränderungen hervorbringen, sind
nun höchst mannigfaltiger Natur. In erster Linie sind es hohe Tem-
peraturen, welche hier in Betracht kommen. Die ersten klassi-
schen Untersuchungen hierüber, welche die morphologische Seite des
Gegenstandes mit einem Schlage fast völlig erschöpften, hat Max
Schultze[1]) an seinem heizbaren Objecttisch angestellt. Schultze
fand, dass die verschiedensten Blutsorten bei Erwärmung auf 50 bis
52° C. amöboide Beweglichkeit und kugeligen Zerfall ihrer rothen
Elemente zeigten. Es ist dies eine so sichere organische Reaction,
dass in der That niemals gegen die Grundthatsache, dass Blut durch

1) Archiv f. mikr. Anat. I. S. 1.

3

ÜBER DEN ZUSAMMENHANG

VON

HERZ- UND NIEREN-KRANKHEITEN.

VON

DR. L. TRAUBE.

BERLIN, 1856.

VERLAG VON AUGUST HIRSCHWALD.

** Unter den Linden, Ecke der Schadow-Str.

Fig. 1. Frontispiece of Senator's textbook [6].
Fig. 2. Original report of Gumprecht on fragmentation of erythrocytes in hematuria of renal origin [7].
Fig. 3. Frontispiece of Traube's monograph [9].

Further refinement of diagnostic procedures had to await the introduction of light microscopy which led to a sudden burst of activity. Within a few years, the reports of Simon [1], Nasse [2], Henle [3] and particularly the monumental monograph *Die Bright'sche Nierenkrankheit* by Frerichs [4] led to recognition of the major constituents of urinary sediment. The early authors correctly assumed that clots arose by precipitation of protein and fibrin (so-called Faserstoff), which gelled within the tubules and trapped tubular cells, cellular debris and erythrocytes [4, 5]. By 1896, Hermann Senator, the forerunner of Franz Volhard, had produced his famous standard textbook *Die Erkrankungen der Nieren (The Diseases of the Kidney)* [6]. Senator was born in Gnesen (then Polish Prussia), had trained with the physiologist Johannes Müller and with Schönlein and Traube, and became director of the famous Charité Hospital in Berlin. In his textbook (fig. 1) he wrote:

'All cylinders in urine owe their shape to the transit through the tubules. They are derived from the kidney and are indicative of renal disease ... The cells which constitute the cylinders are mostly the tubular epithelial cells and the red blood cells. White blood cells are only infrequently the sole constituents of cylinders, but they are very often found as admixture to other types of epithelia, because they stick easily to the viscous substrate.'

A lucid comment on hyalin cylinders is particularly illustrative:

'There remain only two potential sources for the protein substance in hyalin cylinders namely protein from blood serum and from epithelial cells of the tubules.'

From several lines of reasoning, Senator concluded that coagulation of the proteins of blood serum cannot be the cause of hyalin cylinders. He then proceeded to state that:

'The epithelia through some kind of secretion provide the material for the formation of hyalin cylinders.'

It is only necessary to add the word Tamm-Horsfall glycoprotein to reach the present-day concept.

In connection with the recent interest in dysmorphic erythrocytes, it is worth mentioning Senator's statement:

'A very important sign of renal hematuria according to Gumprecht is fragmentation of red blood cells which is not found in hematuria arising from below the kidney' (fig. 2) [7].

By the end of the 19th century not only morphologic, but also chemical analysis of urine had greatly advanced. For example, in 1892 Salkowsky and Leube stated in their famous textbook *Lehre vom Harn* [8]:

'Examinations yielded the result that it is not only serum albumin which transits into urine, but also the second protein in blood serum, the serum globulin, which appears in protein-containing urine ... Furthermore, in each normal urine one finds a mixture of two substances one a protein and one a carbohydrate body *[eines saccharifizierenden Körpers].*'

Again, if the words albuminuria, non-selective proteinuria and Tamm-Horsfall glycoprotein are added, the modern concept is reached.

Relationship between Blood Volume and Blood Pressure: Application of Physiologic Methodology to Clinical Problems

Recognition of the volume-pressure relationship may well be the most brilliant achievement relating to renal disease in 19th century Germany. Ludwig Traube was born in Silesia, and he trained with Purkinje, Müller, Skoda, Rokitansky and Schönlein. He became Professor in Berlin in 1857, and was the first Jewish physician to be employed as a Professor by the state of Prussia after the revolution of 1848.

Traube's main contribution was his monograph *Über den Zusammenhang von Herz- und Nierenkrankheiten (On the Relationship between Cardiac and Renal Diseases)* (fig. 3) [9]. He was not only an accomplished clinician, but also a brilliant experimental investigator who adapted the methodology and the concepts of Carl Ludwig's laboratory to the exploration of clinical problems. Figure 4 is an illustration of techniques used in his laboratory to study cardiovascular problems [10]. Although he made numerous discoveries, his recognition of the relationship between perfusion pressure and urinary solute excretion is the focus here, because it became the basis of the concept of the pressure-natriuresis relationship of Guyton.

Traube had been unaware of the work of Richard Bright [11] when he independently observed that renal disease was linked to hypertrophy of the heart, particularly of the left ventricle. He stated:

'It goes without saying that with shrinking of renal parenchyma the number of small blood vessels passing through it decreases as well ... The shrinking of renal parenchyma has therefore two consequences. It acts first by decreasing the blood volume which flows out in a given time from the arterial system into the venous system. It will secondly act by decreasing the amount of liquid which at the same time is removed from the arterial system as urinary secretion ... As a result of both these conditions, particularly because of the latter, the mean pressure of the arterial system must increase. Consequently

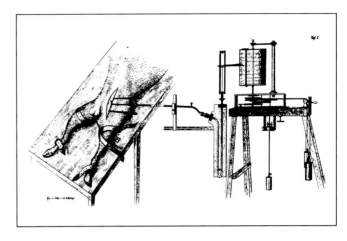

Fig. 4. Experimental apparatus for studying cardiovascular problems, as described by Traube [10].

again, an increase in resistance is produced which opposes the emptying of the left ventricle. It becomes enlarged and the enlargement is accompanied gradually by an increase in the primitive muscle bundles constituting the wall' [10].

The clear logic of his reasoning is illustrated by the following argument:

'... a priori two interpretations are possible. First, that the renal degeneration is a product of the cardiac affection. Second, that both diseases are the common result of an unknown cause.'

He gives reasons against the second possibility and ends by saying:

'This explanation is also inconsistent with the fact that often only the left ventricle is affected [as he had astutely noted]. According to our view one should expect that hypertrophy and dilatation of the left ventricle act in a compensatory manner.'

He had clearly recognized that ventricular hypertrophy maintained circulatory homeostasis at a higher level of pressure. Traube then gives a case report and ends by stating:

'With the increase of the work capacity of the left ventricle, the pressures of the arterial system rose. With this tension the amount of blood flowing off into the venous system and what is more important, the amount of urine increased.'

This is not far from the concepts of Guyton and Hall.

Heterogeneity of Bright's Disease: The Emerging Concept of Glomerulonephritis

Finally, it is worth pointing to the conceptual changes undergone by the notion of 'nephritis' in Germany in the 19th century. Both Bright [12] and Pierre François Rayer [13] had recognized and described renal disease on a macroscopic level, but little was known of the nature of the renal and glomerular lesions at the light microscopic level. With technical progress, particularly the introduction of the microscope as an investigative tool and technologies for tissue staining, an explosion occurred within 1–2 decades. To the authors' knowledge, Gluge [14] was the first to find *Entzündungskugeln,* or inflammatory granules, which he identified as the inflamed Malpighian bodies or glomeruli. He felt that the microvasculature was the primary site of injury and inflammation. This conclusion found support in the later observations of Valentin [15], and in rapid succession important contributions were made by Hecht [16], Henle and Pfeufer [3] and particularly by Reinhardt [17] in the Charité.

It is scarcely surprising that the primary site of injury was a matter of contention, as investigators had to rely on their acumen to reconstruct the sequence of events leading to the findings at autopsy. Interstitial fibrosis was felt to be the *primum movens* in Bright's disease by Henle and Pfeufer [3], as was also taught across the channel by Toynbee [18]. Henle was born in Fürth, was first Professor in Zürich, then had the good judgement to go to Heidelberg and finally worked in Göttingen. He was the founder of the famous *Zeitschrift für Rationelle Medizin,* which introduced science into medicine at a time when this was still felt to be revolutionary. In the first issue of this journal, he and Pfeufer described a 25-year-old woman who died with anasarca. They stated:

'One saw fatty vacuoles in long streaks along the tubules. In addition, one saw pale smooth fibers with a fusiform nucleus. Where the fibers accumulated in large masses the contours of the tubules became indistinct.'

This is followed by the gigantic blunder: 'The Malpighian bodies were not changed' – undoubtedly the result of the poor quality of the microscopes at that time.

Rudolf Virchow, who did not have an all-consuming interest in the kidney, felt that the tubular parenchyma was the site of primary injury [19], a view violently attacked by Traube [20], who still felt years after Henle that the interstitial lesion came first.

An entirely different view was introduced by Reinhardt in the Charité [17] and subsequently by Friedrich Theodor Frerichs [4]. Frerichs was born in East Frisia, was Professor in Göttingen and Breslau and was finally the successor of Schönlein in Berlin. In his main work, the monumental monograph *Die Bright'sche Nierenkrankheit und deren Behandlung,* he gave a lucid analysis of glomerulonephritis, based on histologic studies. In the introduction he stated:

'There are few items in pathology where anatomic analysis was tried with less success than in Bright's disease.'

He ascribed this to the lack of insight into 'innere genetische Zusammenhänge' or (loosely translated) into causal relationships. He obtained remarkable insights by interpreting anatomy in the light of putative changes in glomerular physiology. He reasoned that:

'The composition of the filtrate must depend on the height of the hydrostatic pressure as well as on the quality and the pore size of the glomerular capillary wall ... When the Malpighian body is inflamed one would expect first increased filtration *[vermehrte Durchschwitzung],* subsequently permeation of substances which fail to permeate under conditions of normal pressure, initially proteins, later fibrinogen *[Faserstoff].* Finally the walls of the capillaries rupture and blood as such will leave the vessels.'

This analysis of events would not be out of place in a modern textbook. To return to the topic of the primary site of injury, he also reasoned that this was the glomerulus with a remarkable argument:

'The disturbances of transudation will be observed first in that part of the renal capillary system which under normal conditions has to withstand the highest pressure, i.e. the vascular Malpighian bodies.'

This observation could be interpreted as an early insight into the concept of glomerular capillary hypertension. Frerichs recognized that the different microscopic appearances of Bright's disease represent stages of an evolving process. He distinguished the stage of hyperemia and exudation, followed by the stage of metamorphosis of the exudate, and finally the stage of atrophy.

The term glomerulonephritis was apparently first coined by Klebs in Bern [21]. Born in Königsberg, Klebs became Professor in Bern, Würzburg, Prague, Zürich and finally worked in Chicago's Rush Medical College. At approximately the same time, his colleague Langhans lucidly described the glomerular lesions in the 'acute nephritis' of infectious disease [22].

Limitations of space do not permit a detailed description of the various efforts to classify Bright's disease, or glomerulonephritis as it was later called following the suggestion of Klebs. Suffice it to mention the classification of nephritis adopted by 1896 in the textbook on *Diseases of the Kidney* by Senator [6], in which 'Die hämatogene, nicht eitrige Nierenentzündung "Bright'sche Nierenkrankheit"' (hematogenous non-purulent renal inflammation) was subdivided into the categories of acute nephritis, chronic diffuse non-indurative and chronic indurative nephritis (*Schrumpfniere* or contracted kidneys). It is easy to see that this classification directly led to the ideas that crystalized into the famous monograph by Franz Volhard and Theodor Fahr in 1914 – *Die*

Bright'sche Nierenkrankheit – Klinik, Pathologie und Atlas' [23].

There is no better way to pay tribute to the genius of our predecessors in the last century, who under the most primitive technical conditions achieved insights of lasting value, than to quote Arthur Schopenhauer, according to whom the creative intellect is distinguished by the ability:

'to think something which no one has ever thought of before, whilst seeing something which everyone is able to see *(etwas zu denken, was niemand zuvor gedacht hat, wenn er etwas sieht, das jeder sieht).*'

References

1 Simon JF: Über eigentümliche Formen im Harnsediment bei M. Bright. Arch Anat Physiol Wiss Med 1843;28–30.

2 Nasse: Med Congress Blatt Rhein Westf Ärzte 1843.

3 Henle J, Pfeufer C: Morbus Bright, klinische Mitteilungen. Z Rationelle Med Zürich 1844.

4 Frerichs FT: Die Bright'sche Nierenkrankheit und deren Behandlung. Braunschweig, Vieweg, 1851.

5 Heller F: Die pathologisch-chemische Untersuchung zur medizinischen Diagnose; in Van Gaalen G (ed): Physikalische Diagnostik. Vienna, vol 2, 1845, table 1.

6 Senator H: Die Erkrankungen der Nieren. Spezielle Pathologie und Therapie. Vienna, Hrsg. Hofrath Nothnagel, 1896, 19 Band I.

7 Gumprecht F: Die Fragmentation der rothen Blutkörperchen und ihre Bedeutung für die Diagnose der Hämaturie. Dtsch Arch Klin Med 1894;11:53, 45.

8 Salkowski E, Leube W: Die Lehre vom Harn; in Hirschwald A (ed): Berlin, 1892.

9 Traube L: Über den Zusammenhang von Herz- und Nierenkrankheiten. Berlin, August Hirschwald, 1854.

10 Traube L: Zur Pathologie der Nierenkrankheiten. Ges Beitr 1870;2:966 (originally published in Allge Med Centralzeitung, 29 February 1860).

11 Ritz E, Zeier M, Lundin P: French and German nephrologists in the mid 19th century. Am J Nephrol 1989;9:167–172.

12 Bright R: Reports of Medical Cases Selected with a View to Illustrating the Symptoms and Cure of Diseases by a Reference to Morbid Anatomy. London, Longman Green, vol 1, 1827.

13 Rayer PFO: Traité des Maladies des Reins. Paris, Ballière, 3 vols and atlas, 1837–1840, vol 2, Passini.

14 Gluge F: Anatomisch-mikroskopische Untersuchungen zur allgemeinen und speziellen Pathologie. Jena, vol 2, 1842, pp 126–131.

15 Valentin F: Repetitorium für Anatomie und Physiologie. Bern, Huber, vol 2, 1837, pp 290–291.

16 Hecht: De Renibus in Morbo Brightii Degeneratis. Dissertatio Inauguralis Medica. Berolini, 1839.

17 Reinhardt B: Zur Kenntnis der Bright'schen Krankheit. Ann Charité-Krankenhauses Berlin 1850;1:S185.

18 Toynbee J: On the intimate structure of the human kidney and on the changes of its several component parts under Bright's disease. Med Chir Trans 1846;29:304–326.

19 Virchow R: Über die parenchymatöse Entzündung. Virchows Arch Pathol Anat Physiol 1852;4:260–324.

20 Traube L: Über die Speckentartungen der Nieren. Spezielle Pathologie und Therapie, gesammelte Beiträge. Allge Med Centralzeitung 1858;27:S373–377.

21 Klebs E: Handbuch der pathologischen Anatomie. Berlin, August Hirschwald, 1868, vol 1.

22 Langhans TH: Über die entzündlichen Veränderungen der Glomeruli und die akute Nephritis. Arch Klin Med 1885;99:193–250.

23 Volhard F, Fahr T: Die Bright'sche Nierenkrankheit. Klinik Pathologie und Atlas. Berlin, Springer, 1914.

Am J Nephrol 1994;14:448–451

Natale Gaspare De Santo [a]
Maria Gaetana Lamendola [b]

[a] Chair of Nephrology, Department of
Pediatrics, 2nd University of Naples,
Naples,
[b] Institute of Morbid Anatomy,
2nd University of Naples, Naples, Italy

Luciano Armanni

Key Words
Armanni-Ebstein lesion
Diabetes mellitus
Tuberculosis
Caseous lesion
Renal disease

Abstract

Luciano Armanni (1839–1903) worked as an assistant to Schrön in Naples after graduating in medicine. He was later appointed as Professor of Histopathology, and in 1887 became a full professor. During his life he was Dissector of the Anatomic Institute of the Ospedale degli Incurabili and later director of this hospital. He founded many institutions, including the Cotugno Hospital, but died poor and suffering from diabetes mellitus and tuberculosis, contracted during a post-mortem examination. Armanni is given credit for discovering the contagious nature and specificity of the lesions due to caseous material in tuberculosis, and also the renal lesion in diabetes mellitus that now bears his name (Armanni-Ebstein lesion).

Introduction

In their chapter on diabetic nephropathy, Arieff and Myers state that the only specific tubulointerstitial lesion is the Armanni-Ebstein lesion [1]. This lesion is characterized by pale-staining, glycogen-rich cells in the pars recta of the proximal tubule. Although this was a common autopsy finding in the pre-insulin era, it is seldom seen today [2]. This paper gives a brief profile of the man who discovered the lesion in 1872.

The Life of Luciano Armanni

Luciano Armanni (fig. 1) was born in Naples on 7 March 1839. He first studied at the Scolopi and then as a private student [3]. At the age of 15 years he graduated in literature at the University of Naples. Subsequently, he enrolled in the Faculty of Medicine, graduating in 1861.

From 1864 to 1867 he was an assistant of Otto von Schrön. Of German origin, Schrön (fig. 2) had moved to Italy from his native Hoff after studying under the guidance of Rassirt, Kussmaul and Thiersch, graduating in Munich in 1863. After spending 1 year in Turin, he moved to Naples where the Honorary Chair of Pathologic Anatomy was conferred on him in 1864. Schrön's lectures were said to have attracted the Neapolitan medical profession as well as medical students.

Because of lack of space, the Italian Government rented a 6-room flat in the same building where Schrön lived, and in this flat he worked with 2 assistants and 2 technicians. In 1865, while working as chief technician with Schrön, Armanni founded the Society for Physicians and Naturalists in Naples and became director of its journal, which represented an important forum for the cultural meeting of Neapolitan biology and medicine. This society is still active in Naples today under the name of Societa di Scienze, Lettere ed Arti.

Natale Gaspare De Santo, MD
University of Naples
Policlinico Cappella Cangiani
Via Pansini 5
I–80131 Naples (Italy)

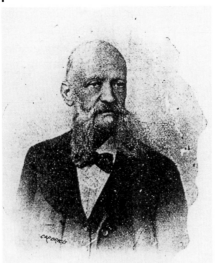

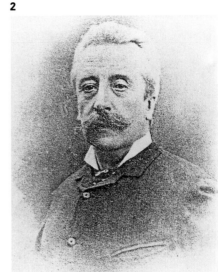

Fig. 1. Luciano Armanni [3].
Fig. 2. Otto von Schrön [3].

In 1867, encouraged by Schrön, Armanni went to Germany, first to Munich with Pettenkofer and then to Berlin with Virchow. On his return to Naples, the Faculty of Medicine in Naples nominated him as Professor of Histopathology with an annually renewable contract. This post was held by him until 1887, when he was officially appointed Full Professor of Histopathology. It should be mentioned that in 1883 Armanni received an invitation to the Chair of Histopathology at the University of Palermo, which he declined.

Armanni was also Dissector of the Anatomic Institute of the Ospedale degli Incurabili (fig. 3) and subsequently became director of this hospital [3]. The Ospedale degli Incurabili is a very old and famous institution in Naples, and is where Professor Moscato, who was canonized by Pope John Paul II, worked.

During his lifetime Armanni discharged many public duties. He founded the Cotugno Hospital, the Health Office and the Institute for Chemical and Bacteriologic Control of the city of Naples. He was also President of the College Vittorio Emanuele II, a member of the National Committees for Universities and for Hospital Control and recipient of many awards. He died a poor man, however, suffering from diabetes mellitus and tuberculosis, contracted during post-mortem procedures on 15 March 1903.

Although he had instructed that on his death there should be 'neither flowers, nor speeches', his funeral was attended by vast crowds with speeches delivered by great personalities from the world of science and politics, and several dedicatory marble busts were erected at the Acad-

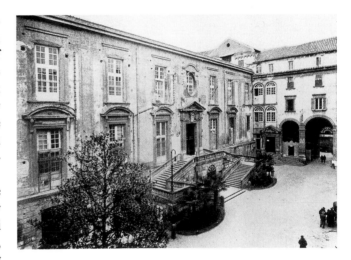

Fig. 3. The Ospedale degli Incurabili in Naples [8].

emy, the Ospedali Riuniti and the Ospedale degli Incurabili. A hospital ward at the Cotugno Hospital was named after him, as also was a public school [4].

Among his obituaries must be recorded the one of Marussia Bakunin [5], a participant in the intellectual life of Naples. Bakunin wrote of him:

'Rebel against factious organizations, fruit of partisan strife: rebel scientist, bringing to an old world the spirit of innovation and geniality which is present in every one of his works. Each of them would deserve careful examination for its insight, the admirable technique it followed, for the severe criticism of the results of his own experiments, for his kindly judgement of other people's experiments, and for the wonderful intuition for truth.'

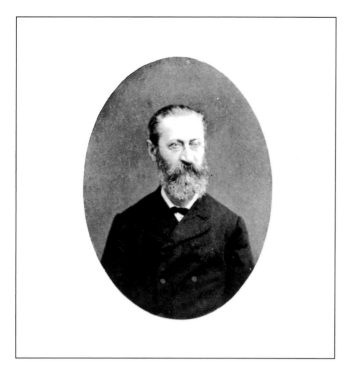

Fig. 4. Arnaldo Cantani.

In 1971, during the centenary of his research into tuberculosis, a meeting was convened in his honor [6] at which numerous tributes were paid to his work and person. Among the most interesting is the one by Califano, Dean of the Faculty of Medicine in Naples, who wrote:

'What a scientist cannot discover is sooner or later discovered by others. Creative works on the other hand are for evermore associated with the name of the artist, who indeed becomes personified by them. Hence, the twin name Gioconda–Leonardo, Dante–Comedy, etc. Thus a scientist who has made a great discovery is inexorably linked with oblivion. It is true, however, that today one feels a moral obligation for the cultural debt, and the heroes of knowledge are often venerated and their memory perpetuated.'

The Contributions of Armanni to Science

Armanni is given credit for 2 great discoveries. First, he showed the contagious nature and the specificity of the lesions due to caseous material from patients who died from tuberculosis [7]. The results were obtained in guinea-pig cornea and lent support to Villemin, who had been

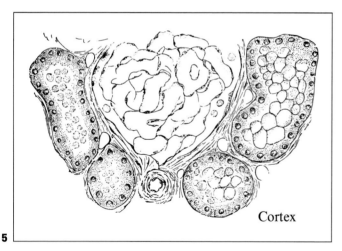

5

Fig. 5, 6. '(1) The cortex of the Bowman capsule undergoes an almost twofold enlargement. The glomerular tuft is also enlarged, and consists of dilated capillaries showing a diameter three times greater than that of normal people; (2) In the medulla, the pars recta of the tubules undergoes peculiar changes. The cells appear dilated with thickened membranes and undergo a process of hypertrophy. Finally, they appear as large, polygonal, epithelial cells filled with hyaline material' [2, 9].

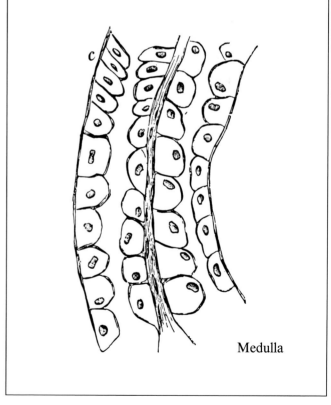

6

severely criticized when he had proposed such a hypothesis.

Secondly, the name of Armanni, who made the 1st discovery of the renal lesion in diabetes mellitus (1872), is linked to that of Ebstein, who observed the cells in 1882 (Armanni-Ebstein lesion), and to that of Ehrlich, who saw them in 1893, so that it was formerly known as the Armanni-Ebstein-Ehrlich lesion. Armanni's discovery was made under rather fortunate circumstances. The diabetic lesion was described by Armanni as a result of his autopsy studies performed on 20 February, 11 and 14 March 1872. He had been asked to perform the post-mortem examinations of patients who had died at the Department of Medicine directed by Professor Arnaldo Cantani (fig. 4), who greatly appreciated his work. Cantani was already a famous internist [8], well-known abroad through the German translations of his textbooks. When the autopsy results were available, Cantani asked Armanni to discuss his findings with the students of the internal medicine course. In the following year, a description appeared in Cantani's textbook (figs. 5 and 6) [2].

The primacy of this discovery is attributed to Cantani in Charcot's textbook.

The cells were more recently described by Richtie and Waugh [10] as having cytoplasmic inclusions of glycogen. Zollinger and Mihatsch in 1978 observed Armanni-Ebstein cells in patients who died from diabetes mellitus while their blood glucose level was above 500 mg/dl [11]. In their experience, the cells were high, clear, polygonal and with a foamy cytoplasm. In addition, the cells were full of glycogen, which it was possible to demonstrate with specific stains. On electron microscopy, giant cystic lysosomes rich in glycogen were shown by autoradiography. Glycogen was also shown as a free cytoplasmic inclusion by Ditscherlein and Marx [12] in cells which after removal of glycogen appeared empty.

References

1 Arieff AI, Myers BD: Diabetic nephropathy; in Brenner BM, Rector F (eds): The Kidney, 2nd ed. Philadelphia, Saunders, 1981, pp 1909.

2 Armanni L: Di alcune lesioni nel diabete. Analisi istologica; in Cantani A (ed): Patologia e Terapia del Ricambio Materiale. Milan, Vallardi, 1875, pp 301–310.

3 Miraglia B: L'anatomia patologica nella scuola medica napoletana. Ann Med Navale Tropicale 1956;61:1–8.

4 Associazione Napoletana di Medici e Naturalisti: Studii e Ricerche del Prof. L Armanni. Naples, G ed A Morano, 1904.

5 Bakunin M: Luciano Armanni. Atti Accademia Pontaniana 1906;36:3–8.

6 Blasi A, Catena E: Il Contagio nella Tubercolosi all'Epoca Attuale. Naples, November 1971.

7 Armanni L: Specificità e virulenza delle sostanze caseose e tubercolosi; in Movimento Medico Chirurgico. Naples, A Trani, 1872, pp 1–44.

8 Cutolo A: Storia dell'Università di Napoli. Verona, Mondadori, 1923.

9 Giordano C, De Santo NG, Lamendola MG, Capodicasa G: The genesis of the Armanni-Ebstein lesion in diabetic nephropathy. J Diabetic Complications 1987;1:2–3.

10 Richtie S, Waugh D: The pathology of the Armanni-Ebstein lesion in diabetic nephropathy. Am J Pathol 1957;31:1035–1040.

11 Zollinger HU, Mihatsch MJ: Renal Pathology in Biopsy. New York, Springer, 1978.

12 Ditscherlein G, Marx I: Feinstruktur der Armanni-Ebstein-Zellen. Z Mikrosk Anat Forsch 1969;80:485.

Am J Nephrol 1994;14:452–457

Giovanni B. Fogazzi[a]
J. Stewart Cameron[b]
Eberhard Ritz[c]
Claudio Ponticelli[a]

[a] Division of Nephrology and Dialysis, Ospedale Maggiore, IRCCS, Milan, Italy;
[b] Guy's Campus, United Medical and Dental Schools, London, UK;
[c] Renal Unit, Department of Internal Medicine, Ruperto Carola University, Heidelberg, Germany

The History of Urinary Microscopy to the End of the 19th Century

Key Words
Urinalysis
Urinary sediment
Urinary microscopy

Abstract
In the 17th and 18th centuries, several authors performed urinary microscopy occasionally and were often unable to give their observations a practical diagnostic application. Such men included De Peiresc, Boerhaave, Ledermüller and Galeazzi. In the 1st half of the 19th century, however, urinary microscopy began to be used systematically. Rayer and Vigla identified for the first time elements other than crystals in urine and contributed to the methodology of handling samples for microscopy. Becquerel described dysmorphic erythrocytes, and Simon and Henle observed casts in urine and in histological preparations. In contrast, Bird mentioned casts only in passing, though he described many other elements and published the first complete book on urinary microscopy. The 2nd half of the 19th century was characterized by further advances, and in the book of Beale tubular cells were distinguished from other epithelial cells. Different types of casts were also linked with different renal diseases. By 1875 the classification of casts was complete. The work of the 19th century microscopists culminated in Rieder's book on clinical microscopy, which described each element of urinary sediment through 36 beautiful chromolithographic plates.

Introduction

The only available study devoted to the history of urinary microscopy was written by one of the present authors as an introduction to a recent book on urinary sediment [1]. The present paper, which is an interim account of research not yet completed, arose from that brief work.

Even though the history of urinary microscopy, like every other history, developed as a continuum, the material has been assembled into three distinct sections. Each deals with a different historical period, which in turn reflects a different approach to urinary microscopy.

17th and 18th Centuries: the Unaware Pioneers

This section includes early authors who performed urinary microscopy occasionally rather than in a framework of systematic studies, and who were often unable to give to their observation(s) practical diagnostic application (table 1).

Nicholas Claude Fabri de Peiresc (1580–1637)

This Provençal amateur of science and art had several cultural interests ranging from astronomy to anatomy, but he was not a physician or a surgeon [2]. Despite this, how-

Giovanni B. Fogazzi, MD
Divisione di Nefrologia e Dialisi
Ospedale Maggiore, IRCCS
Via Commenda 15
I–20122 Milano (Italy)

ever, he was probably the first to use a microscope to examine urine. This information is found in the biography of De Peiresc written by his close friend, the philosopher Pierre Gassendi [3]. Peiresc was able to see that 'calcolous sand' observed in a urine specimen appeared 'like a heap of rhomboical bricks' under the microscope. Very brilliantly, he also observed that because the bricks had acute angles, they might cause irritation and pain in their passage with urine.

Hermann Boerhaave (1668–1738)

This celebrated Hippocratic Dutch doctor also examined urine under the microscope in order to determine whether or not the urine of normal subjects contained the 'rudiments' of urinary stones [4]. The urine was carefully examined at different intervals after micturition, and with different types of microscope. 'Corpuscles similar to little flocks of wool' were first seen, followed by: 'streaks similar to those observed when wine is added to water,' and then by: 'extremely minute shining concreted little crumbs'. After standing for 24 h, rhomboidal crystals finally appeared at the bottom of the tube. These observations enabled Boerhaave to conclude that all the elements of urinary stones are contained in normal urine, and that crystals are the very core of stones [5].

Martin Frobenius Ledermüller (1719–1769)

Obviously, urine could not escape the curiosity of the early 18th century microscopists. Thus, Ledermüller, a German born in Nuremberg and author of several books on microscopy [6], analysed urine. He presented his findings in table XV titled *Ein Tropfen Urin (One drop of urine)* of his *Mikroskopischer Gemüts und Augen Ergötzung,* which was published in 3 volumes in 1760–1762 (fig. 1) [7]. Interestingly, Ledermüller commented that the 'salts' he saw were not always the same, and this depended on what the subject had been drinking. He also noted that different elements could be observed in the same subject at different times.

Domenico Gusmano Galeazzi (1686–1775)

Urinary microscopy was also used to study diseases, as in the case of an Italian woman, who presented with black urine and sweat and black skin (a case of alkaptonuria?). The case was beautifully described by Galeazzi, who was a distinguished anatomist [8]. Microscopy was performed by a colleague of his, Benedetto Donelli, who saw in the urine: 'extremely minute globules, mingled with acicular saline crystals'.

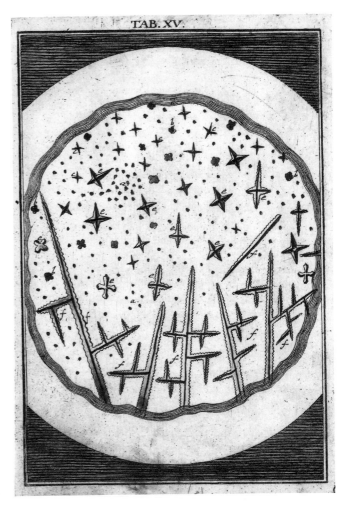

Fig. 1. Table XV from Ledermüller's book [7]. It shows several types of crystals and the transformations they underwent under the microscope. With permission from the Biblioteca Braidense, Milan.

Table 1. Urinary microscopy in the 17th and 18th centuries

Author	Year	Country	Urine	Finding
De Peiresc	1630	France	Sandy	'Rhomboidal bricks'
Boerhaave*	1743	Holland	Normal	'Grains of the figure of rhombi'
Ledermüller	1760	Germany	Normal	Crystals
Galeazzi	1783†	Italy	Black	Globules and crystals

* Boerhaave died in 1738, but the book quoted in the text (reference 5) appeared in 1743.

† Galeazzi died in 1775, but the paper quoted in the text (reference 8) only appeared in 1783.

Table 2. The main contributions to urinary microscopy in the 1st half of the 19th century

Author	Year	Country	Contribution
Vigla and Rayer	1837–38	France	Foundation of clinical urinary microscopy
Becquerel	1841	France	'Irregular' erythrocytes in Bright's disease
Simon	1842	Germany	Casts in Bright's disease
Henle	1842	Germany	Casts in both urine and tubules in Bright's disease
Bird	1844	England	First book devoted to urinary deposits
Johnson	1846	England	Lipid particles in Bright's disease

Table 3. Some of the main contributions to urinary microscopy in the 2nd half of the 19th century

Author	Year	Country	Contribution
Frerichs	1854	Germany	Leucine and tyrosine crystals in acute liver atrophy
Beale	1869	England	Cholesterol crystals in fatty degeneration of the kidney
Harley	1872	England	'Nucleated' erythrocytes in Bright's disease
Rovida	1870	Italy	'Albuminoid' nature of the casts
Tyson	1880	USA	Scanty urinary sediment in renal amyloidosis
Rieder	1898	Germany	Comprehensive book on urinary microscopy

1st Half of the 19th Century: the Founders of Scientific Urinary Microscopy

This section concerns the authors who first used urinary microscopy systematically and/or routinely. This enabled them to identify several new elements and to outline classifications of their urinary findings, which were then correlated with the clinical features of the patients. The main discoveries came over a very short period of time, indicating a burgeoning of studies in the field of urinary microscopy, spreading through different European countries (table 2).

Pierre Rayer (1793–1867) and Eugène Napoléon Vigla (1813–1872)

Credit must be given to Rayer and Vigla, who worked in Rayer's group, for being the first to perform urinary microscopy routinely for the patients they saw at the Hôpital la Charité in Paris [9]. Their findings, reported both in the *Traité des Maladies des Reins* [10] and in journals [11] in the late 1830s, are relevant for many reasons. They identified for the first time elements other than crystals in the urine, e.g. epithelial scales, mucous globules, pus cells, blood corpuscles and lipid, and described microscopic haematuria and urinary findings in physiological and pathological conditions, e.g. acute and chronic albuminous nephritis and acute and chronic pyelitis. Moreover, they made important methodological contributions by indicating how to handle urine samples and how to examine them under the microscope, and by suggesting that the microscopic findings should always be matched with chemical tests and vice versa.

Alfred Becquerel (1814–1866)

Again in France, and only a few years after the papers of Rayer and Vigla, Becquerel published an important book on urine [12]. Microscopy and physicochemical studies were routinely applied to a large spectrum of disorders, for most of which Becquerel had personal data. Special emphasis was placed on Bright's disease, and interestingly, Becquerel noted that in this condition urinary erythrocytes are: 'presque toujours irréguliers, déformés' ('almost always irregular, deformed'). This probably represents the first report of dysmorphic erythrocytes in glomerular diseases.

Johann Franz Simon (1807–1843) and Jacob Henle (1809–1885)

The authors do not yet know exactly who first described casts in urine [1], but Simon was surely among the very first. He described them in a book devoted to animal chemistry, which contains a large chapter on urinalysis, and which was published in Berlin in 1842 and translated into English in 1845–1846 [13]. It may be relevant to his discovery that Simon, a chemist but not a physician, was a constant attendant at Schönlein's ward at the Charité Hospital in Berlin, where his services were highly valued [14]. Simon distinguished 'amorphous', 'granular', and 'cellular' casts (fig. 2) and noted that very commonly they were: 'contemporaneous with a certain amount of albumin in the urine'. In the same period, another important contribution was that of Jacob Henle, who observed casts not only in urine but also in histological preparations [15].

John William Griffith (1819?–1901) and Golding Bird (1814–1854)

Griffith included 2 tables of urinary microscopy (not mentioning casts, however) in his booklet devoted to blood and other secretions, which appeared in 1843 in England [16]. Interestingly, this book was dedicated to Bird, a physician at Guy's Hospital in London and the author of the first complete book on urinary microscopy, which was published in 1844 [17]. Bird described a long list of elements: crystals, blood corpuscles, pus and mucous globules, epithelium, milk, fatty matter, spermatozoa, torulae and vibriones. Moreover, he saw: 'large and small organic globules', the exact nature of which was unclear to him (as well as to the present authors!), but which stimulated subsequent research [18]. Casts, by contrast, were only incidentally mentioned as a discovery of Simon's.

George Owen Rees (1813–1889)

Rees also worked at Guy's Hospital and dealt with urinary microscopy. This appeared, however, only in the 1845 edition of his book on the analysis of blood and urine [19], while urinary microscopy was not mentioned in the 1st edition, which appeared in 1836. This fact shows clearly that the historical watershed for urinary microscopy may be defined as 1835–1840 and probably resulted from the publication of the French studies.

George Johnson (1818–1896)

Rees was one of Richard Bright's team, as also was Johnson [20, 21], who described lipid particles in the urine of patients with renal disease in 1846 [22]. Thus, even though the celebrated Bright did not mention urinary microscopy in his classical works on renal disease, it is likely that he knew about it from the 2nd half of the 5th decade.

Mark Aurelius Hoefle (?–1855)

From a book on the role of *Chemistry and Microscopy at the Patient's Bedside,* written by the German Hoefle and published in 1850, it can be discovered that by that time casts were considered a typical finding in Bright's disease, even though they could also be found in other disorders [23].

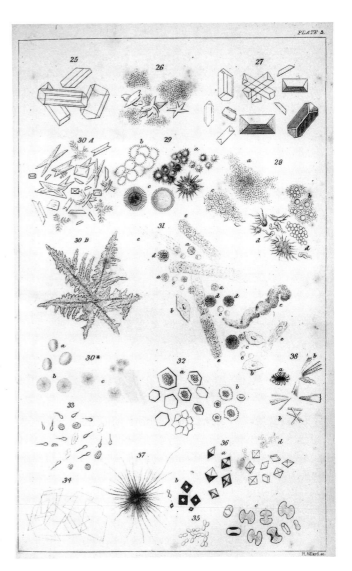

Fig. 2. Different types of casts (31e) shown, probably for the first time, in plate 3 of Simon's book [13]. With permission from the Wellcome Institute Library, London.

2nd Half of the 19th Century: Towards Definition

This period was characterized by further advances in urinary microscopy. Microscopes improved greatly and allowed a better examination of urine. The classification of the formed elements of urine became more and more similar to what is known today, even though the nature of some elements remained unclear. The correlations between the urinary abnormalities and the other clinical parameters became more and more evident (table 3).

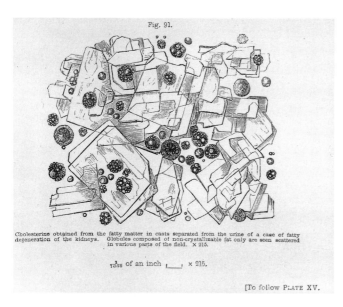

Fig. 91.

Cholesterine obtained from the fatty matter in casts separated from the urine of a case of fatty
degeneration of the kidneys. Globules composed of non-crystallizable fat only are seen scattered
in various parts of the field. × 215.

$\frac{1}{1000}$ of an inch ⌐___⌐ × 215.

[To follow PLATE XV.

Fig. 3. Cholesterol crystals as seen in fatty degeneration of the kidney. From plate XVI of Beale's book [24]. With permission from the Wellcome Institute Library, London).

Lionel S. Beale (1828–1906)

Beale devoted several parts of his book of 1869 on kidney diseases to urinary microscopy [24]. Fine details about the use of the microscope and the handling of urine were given and a very extensive list of elements, all superbly illustrated (fig. 3). Tubular cells, unlike previous descriptions, were distinguished from other epithelial cells. Different types of casts were recognized in different renal disease, e.g. epithelial casts and casts containing blood globules in acute nephritis, granular casts in chronic nephritis, and 'oily' casts in fatty degeneration of the kidney.

Other Workers

Similar findings were reported by George Harley (1829–1896) in his book on urine, published in 1872 [25]. Interestingly, Harley gave credit to Beale for being the first to describe 'cholesterin' in fatty degeneration of the kidney, and to Friedrich Theodor Frerichs (1819–1885) for being the first to recognize the diagnostic value of leucine crystals in the urine of patients with acute liver atrophy. Frerichs described this finding in a paper which appeared in 1854 [26]. Harley, moreover, while reporting on the urinary sediment findings in Bright's disease, described 'nucleated blood corpuscles', which clearly correspond to dysmorphic erythrocytes and acanthocytes as seen in the urine of patients with glomerular disease.

In 1875 the classification of casts was quite complete (and very similar to the present day), and it was well recognized that they were formed in the tubules of the kidneys. Their nature, however, was very unclear. Henle considered casts to be the result of fibrinous intratubular coagulation, while others, e.g. the Italian Carlo Rovida (1844–1877), considered them to be 'albuminoid' elements [27]. This problem continued unresolved for many years afterwards, as the main constituent protein of the casts was discovered by Tamm and Horsfall only in 1950 [28].

The North American James Tyson (1841–1919), who had by 1880 accumulated a 15-year experience on urinary microscopy, extended urinary investigation beyond Bright's disease and found scanty sediments, containing only a few casts, in 'lardaceana or amyloid degeneration of the kidney' and in patients with mild isolated proteinuria [29]. This is still considered to be true today.

At the turn of the century, in 1898, Hermann Rieder (1858–1932) published a valuable book on the clinical microscopy of urine [30]. Through 36 beautiful chromolithographic plates, each element of the urinary sediment was clearly described, and the patterns seen in the main diseases of the urinary tract were identified, forming the culmination of 19th century investigations.

Then the 20th century came. No wonder that with these solid foundations, it also brought further improvements and new ideas, and with them the awareness that urinary microscopy is a simple but valuable tool for the study of urinary tract diseases.

Acknowledgements

We would like to thank Professor Gabriel Richet for assistance in the gathering of material for this paper.

References

1 Cameron JS: Introduction; in Fogazzi GB, Passerini P, Ponticelli C, Ritz E (eds): The Urinary sediment. An Integrated View. London, Chapman and Hall, 1994, pp 1–10.

2 Brown H: Peiresc Nicholaus Claude Fabri de; in Gillispie CC (ed): Dictionary of Scientific Biography. New York, Scribner, 1974, vol 10, pp 488–492.

3 Gassendus P: Viri Illustris Nicolai Claudii Fabricii de Peiresc, Senatoris Aquisextiensis Vita, per Petrum Gassendum, Philosophum et Matheseos Professorem Parisiensem. Hagae Comitis, Adriani Vlach, 1651, p 150.

4 Van Swieten G: The Commentaries upon the Aphorisms of Dr Hermann Boerhaave, the Late Learned Professor of Physics in the University of Leiden, Concerning the Knowledge and Cure of Several Diseases Incident to Human Bodies. Translated into English. London, R Horsfield and T Longman, 1773, p 105.

5 Boerhaave H: Praelectiones Publicae de Calculo. In Consultationes Medicae (sive Sylloge Epistolarum cum Responsis Hermanni Boerhaave in Britannia Primum Editae nunc Aliquot Exemplis Auctiores, Adcesserunt eiusdem Introductio ad Praxim Clinicam et Praelectiones de Calculo). Editio Göttingensis Altera Aucta et Amendata. Göttingen, A Vandenhoeck, 1752, vol 2, pp 143–147.

6 Gurlt E, Wernich A, Hirsch A (eds): Biographisches Lexicon der hervorragenden Ärzte aller Zeiten und Völker. Munich, Urban and Schwarzenberg, 1962, vol 3, p 714.

7 Ledermüller MF: Mikroskopischer Gemüts und Augen Ergötzung. Nuremberg, C De Launcy, vol 1, 1760–1762, pp 27–28.

8 Galeazzi DG: De Morbo quodam Sudoribus, Urinisque Nigerrimis Insigni. De Bononiensi Scientiarum et Artium Institutio atque Academia Commentarii. Bononiae, Typographia Laelii A Vulpe, vol 6, 1783, pp 60–63.

9 Richet G: From Bright's disease to modern nephrology: Pierre Rayer's innovative method of clinical investigation. Kidney Int 1991;39: 787–792.

10 Rayer PFO: Traité des maladies des reins etc. 3 vols and atlas. Paris, JB Baillière, 1839–1841. Vol 1: Preface VIII–IX; and pp 58, 99, 105, 114, 116–117, 122, 133, 152–154, 178, 207; vol 2: pp 105–107, 112–116; vol 3: pp 3, 6–8.

11 Vigla EN: Etude microscopique de l'urine, éclairée par l'analyse chimique. L'Expérience 1837;12:177–190; and 1838;13:193–204.

12 Becquerel A: Séméiotique des Urines, ou Traité des Altérations de l'Urine dans les Maladies; Suivi d'un Traité de la Maladie de Bright aux Divers Ages de la Vie. Paris, Fortin, Masson, 1841.

13 Simon JF: Animal Chemistry with Reference to the Physiology and Pathology of Man. London, Sydenham Society, vol 2, 1845–1846, p 235.

14 Simon JF: Editor's preface, in Animal Chemistry with Reference to the Physiology and Pathology of Man. London, Sydenham Society, vol 1, 1845.

15 Henle FGJ: In Pfeufer C. Morbus Bright. Klinische Mitteilungen. Z Rat Med 1844;1:57–60.

16 Griffith JW: A Practical Manual, Containing a Description of the General, Chemical and Microscopical Characters of the Blood and Secretions of the Human Body etc. London, Taylor, 1843.

17 Bird G: Urinary Deposits. Their Diagnosis, Pathology, and Therapeutical Indications. London, Churchill, 1844.

18 Balfour G: On the diagnostic value of albumen in the urine. Edinb Med J 1856;1:606–624 (note 1, p 617).

19 Owen Rees G: On the Analysis of the Blood and Urine in Health and Disease; and on the Treatment of Urinary Diseases, 2nd ed. London, Longman, Brown, Green and Longman, 1845.

20 Bright P: Dr Richard Bright 1789–1858. London, Bodley Head, 1983, pp 164, 193, 196, 221, 225, 274.

21 Berry D, Mackenzie C: Richard Bright 1789–1858. Physician in an Age of Revolution and Reform. London, Royal Society of Medicine Services Ltd, 1992, pp 133, 156, 179, 202, 217, 233.

22 Johnson G: On the minute anatomy and pathology of Bright's disease of the kidney and on the relation of the renal disease to those diseases of the liver, heart and arteries with which it is associated. Med Chir Trans 1846;29:1–43.

23 Hoefle MA: La Chimica e la Microscopia al letto dell'Ammalato. Pavia, Fusi, 1856, pp 694–695 (translated from the 2nd German ed, 1850).

24 Beale LS: Kidney Diseases, Urinary Deposits, and Calcolous Disorders: Their Nature and Treatment, 3rd ed. London, Churchill, 1869, pp 95–99, 282–297, 317–396.

25 Harley G: The Urine and its Derangements, with the Application of Physiological Chemistry to the Diagnosis and Treatment of Constitutional, as well as Local Diseases etc. London, Churchill, 1872.

26 Frerichs FT, Staedeler G: Über das Vorkommen von Leucin und Tyrosin in der menschlichen Leber. Arch Anat Physiol Wiss Med 1854;382–392.

27 Bartels C: Handbuch der Krankheiten des Harnapparatus. Leipzig, Vogel, vol 1, 1875, pp 66–86.

28 Tamm I, Horsfall FL: Characterization and separation of an inhibitor of viral hemagglutination present in urine. Proc Soc Exp Biol Med 1950;74:108–114.

29 Tyson J: A Guide to the Examination of Urine for the Use of Physicians and Students, 3rd ed. Philadelphia, Lindsay and Blakiston, 1880, pp 167–168.

30 Rieder H: Atlas der klinischen Mikroscopie des Harnes. Leipzig, Vogel, 1898.

Am J Nephrol 1994;14:458–460

Giovanni Chieffi

Dipartimento di Fisiologia Umana e
Funzioni Biologiche Integrate,
2nd University of Naples, Italy

Osmoregulation at the Zoological Station of Naples at the End of the 19th Century

Key Words
Osmoregulation
Marine animals
Aquatic animals

Abstract

The Zoological Station of Naples was founded in 1872 by Anton Dohrn as a research institute for zoology and comparative anatomy. Although the original fields of interest were the morphology of vertebrates and comparative embryology, a department of physiology was added to the station in 1888. Osmoregulation in marine organisms has been extensively studied, notably by Bottazzi, who investigated chemical composition, electrical conductivity, surface tension, osmotic pressure and extracellular viscosity in circulating fluids in man and lower animals. Bottazzi classified aquatic animals into 2 groups, a distinction that is accepted today. More recent workers at the station include Bern, who made important contributions to the study of the essential role played by prolactin in regulation of hydromineral metabolism in euryhaline teleost fish in a freshwater environment.

Introduction

The Zoological Station of Naples was established in 1872 [1] as a research institute for zoology and comparative embryology. Its founder and director, Anton Dohrn, was a zoologist and his original fields of interest were the morphology of vertebrates and comparative embryology. Dohrn published a series of papers under the general title *Studies on the Origin of the Vertebrate Body*. In 1876, Dohrn added a department of botany.

Dohrn persevered in his morphologic research until the end of his life. He was attracted by novel scientific fields, however, particularly comparative physiology and physiologic chemistry, which in Germany benefitted from the outstanding leadership of scientists like Johannes Müller and Justus von Liebig. Thus it was that in 1888 Dohrn built a new Department of Physiology in the City Garden of Naples, connected to the older building by a footbridge. To this was added another larger building, which was finished in 1906. Two subdepartments of physiologic chemistry and animal and comparative physiology were established within the Department of Physiology. On this occasion the municipality of Naples, which leased out the land, recognized that the Zoological Station was the 'fame and credit of Naples'. With the new physiologic laboratories, Dohrn demonstrated his awareness of

Giovanni Chieffi, MD
Dipartimento Fisiologia
Via San Andrea Delle Dame 8
I–80138 Naples (Italy)

the importance of the new directions in scientific research.

Dohrn died in 1909, after giving a tremendous impetus to the scientific activities of the Zoological Station. The result of his efforts was its transformation into a 'permanent zoological congress'.

Research into Osmoregulation

Although no specific research on the kidney has been carried out at the Zoological Station, osmoregulation in marine organisms has been extensively studied. The following are a few thoughts on the great contribution of the Zoological Station of Naples to the advancement of comparative physiology and its constant adaptation in view of progress in biologic research.

Filippo Bottazzi

Bottazzi was an active visitor to the Physiology Department at the end of the 19th century. As a human physiologist, he was well aware of the great importance of the expanding new disciplines of comparative physiology and physiologic chemistry. Bottazzi carried out his well-known experiments on osmoregulation in marine animals in Naples. This line of research originated from the concept of the *milieu intérieur* formulated years earlier by Claude Bernard.

Physiologic chemistry – as Bottazzi said – concerns the analytic study of those substances that make up living beings, and also the study of the possible transformations that these substances, when introduced into organisms, can undergo during digestion and metabolism in normal and pathologic conditions. Starting from this point, he investigated circulating fluids in man, included studies on chemical composition, electrical conductivity, surface tension, osmotic pressure and extracellular viscosity. He also extended his research to lower terrestrial and aquatic animals. As a result of his studies on osmoregulation in aquatic animals, a new line of research in comparative physiology commenced.

Bottazzi's 1st publication on osmoregulation dates to 1896 [2], and was followed by many others. On the basis of his results, Bottazzi classified aquatic animals into 2 groups – omeosmotic and pecilosmotic – a distinction that is accepted today but with the modern designations of osmoconformers and osmoregulators.

Osmoregulation in Aquatic Animals

Osmotic balance is the simplest and most common state to be found in all marine invertebrates. As the osmotic pressure of the water varies from one region to another, so it can be presumed that in the invertebrates osmotic pressure also varies according to their natural habitat. These organisms are therefore able to adapt themselves to habitats that are osmotically different.

Bottazzi maintained that aquatic organisms whose circulating fluids have low or high osmotic pressure, e.g. animals living in fresh water or in salt pans, do not exhibit osmotic balance. This means that the body surface of these animals must be able to prevent the passage of water and salts from outside to inside and vice versa. These observations led Bottazzi to pursue his studies in this direction, particularly on the permeability of the plasma membrane.

In more recent years osmoregulation has again been the object of research by visitors to the Zoological Station, including Howard Bern [3]. Bern made important contributions to the study of the essential role exerted by prolactin on regulation of hydromineral metabolism in most euryhaline teleost fish in a freshwater environment. These studies commenced in the context of work by Pickford and others, who demonstrated the essential involvement of prolactin in the survival in fresh water of *Fundulus heteroclitus* and several other teleost species. It has become clear that osmoregulation is a major action of prolactin in teleosts. Bern and his associates concentrated on the evolution of prolactin and its actions and on regulation of its synthesis and release.

Osmoregulatory problems vary in different vertebrate species. It is therefore not surprising that different hormones may assume different degrees of importance in different vertebrate groups. In fresh water the body fluids of these animals are salty compared with the external environment, and the answer to the osmotic challenge is to drink little and to excrete large quantities of dilute urine. Seawater animals are in the opposite situation. Their body fluids are much less salty than the external environment, and they are faced with the problem of exosmosis and constant influx of ions across permeable body membranes. The solution in seawater species is to drink sea water, absorb sodium chloride and excrete the excess sodium chloride by the development of accessory structures in addition to the kidney. Thus, in fishes and other seawater vertebrates, e.g. turtles and marine birds, adrenal corticosteroids, e.g. cortisol, are important regulators, largely because they stimulate salt secretion by certain cells (the so-called salt cells of the nasal gland of marine birds, of the rectal gland of elasmobranchs and the harderian gland of turtles). In freshwater species the most active hormone is prolactin. Hypophysectomized teleosts can be kept alive in fresh water only by giving them prolactin, and for this reason this hormone has been called 'freshwater survival factor'. The primary, but not exclusive sites of action of prolactin are the gut epithelium and the kidney.

Some of this research has been carried out at the Zoological Station by the author's research team [4], particularly on the role played in osmoregulation by the harderian gland of the terrapin.

References

1 Dohrn A: The Foundation of the Zoological Station. Nature 1872;5:277–280, 437–440.
2 Bottazzi F, Ducceschi V: Résistance des érythrocytes, alcalinité du sang et pression osmotique du sang dans les différent classes des vertébrés. Arch Ital Biol 1896;26:161–172.
3 Bern HA, Nicoll CS: The comparative endocrinology of prolactin. Recent Prog Horm Res 1968;24:681–696.
4 Chieffi G, Chieffi Baccari G, di Matteo L, d'Istria M, Marmorino C, Minucci S, Varriale B: The harderian gland of amphibians and reptiles; in Webb SM, et al (eds): Harderian Glands. Berlin, Springer, 1992, pp 91–108.

Am J Nephrol 1994;14:461–466

Robert L. Chevalier

Genentech Professor and Vice-Chair,
Department of Pediatrics, and Director of
Research and Development, Children's
Medical Center, Charlottesville, Va., USA

Kidney and Urologic Disorders in the Age of Enlightenment

Key Words

Age of Enlightenment
Renal anatomy
Renal physiology
Urinary disorders
Urinary calculi

Abstract

The Enlightenment, a unique period in the history of Europe, was founded in the scientific and intellectual revolution of the 17th century. Renal anatomy and physiology advanced through the work of men like Eustachio, Malpighi, von Rosenstein and Cotugno, who described both normal and pathologic structures. Despite the earlier discovery of renal tubules and glomeruli, their anatomic and physiologic relationship remained unclear during the 18th century. The definitive explanation would not come until the work of Bowman and Bright in the 19th century. Similarly, the role of renal nerves would not emerge until the 19th century, when Claude Bernard elucidated their role in controlling urine flow in the dog. A key figure was Morgagni (1682–1771), who provided highly precise descriptions of a number of urinary tract anomalies and forms of obstructive nephropathy and developed many insights into renal pathophysiology by pure deductive reasoning. He gave a remarkably accurate description of the basis of reflux nephropathy and recognized that urinary calculi could have many etiologies. Lithotomy was performed as a last resort, and Cheselden reduced the mortality to 17% with a perineal approach; Baseilhac designed a new instrument to facilitate the suprapubic approach. Despite the high quality of men such as Morgagni, physicians had a reputation for quackery and rapacity, and most of their efforts met with little success.

Introduction

The Enlightenment, a unique period in the history of Europe, was founded in the scientific and intellectual revolution of the 17th century. This new secularism was embodied in the works of Bacon, Descartes, Locke and Newton, and led to the development of 'natural law' and the concept of progress by the acquisition of knowledge through experience and reason. Whereas previously the knowledge of the Ancients had been venerated, the discoveries of the Moderns gleaned by the empiric approach assumed greater importance: general rules could be formulated from the meticulous examination of particulars.

Anatomy and Physiology in the Enlightenment

An understanding of disorders of the urinary tract is necessarily dependent on an understanding of normal anatomy and physiology. Through a quirk in the history of publication, the detailed illustrations of the great anatomist Bartolomeo Eustachio (about 1500–1574) were lost until their rediscovery in the 18th century, when they were published by Lancisi in 1714. These plates, along with Eustachio's original descriptions of 1564, clearly indicate the identification of renal tubules a century before Bellini in 1662 [1]. Eustachio was also aware of variations and abnormalities in human renal anatomy: in

Robert L. Chevalier, MD
Department of Pediatrics
Box 386
University of Virginia Health Sciences Center
Charlottesville, VA 22908 (USA)

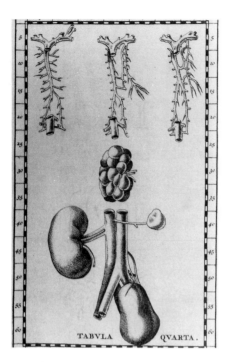

Fig. 1. Top: connection of the thoracic duct and the central venous circulation. Middle: bear kidney showing multiple lobulation. Bottom: left pelvic kidney. From the *Tabulae Anatomicae* of Bartolomeo Eustachio, originally engraved in the 16th century and rediscovered and published by Lancisi [2].

Plate 4, the appearance of a lobulated bear kidney is portrayed, as well as that of a human pelvic kidney (fig. 1).

Additional observations of renal anatomy were made by another brilliant Italian morphologist, Marcello Malpighi (1628–1694). Characteristic of the Enlightenment, Malpighi availed himself of the latest technology, the microscope, in describing the glomeruli for the first time. In his introduction to *De Renibus* (1666), he wrote:

'Do not stop to question whether these ideas are new or old, but ask, more properly, whether they harmonize with Nature. And be assured of this one thing, that I never reached my idea of the structure of the kidney by the aid of books, but by the long, patient, and varied use of the microscope. I have gotten the rest by the deductions of reason, slowly, and with an open mind, as is my custom' [3].

Malpighi understood, however, that not all urinary abnormalities are due to structural renal disease:

'For the most part the abnormalities appearing in the urine spring from disease of the blood coming to the kidneys, and particularly those hereditary diseases whose diathesis is not developed in the structure of the kidney, but is in the blood' [3].

A century later, in 1764, 2 physicians at the northern and southern extremes of Europe published descriptions

of acute glomerulonephritis and nephrotic syndrome. In Sweden, Nils Rosen von Rosenstein (1706–1773), a student of Boerhaave, published *The Diseases of Children and Their Remedies*, which was subsequently translated into 8 languages [4]. In a detailed description of scarlet fever, he wrote:

'... but some others began to look low-spirited between the eighteenth and the twenty-second day when the disease was supposed to be quite cured ... very little urine was discharged and it is said to have been bloody' [4].

Meanwhile in Naples, Domenico Cotugno (1736–1822), a student of Morgagni, described a 28-year-old soldier who:

'... was suffering at this time with immense watery swellings of his whole body ... For with two pints of this urine exposed to the fire, when scarcely half evaporated, the remainder made a white mass like egg albumen' [5].

Despite the earlier discovery of the renal tubules by Eustachio and Bellini, and the description of the glomeruli by Malpighi, there remained during the 18th century a lack of understanding of their anatomic and physiologic relationship. In his *First Lines of Physiology* published in 1747, the pre-eminent physiologist of the age, Albrecht von Haller, stated:

'That [uriniferous tubuli] are continuous with the arteries, or at least that they receive their branches into them, we know, from experiments which show that water, or even air, passes easily from the arteries of the kidneys into the ureter; and lastly, from diseases, in which the blood itself takes the same course' [6].

Haller and his contemporaries attempted to integrate the anatomic, physiologic and pathophysiologic knowledge available. The definitive explanation of these interrelations would not come, however, until the following century and the work of Bowman and Bright.

Although Malpighi did not publish figures to illustrate his descriptions of the glomeruli:

'... in spite of many attempts (but in vain) [he] could not demonstrate the connection of the glands and the urinary vessels' [3].

This connection remained unclear throughout the 18th century. The greatest publishing enterprise of the Enlightenment, the *Encyclopédie ou Dictionnaire Raisonné des Sciences, des Arts, et des Métiers* (1751–1772), edited by Diderot and d'Alembert, was a compendium of scientific, technical and historical knowledge aimed at the nobility and newly educated bourgeoisie. Of particular interest are

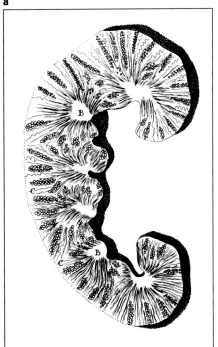

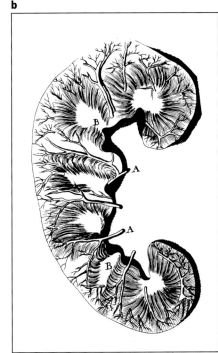

Fig. 2. Details of Anatomie Plates X and XX of the *Encyclopédie* of Diderot and d'Alembert (Paris, 1762–1777). **a** Sagittal section of kidney showing glomeruli and tubules. **b** Sagittal section of kidney showing intrarenal vasculature. **c** Sympathetic innervation and the kidneys. Reproduced with permission from [7].

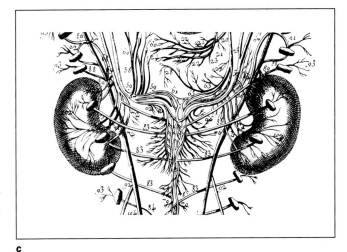

the anatomic plates, which show glomeruli in relation to tubules (fig. 2a) rather than to vessels (fig. 2b). No detail is provided, however, and glomeruli are depicted simply as clusters of circles.

Another example of anatomic inference regarding the kidney is Malpighi's description of renal nerves:

'About the nerves there will certainly be no difficulty, for it is commonly observed that these are carried throughout the interior of the kidney, whence it is probable that they are led to the glands along with the other vessels, as is seen in like conditions in other organs' [3].

The renal nerves are clearly depicted in the *Encyclopédie* (fig. 2c), which is a plate taken from the work of Vieussens (1685) [8]. Haller states:

'The nerves of the kidneys are small, but numerous; arising from a considerable plexus, mixed on each side with ganglions, which is generated by branches of the great semilunar ganglion, joined with others coming from the intercostal trunk ... As these nerves are small, they give but a small degree of sensibility to the kidney' [6].

As with glomerular filtration, the role of renal nerves would not emerge until the 19th century, when Claude Bernard elucidated their role in controlling urine flow in the dog [9].

Urinary Disorders in the Age of Enlightenment

One of the key figures providing a bridge between the early observations and the scientific explosion linked to the Industrial Revolution of the 19th century was another Italian giant in the history of medicine, Giovanni Battista Morgagni (1682–1771). At 15 years of age, he studied in Bologna with Valsalva (a pupil of Malpighi), and at 33 years old assumed the Chair of Anatomy at Padua. In his monumental *The Seats and Causes of Diseases Investigated by Anatomy* (1761), he described hundreds of autopsy studies arranged by organ system, and related his

Table 1. Renal disorders described by Morgagni [10]

Renal anomalies	Obstructive nephropathy
Renal agenesis	Calculi
Fetal lobulation	Worms
Renal cysts	Tumors
Duplicated collecting system	Gravid uterus
Vesicoureteral reflux	Prostatic hypertrophy
Ureteral valves	

findings to the clinical case histories preceding the death of the patients [10]. In addition to highly precise descriptions of a number of urinary tract anomalies and forms of obstructive nephropathy (table 1), he developed many insights into renal pathophysiology by pure deductive reasoning. In a remarkably accurate description of the basis of reflux nephropathy, Morgagni elaborated:

'For the orifices of the ureters being very much enlarg'd also, together with the ureters themselves, where they open into the bladder; no part of them now remains to pass obliquely betwixt the coats of the bladder ... the urine, and therewith pus, if it happens to be in the bladder, may easily be driven up through the ureters quite to the kidnies; especially if the patient lies down while attempting to make water.' Book III, letter XLII, article 23 [10].

Compensatory Renal Growth

A particular clinical problem that continues to intrigue nephrologists is compensatory renal growth. Morgagni wrote:

'Eustachio, moreover, having found, in Bonifacio Corneo, one of the kidnies to be scarcely equal to a small chestnut in magnitude, and the other large ... What blood, therefore, cannot now be carried into this kidney, is diverted into the other by the opposite artery; and, by this unusual flow of blood, the opposite kidney is distended.' Book III, letter XL, article 14 [10].

The concept of a hemodynamic basis for compensatory hypertrophy has persisted and is supported by more recent experimental evidence [11]. Morgagni also recognized the functional adaptation of the contralateral kidney:

'But as we see it so often happen, that one kidney not secreting, or not emitting urine, by reason of its being corrupted, on account of obstructing calculi, is supplied by the other, and that this is confirmed by the very increase of it.' Book III, letter XL, article 15 [10].

Morgagni did not stop here with his inquiry. He also considered the differing processes of renal atrophy and agenesis:

'I have a suspicion that the kidney has been contracted by disease, and even so attenuated, and consum'd; in those who have labor'd under pains of the kidney, from calculi, and other disorders; as to make learned men think that they were originally deficient.' Book III, letter XL, article 15 [10].

In contrast to the effects of disease on renal size, Morgagni recognized that congenital renal agenesis may account for the presence of a single kidney:

'But I should suppose that kidney to have been deficient from the original formation, as Aristotle observ'd even formerly, in those persons where no disorders of the kidnies have preceded; and no vestige of traces, either of its emulgent vessels, or the ureter, exists.' Book III, letter XL, article 15 [10].

Anuria

In view of the selection of subjects for dissection, it is perhaps not surprising that Morgagni did not identify any patients with ureteropelvic junction obstruction, which is now the most common cause of congenital urinary tract obstruction. He certainly recognized, however, that anuria due to obstruction necessarily involves both kidneys:

'Although the total defect of a urinary discharge happens either from a disorder of the kidnies and ureters, or of the bladder itself, and urethra; yet it has never happen'd either to Valsalva, or to me, to dissect the bodies of those who died from the former cause only. Nor is it to be wonder'd at, since the kidnies and ureters are double; so that if their office should happen to be suspended in one side, the defect is supplied by the other.' Book III, letter XLI, article 1 [10].

It is evident from this passage that Morgagni did not recognize the lethal consequences of renal parenchymal failure. Indeed, the naïve concept of uremia in the 18th century is illustrated by additional case histories:

'A virgin of Padua ... whereas not only the natural discharges of the kidnies were suppress'd, but the natural discharges of the intestines also. And even insensible perspiration seems to have supplied this defect, in a young woman, who; which is a very extraordinary instance, though well-known at Verona; had not excreted a drop of urine for two and twenty months ... for in the bed-chamber of this woman an odor of urine was perceiv'd.' Book III, letter XLI, article 8 [10].

Urinary Calculi

As in earlier times, kidney and bladder stones constituted one of the most common and troublesome urinary tract disorders during the Age of Enlightenment. Malpighi believed that stones were formed in the renal tubules and resulted in progressive renal damage:

'Now it frequently happens that small stones are held in these membranous ducts and are enlarged by the accretion of tartar, so that they injure the delicate membrane of the vessels and consequently the flesh of the kidneys is often observed to be destroyed' [3].

The premier English physician, John Hunter (1728–1793), understood that stone formation was a process similar to the calcification of an egg shell and that crystallization was involved [12]. During the 2nd half of the 18th century, the chemical basis of stone formation was emerging. DeMargraff identified phosphate in the urine, while Scheele found uric acid in stones and Woolaston described calcium oxalate, ammonium magnesium phosphate and cysteine as components of stones.

Morgagni recognized that stones could have many etiologies, including congenital:

'And that there are urines which deposit these particles sooner, and more readily, [Brendelius] does not at all doubt, where he mentions the cases of two infants; one but just two days old, and the other about eight; who not only discharg'd calculi before death, but had calculi found within them when dead.'
Book III, letter XLII, article 18 [10].

The beneficial effects of a high urine volume on stone formation was also known to Morgagni, who reasoned:

'In summer the calculous matter is much less diluted by the watery matter, which then goes off, through the skin, in a very considerable portion: and this seems to me another reason why, if it is in our power to choose, the excision of the calculus should be put off from autumn to spring, rather than from spring to autumn.'
Book III, letter XLII, article 19 [10].

Lithotomy was one of the few operations that could be performed in the 18th century without unacceptable rates of mortality. In view of the lack of anesthesia and sterile technique, however, excruciating pain and common septicemia understandably made the procedure one of last resort. One of the most famous lithotomists of the age was William Cheselden (1688–1752), who could perform the operation in less than 1 min and reduced the mortality to a record low of 17% [12]. Complications of the usual perineal incision included fecal or urinary incontinence, impotence, fistula and ruptured bladder [13]. To avoid these, the suprapubic approach was championed by Jean Baseilhac (1703–1781), otherwise known as Frère Come. He developed his *sonde à flèche* (fig. 3), a curved, hollow, silver catheter containing a pointed stylet, which was introduced through a perineal urethrostomy to guide the insertion of a trochar via a suprapubic incision through which the stone was removed [13, 14]. Frère Come's expertise with this technique was so famous that King

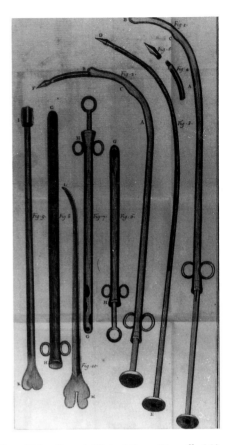

Fig. 3. Jean Baseilhac (Frère Come). Plate 1 from *Nouvelle Méthode pour Extraire la Pierre de la Vessie Urinaire par-dessus le Pubis*, Yverdon, 1779 [14]. Shown as Figs. 1–5, sonde a flèche or arrowhead catheter, used to localize a suprapubic incision from within the bladder. Shown as Figs. 6–8 are silver cannulas to drain urine and foreign matter via the urethra in females or a perineal cystostomy in males. Shown as Fig. 9 is a stylet to clean the cannula, and Fig. 10 is a guide for insertion of the perineal cannula.

Louis XIV reportedly said that if he were to have a stone, he would refuse to be operated on by anyone else.

A particularly poignant case study reported by Morgagni is that of:

'a country girl ... died in her fourteenth year. For having introduc'd a brass hair-bodkin, notwithstanding it was bent in the middle, very high into the urethra, ... she was silent as to the true cause of the pains. For even the bodkin could not be extracted, by reason of a calculus that was form'd upon it. But the ureters, and the kidneys themselves, were in a very bad condition indeed.'
Book III, letter XLII, article 20 [10].

Bladder stones resulting from foreign bodies introduced through the urethra were apparently not uncommon at that time, and often resulted in infection, chronic

465

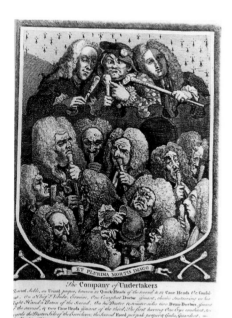

Fig. 4. William Hogarth's *The Consultation of Physicians or the Company of Undertakers*, published in 1761. Above the 12 physicians are 3 specific caricatures, depicting on the left John Taylor (a quack oculist), in the center 'Crazy' Sally Mapp (a quack bone-setter) and on the right, Joshua 'Spot' Ward (a quack vendor of pills and fever powders).

pyelonephritis and death from uremia. Most interesting are Morgagni's comments regarding the public health implications of this entity, and the physician's responsibility in ferreting out the history to allow early intervention:

'Yet such instances ought not to be pass'd over in silence, that physicians, being admonish'd by the frequency of them, may, if any girl begin to complain of a difficulty of making water, inquire very narrowly into every circumstance; and, by a cautious dexterity, force

out the truth, while it is as yet possible to administer relief ... More examples would be extant ... if shame did not oblige most women to conceal the true cause of their disease.'

Book III, letter XLII, Article 27 [10].

Status of Doctors in the 18th Century

Not all physicians of the 18th century shared Morgagni's integrity or his concern for understanding his patients' disease processes. Physicians had a reputation for rapacity and quackery that was caricatured mercilessly by William Hogarth (1697–1764) in his engraving *The Consultation of Physicians or the Company of Undertakers* published in 1761. In figure 4 are shown 12 'quack heads' in periwigs, 1 of whom has his finger in a urinal (a reference to the pseudo-science of uroscopy), while the others are solemnly clasping their cane heads, the symbol of the physician. This cynical view emphasizes the futility of most physicians' efforts at the time, and the pretentiousness with which ignorance was hidden. Morgagni was careful to dissociate himself from this majority of physicians by his reliance on the autopsy examination and his keen powers of observation and reasoning. In the finest spirit of the Enlightenment, he wrote:

'For those who have dissected or inspected many, have at least learned to doubt, when the others, who are ignorant of anatomy, and do not take the trouble to attend to it are in no doubt at all.'

Book I, letter XVI, article 25 [10].

Acknowledgments

The assistance of Danièle Calinon of the Institut Universitaire d'Histoire de la Médecine et de la Santé Publique, Lausanne, Switzerland, and of Joan Echtenkamp Klein of the Historical Collections and Services, Health Sciences Library of the University of Virginia, Charlottesville, Va., USA, is gratefully acknowledged.

References

1 Fine LG: Eustachio's discovery of the renal tubule. Am J Nephrol 1986;6:47–50.
2 Eustachii B: Tabulae Anatomicae. Amsterdam, Weststenios, 1722.
3 Hayman JM Jr: Malpighi's 'Concerning the structure of the kidneys'. Ann Med Hist 1925; 7:242–263.
4 Rosenstein NR von: The Diseases of Children and Their Remedies. A Sparrman (translator). London, Cadell, 1776.
5 Cotugno D: De Ischiade Nervosa Commentarius. Naples, apud Frat. Simonios, 1764.

6 Haller A von: First Lines of Physiology. Troy, Penniman, 1803.
7 Diderot D: Diderot's Encyclopedia: the Complete Illustrations 1762–1777. New York, Abrams, 1978.
8 Vieussens R: Neurographia Universalis. Lyons, Jean Certe, 1685.
9 Bernard C: Leçons sur les Propriétés Physiologiques et les Altérations Pathologiques des Liquides de l'Organisme. Paris, Baillière, 1859.
10 Morgagni JB: The Seats and Causes of Diseases Investigated by Anatomy. New York, Hafner, 1960.

11 Krohn AG, Peng BBK, Antell HI, Stein S: Compensatory renal hypertrophy: the role of immediate vascular changes in its production. J Urol 1970;103:564–568.
12 Modlin M: A history of urinary stone. S Afr Med J 1980;58:652–655.
13 Beamon CR: Jean Baseilhac (Frère Come) 1703–1781. Invest Urol 1973;10:493–494.
14 Baseilhac J: Nouvelle Méthode pour Extraire la Pierre de la Vessie Urinaire par-dessus le Pubis. Yverdon, 1779.

Am J Nephrol 1994;14:467–472

Johannes Hierholzer[a]
Christel Hierholzer[b]
Klaus Hierholzer[c]

[a] Department of Radiology,
Universitätsklinikum Rudolf Virchow,
[b] Free University of Berlin,
[c] Department of Clinical Physiology,
Universitätsklinikum Benjamin Franklin,
Berlin, Germany

Johann Lukas Schönlein and His Contribution to Nephrology and Medicine

Key Words
Henoch-Schönlein purpura
Favus
Trichophyton schönleinii
Mycology

Abstract
Schönlein published few papers, and most of what is known of his achievements in nephrology comes from notes and publications of his students. It seems, however, that he described the combination of rheumatic fever, affection of internal muscular organs, a typical exanthem and oliguria, coining the name *purpura rubra* to describe this syndrome. Although patients with symptoms of Schönlein's syndrome had been described earlier, Schönlein was the first to describe purpura rheumatica as an entity. Schönlein's greatest contribution was the discovery of the anthropophilic pathogenic fungus *Trichophyton schönleinii* as the cause of the contagious skin condition favus (honeycomb ringworm). This opened a new field – mycology – and allowed therapy to be aimed specifically at the cause of the disease.

Introduction

In 1791 a young man died from a disease that would later be described and recognized as a pathogenetic entity by a physician who would be born 2 years later, in 1793. The young man was Wolfgang Amadeus Mozart [1, 2], the physician was Johann Lukas Schönlein (fig. 1), the disease to be described was rheumatic purpura rubra with renal lesions, i.e. Schönlein's syndrome, or, after Henoch had stressed the intestinal lesions [3, 4], Henoch-Schönlein syndrome, also known as anaphylactoid purpura or rheumatoid purpura.

Schönlein's contribution to clinical medicine in general and to nephrology in particular has been discussed in several reviews. This paper recalls particularly his contributions to nephrology and attempts to define his impact on the development of scientific medicine in the 1st half of the 19th century. A brief synopsis of the life of Schönlein is presented in table 1.

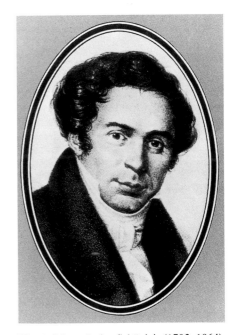

Fig. 1. Johann Lukas Schönlein (1793–1864).

Johannes Hierholzer, MD
Department of Radiology
Universitätsklinikum Rudolf Virchow
Augustenburger Platz 1
D-13353 Berlin (Germany)

Table 1. Curriculum vitae and scientific achievements of Schönlein (1793–1864)

1793	Born in Bamberg, son of an artisan family
1811	Studied philosophy and medicine in Landshut Interested in comparative anatomy, contact with natural (romantic) philosophy (Schelling)
1813–1816	Studied medicine in Würzburg, then traveled to Göttingen, Jena and London (visited Thomas Addison)
1817	Habilitation in Würzburg, on pathologic anatomy
1820–1833	Professor of Pathology and Therapy in Würzburg Classification of diseases on scientific (physiologic) basis Textbook on *Allgemeine und specielle Pathologie und Therapie* published by some of his students on the basis of lecture notes
1833–1839	Professor of Medicine in Zürich Clinical training of students Discovery of fungal infection (favus) initiates mycology
1839–1856	Professor of Medicine in Berlin Introduction of physical, chemical and microscopic methods into clinical research Re-examination of autopsy findings Description of purpura rubra (rheumatism, dermal, articular, intestinal and renal lesions) Foundation of the Berlin School of Scientific Medicine, together with Müller Later incapacitated by hypothyroidism (goiter)
1864	Died in Bamberg

Table 2. Publications of Schönlein

Thesis *Von der Hirnmethamorphose[1]*	Würzburg, 1816
Über Crystalle im Darmkanal bei Typhus abdominalis[1]	Zürich, 1836
Zur Pathogenie der Impetigenes, 1 page [14]	Zürich, 1839
Notes on *Keichhusten* (whooping cough)[1]	1818/1819
Notes on his inaugural lecture in Würzburg[1]	1819
Publications by students *Allgemeine und specielle Pathologie und Therapie nach J.L. Schönlein's Vorlesungen, niedergeschrieben und herausgegeben von einigen seiner Zuhörer* (figure) 5 editions in 9 years, plus translations into English, French, Russian and Italian	1832–1839
Volume of lectures in Zürich	1840
Schönlein's Klinische Vorträge in dem Charité-Krankenhaus zu Berlin [7]	1842

[1] See further reading list.

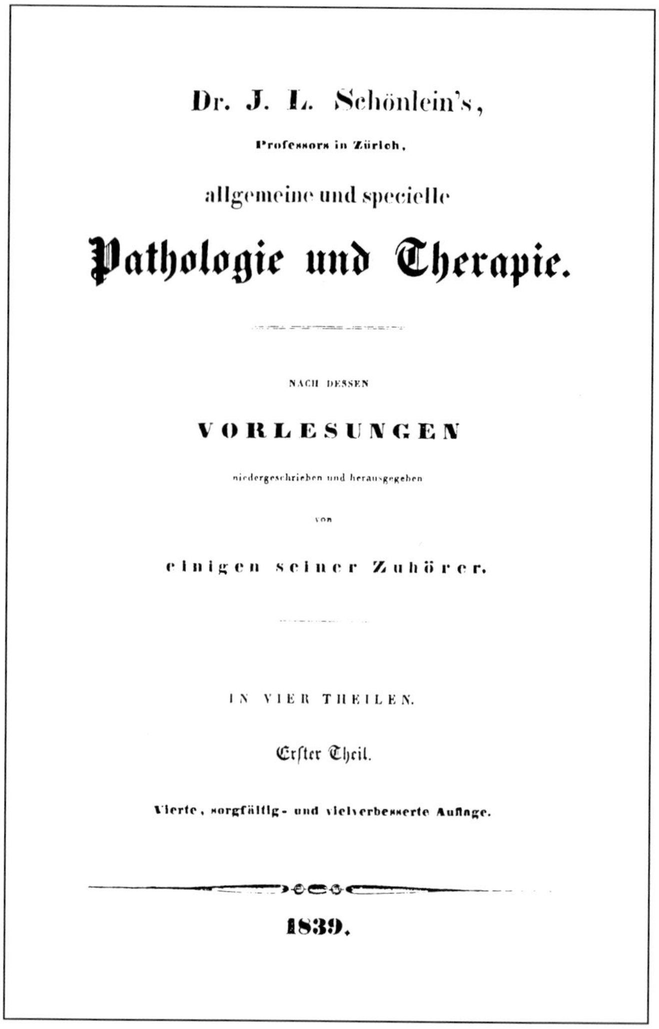

Dr. J. L. Schönlein's,

Professors in Zürich,

allgemeine und specielle

Pathologie und Therapie.

NACH DESSEN

VORLESUNGEN

niedergeschrieben und herausgegeben

VON

einigen seiner Zuhörer.

IN VIER THEILEN.

Erster Theil.

Vierte, sorgfältig- und vielverbesserte Auflage.

1839.

Fig. 2. Cover page of the 1839 edition of notes taken from lectures of Schönlein on pathology and therapy.

Schönlein and Nephrology (Schönlein's Purpura)

It is not easy to evaluate Schönlein's contributions to nephrology, because he himself never published a manuscript in this field (table 2). Indeed, he published only 3 papers in total, as he felt:

'My achievements until now are still too incomplete to be presented to a large audience of physicians' [5].

He assumed that rapid new development would soon render any written communication insufficient. Thus, the pertinent reports dealing with Schönlein's statements on renal disease are limited to texts written, edited and published by some of his students as *Allgemeine und specielle*

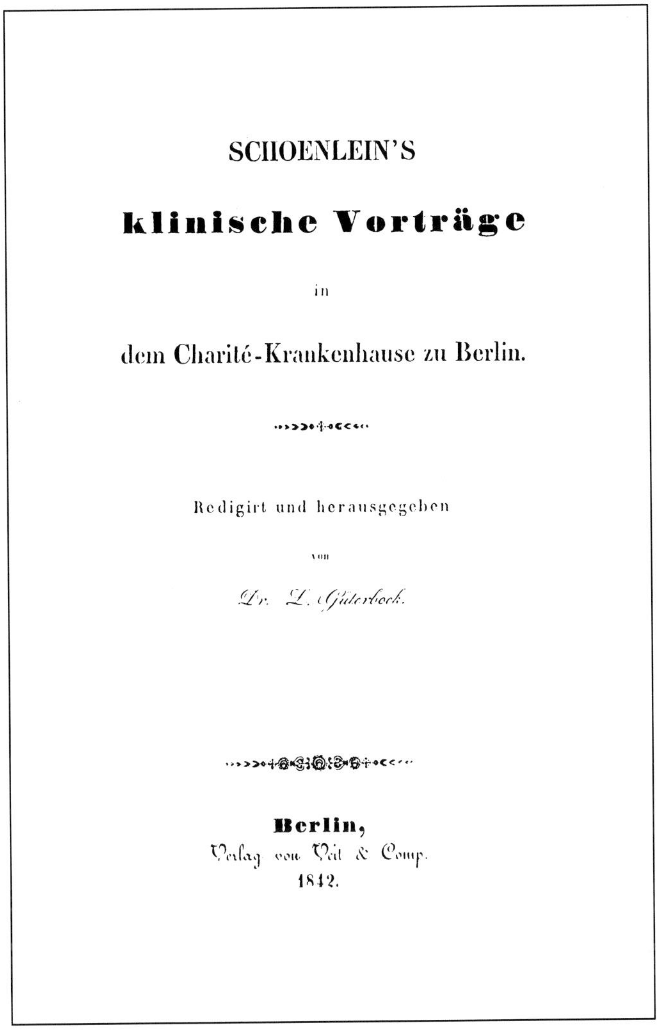
SCHOENLEIN'S

klinische Vorträge

in

dem Charité-Krankenhause zu Berlin.

Redigirt und herausgegeben

von

Dr. L. Güterbock.

Berlin,

Verlag von Veit & Comp.

1842.

Fig. 3. Cover page of Schönlein's clinical lectures in Berlin, published by Güterbock [7].

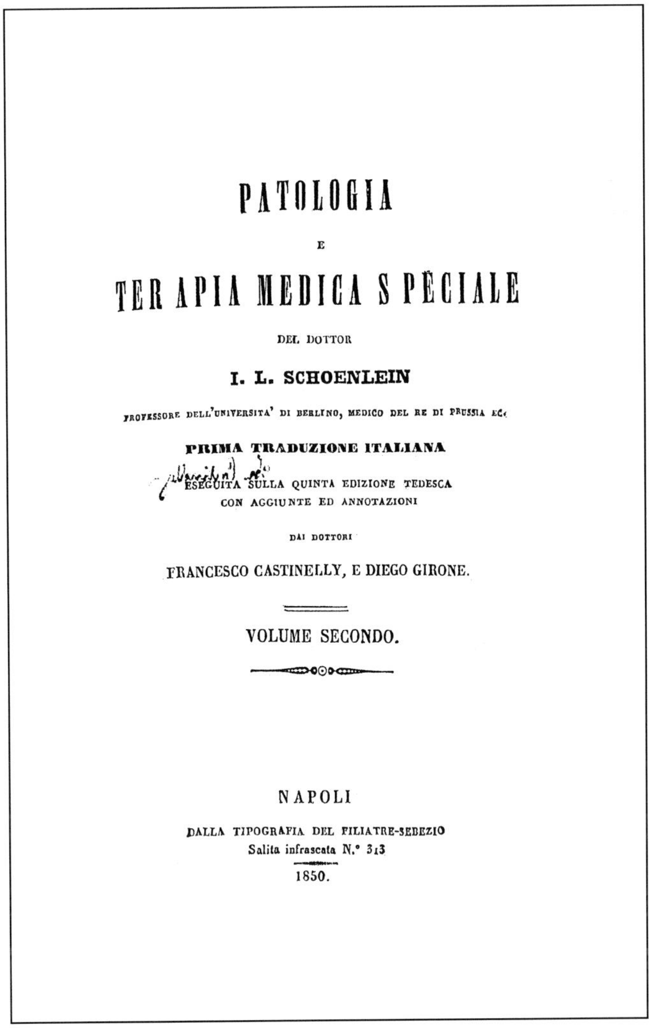
PATOLOGIA

E

TERAPIA MEDICA SPECIALE

DEL DOTTOR

I. L. SCHOENLEIN

PROFESSORE DELL'UNIVERSITA' DI BERLINO, MEDICO DEL RE DI PRUSSIA EC.

PRIMA TRADUZIONE ITALIANA

ESEGUITA SULLA QUINTA EDIZIONE TEDESCA

CON AGGIUNTE ED ANNOTAZIONI

DAI DOTTORI

FRANCESCO CASTINELLY, E DIEGO GIRONE.

VOLUME SECONDO.

NAPOLI

DALLA TIPOGRAFIA DEL FILIATRE-SEBEZIO

Salita infrascata N.° 313

1850.

Fig. 4. Cover page of the Italian translation of the textbook based on Schönlein's notes. (Original in the library of the Institute of History of Medicine, Free University of Berlin.)

Pathologie und Therapie between 1832 and 1841 (fig. 2) [6] and to records of his lectures at the Charité in Berlin, edited by Güterbock (fig. 3) [7]. The text on pathology and therapy received enthusiastic attention, and although not authorized by Schönlein, was soon translated (table 2), in 1850 even into Italian (fig. 4); this edition was published in Naples. Some information can also be obtained from doctoral theses written under the guidance of Schönlein in Würzburg and Zürich. This topic has been extensively discussed by Bleker [8].

In the published lecture notes are several interesting nephrologic observations, e.g. concerning daily variations of urine secretion, pH changes of the urine in various diseases, the measurement of urea concentration in tissues of patients with nephritis and other subjects. In the 1834 edition of *Pathologie und Therapie* (vol. 2, p. 320 onwards) [6] can be found a description of patients with rheumatic fever, affection of internal muscular organs (heart, intestinal tract, uterus) and a typical exanthem (details on p. 321). Schönlein coined the name *purpura rubra* to describe the last symptom, and he pointed to the fact (p. 322) that in this condition:

'... urine is secreted only in small amounts, it is strikingly acid, and contains sediments [precipitations], consisting of rosy or of uric acid material.'

Prognostic signs, according to his experience (p. 327) were:

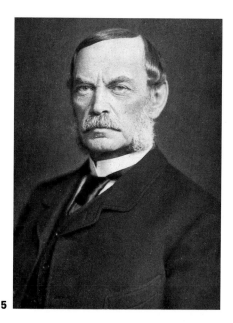

5

6

Fig. 5. Eduard Henoch, who focused attention on intestinal symptoms in Schönlein's purpura.
Fig. 6. Paper of Henoch: 'On a peculiar form of purpura' (1874).

'Amply flowing urine with amber color is advantageous; disadvantageous, however, is when urine flows profusely but is watery clear; worst is when urine is excreted only in small amounts and if it gives rise to thick sediments.'

Schönlein also pointed out (p. 321) that purpura had also been described as *Friesel* and that its appearance could differ:

'The vesicles are very large, filled with clear fluid, and their halo [vicinity] indifferent, then it is a "white Friesel", miliaria s. purpura alba.'

In this connection it is interesting to recall that Mathias von Sallaba, when he visited Mozart in Salzburg shortly before his death, diagnosed 'white Friesel-fever'; this is also the diagnosis which the attending physician, Dr Thomas Franz Closset listed as the cause of death in the official record. Of course *Friesel* at that time may have been a rather general and non-specific dermatologic diagnosis. The subject has recently been reviewed [9].

In the 3rd volume of *Pathologie und Therapie*, Schönlein described a skin disease which, as he pointed out (p. 28), was commonly seen in England – pityriasis rubra. He assumed that: 'most likely this affection goes along with an impairment of the secretion of urine'. According to the *Clinical Lectures* (table 2) [7], he also described further relevant patients (p. 192 onwards) with rheumatic disease and changes of urine excretion that were pathologic in terms of amount and composition (compare also p. 473).

In retrospect, it seems that patients with symptoms of Schönlein's syndrome were also observed and described by Heberden in 1802 [10], Willan in 1808 [11] and Johnson in 1852 [12]. Schönlein, however, without knowing these descriptions (at least there is no evidence that he knew them), was the first to describe purpura rheumatica as an entity. Schönlein stated clearly (1834, p. 320) [6]:

'Miliaria *[Friesel]* ... presents so many characteristic features as to its appearance and course that one cannot doubt any more that it constitutes a specific disease.'

In his lectures he also described intestinal affections connected with miliaria (p. 320). The observation of intestinal lesions, i.e. the coincidence of purpura with intestinal bleeding, was also noted by Henoch (fig. 5), who presented case reports to the Medical Society of Berlin in 1868 and again in 1874 (fig. 6) [3, 4]. The more or less dialectic question as to whether or not Schönlein's syndrome (purpura) should be named Henoch-Schönlein or Schönlein-Henoch syndrome has been discussed previously [13].

Schönlein and Parasitology (Mycology)

The greatest contribution of Schönlein to medicine was the discovery of an anthropophilic pathogenic fungus, later designated *Achorion* (now *Trichophyton*) *schönleinii,* as the cause of the contagious skin disease, favus (also known as tinea favosa, honeycomb ringworm, or *Kipfgrind*). Figure 7 shows a child with the disease, which was not uncommon in Europe in the 19th century, particularly in the valleys of the Swiss Alps. The disease usually lasted throughout life, and as it was apparently contagious, children were often dismissed from school and lived as outcasts.

Schönlein, then Professor of Medicine in Zürich (where he had moved in 1849 following dismissal from Würzburg for being a liberal), was led to the discovery of the cause of the disease by an observation of Agostino Bassi in Milan (1832), who had identified a fungus *(Schimmelpilz)* as the cause of the disastrous silkworm disease [5]. Schönlein had also come across a paper of Unger (1832) which described fungal growth on plant leaves (cited in Schönlein [14]). In Zürich Schönlein had several patients with favus. When he read Bassi's report he considered the possibility that the disease might also be caused by a microorganism, a hypothesis that could easily be tested. Indeed, although Schönlein was not a dermatologist, he could identify structures in the skin lesions of some patients that resembled the structures of the silkworm disease (muscardine). He concluded that favus was caused by a fungus. This preceded the discovery of the bacterial cause of tuberculosis by Robert Koch.

The demonstration that favus was caused by a microorganism not only opened the way for specific therapy aimed at the cause of this particular disease, but much more importantly opened a new field in medicine, specifically that of mycology and in general that of parasitology. The description of *Achorion schönleinii* was the first demonstration of the existence of an anthropophilic pathogenetic microorganism.

Conclusions

It is not only the pioneering work on favus (published on 1 page) or the careful observation of a skin lesion in combination with rheumatism and a subsequent renal lesion that puts Schönlein on a par with leading medical scientists of his time. Schönlein's impact on medicine and its revolutionary development in the 19th century was not only due to his publications, but was particularly due to

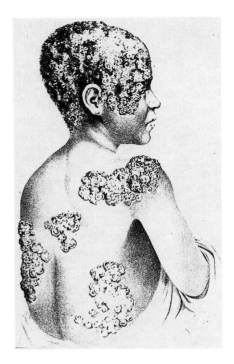

Fig. 7. Child with *Erbgrind* (favus). Illustration from Ferdinand Hebra's *Atlas der Hautkrankheiten* (Vienna, 1856–1876).

the new methods he introduced into clinical medicine. He used physical, chemical and morphologic techniques. He also introduced the native language, instead of Latin, into the lecture halls, and he revolutionized clinical teaching of students on the ward. Advanced medical students, he ordered, should be assigned to special patients whom they should observe and report on daily. They should formulate a tentative diagnosis and propose a therapeutic regimen. Eventually they should also take into consideration autopsy findings. In this connection it is interesting that Schönlein was indirectly in contact with Jacob Henle, then Professor of Anatomy in Zürich. In his *Klinische Vorträge* can be found the statement (p. 480):

'I am glad that my successor in Zürich, Professor Pfeuffer, could follow a number of the cases which I had seen there up to the lethal outcome and subsequently performed autopsies together with Professor Henle.'

Henle was by that time Professor of Anatomy and Pathology in Zürich. The reference refers to patients with 'Rose (Erysipelas)'.

Schönlein as the leading clinician, and Müller as the leading physiologist and anatomist in Berlin, were to establish a new era of scientifically based medicine and physiology. They founded the 'Berlin School' [8], which eventually triumphed over natural philosophy and guided medicine onto the road to natural science. This, however, is beyond the scope of the present discussion.

Acknowledgements

The authors wish to thank Ms. A. Kliesch and Professor R. Winau for help in locating relevant literature, and Professor P. Wolf, Department of Pathology, University of California, San Siego, Calif., USA, who drew attention to sources relating to the death of Mozart.

References

1 Davies PJ: Mozart in Person. His Character and Health. Connecticut, Greenwood Press, 1989.
2 Robbins Landon HC: Chapter 11: The Final Illness; Chapter 12: Mythos and Theories, in Mozart's Last Year, 1791. New York, Schirmer Books, 1988, pp 148–171; pp 171–181.
3 Henoch E: Über den Zusammenhang von Purpura und Intestinalstörungen (Vortrag). Aus den Verhandlungen Ärztliche Gesellschaften, Berliner Medizinische Gesellschaft, Sitzung vom. 11.11.1868. Berl Klin Wochensch 1868; 5:517–519.
4 Henoch E: Über eine eigenthümliche Form von Purpura. (Nach einem in der Berliner medicinischen Gesellschaft am 18. November 1874 gehaltenen Vortrag.) Berl Klin Wochenschr 1874;11:641–643.
5 Nowicki A: Darstellung der Beziehung JL Schönlein R. Remark. (Anhand überlieferten Schriftums. (Erste Schritte auf dem Gebiet der medizinischen Mykologie)). Inaugural-Dissertationsarbeit, Würzburg, 1985.

6 Schönlein JL: Allgemeine und specielle Pathologie und Therapie nach JL Schönlein's Vorlesungen, niedergeschrieben und herausgegeben von einigen seiner Zuhörer. 5 editions and a translation into Italian: 1st edn Würzburg, Etlinger, 1832; 2nd edn Herisau, Literatur-Comptoir, 1834; 3rd edn Freiburg, 1837; 4th edn St. Gallen, Leipzig, Literatur-Comptoir, 1839; 5th edn, Dr. JL Schönleins allgemeine und specielle Pathologie und Therapie nach dessen Vorlesungen niedergeschrieben und herausgegeben von einigen seiner Zuhörer. St. Gallen, Literatur-Comptoir, 1841; translation of 5th edn, Patologia e Terapia Medica Speciale del Dottor IL Schönlein, Prima Traduzione Italiana, Eseguita sulla Quinta Edizione Tedesca con Aggiunte ed Annotazioni dai dottori Francesco Castinelly e Diego Girone. Naples, dalla Tipografia del Filiatre-Sebezio, 1850.

7 Güterbock L: Schönlein's klinische Vorträge in dem Charité Krankenhaus zu Berlin. Berlin, Verlag von Veit, 1842.
8 Bleker J: Die Naturhistorische Schule. IV: Das medizinische Konzept Johann Lukas Schönleins. Stuttgart, Gustav Fischer Verlag, 1981.
9 Robbins Landon HC: Mozart's last year 1791. New York, Schirmer Books, 1988.
10 Heberden W: Commentarii de Morborum Historia et Curatione, chapter 78. London, T Payne, 1802.
11 Willan RW: Die Hautkrankheiten und ihre Behandlung (translated from: Description and treatment of cutaneous diseases, by Friese FG). London, vol 1–3, 1799, 1803, 1806 (sect. 1), 1816 (sect. 2).
12 Johnson G: On the Diseases of the Kidney. London, Parker and Son, 1852.
13 Jones JV: Schönlein versus Henoch. BMJ 1973;4:677–678.
14 Schönlein JL: Zur Pathogenie der Impetigenes. Müllers Arch Anat Physiol Wiss Med 1839;82.

Further Reading

Ackerknecht EH: Johann Lucas Schönlein 1793–1864. J Hist Med 1964;19:131–138.
Ajello L: Milestones in the history of medical mycology: the dermatophytes; in Iwata K (ed): Recent Advances in Medical Veterinary Mycology. Tokyo, University of Tokyo Press, 1977, pp 3–15.
Alkiewicz JA: On the discovery of Trichophyton schönleinii (Achorion schönleinii). Inaugural dissertation, 1966. Mycopathologia 1967;33: 28–32.
Fuhrmann HR: Dr Johann Lukas Schönlein, der Begründer einer neuen Zeit in der Medizin. Inaugural dissertation, Würzburg, 1938.
Gairdner D: The Schönlein-Henoch syndrome (anaphylactoid purpura). Q J Med 1948;17:95–122.
Griesinger W: Zum Gedenken an Johann Lukas Schönlein. Arzt Intell 1864;32:445–551.
Gruby D: Über Tinea Favosa. Müllers Arch Anat Physiol Wiss Med 1842;22–24.
Henoch E: Vorlesungen über Kinderkrankheiten. Ein Handbuch für Ärzte und Studierende. VII, 751 S. Berlin, Hirschwald, 1881.
Knorr M: Johann Lukas Schönlein, Familie, Leben, Persönlichkeit. Ber Phys Med Ges Würzburg 1938;62:108–129.

Knorr M: Dr Johann Lukas Schönlein und sein Einfluss auf die Lehre von den Infektionskrankheiten. Ber Phys Med Ges Würzburg 1938;62:181–189.
Müller F von: Johann Lukas Schönlein, Professor der Medizin 1793–1864. Sonderabzug aus: Lebensläufe aus Franken. Erlangen, Palm und Enke Verlag, 1936, pp 332–349.
Remak R: Gelungene Impfung des Favus. Med Zeitung Berl 1842;11:137.
Schadewaldt H: Anfänge der Medizinischen Mykologie. Mykosen 1981;24:654–667.
Schönlein JL: Von der Hirnmetamorphose. Medizinische Dissertation, Würzburg, Medical Faculty, 1816.
Schönlein JL: Manuskript über den 'Keichhusten' (1818–1819). Handgeschriebenes Original. Universitätsbibliothek Würzburg, Nachlass Sticker F85 (not published).
Schönlein JL: Über Crystalle im Darmkanal bei Typhus abdominales. Aus brieflicher Mittheilung an den Herausgeber. Müllers Arch Anat Physiol Wiss Med 1836;258.
Schönlein JL: Ansprache gehalten am 4. November 1819 bei der Übernahme der medizinischen Klinik in Würzburg; in Ebstein E (ed): Deutsche Ärztereden aus dem 19. Jahrhundert. Berlin, Springer, 1926, pp 6–12.

Schönlein JL: Gutachten über Dr. du Bois-Reymond von 18.8.1855. Berlin, Staatsbibliothek Preussischer Kulturbesitz, 1855.
Schrödel P: Unveröffentlichte Briefe von Johann Lukas Schönlein 1818–1821, in Bayerisches Ärzteblatt. München, Bayerische Landesärztekammer, Sonderdruck aus Heft 2, 3, 4, 6. 1964.
Schrödel P: Johann Lukas Schönlein zum 100. Todestag. Berl Med 1964;15:217–224.
Seeliger HPR: Gedanken zur Entdeckung des Trichophyton (Achorion) schönleinii. Vortrag anlässlich der Eröffnung der XIX. Jahrestagung der Deutschsprachigen Mykologischen Gesellschaft – 'myk85'. Würzburg, 11 October 1985, pp 3–14.
Sigerist HE: Johannes Müller (1801–1858) und Johann Lukas Schönlein (1793–1864), in Grosse Ärzte. Munich, Lehmann, vol 4, 1958, pp 273–285.
Virchow R: Gedächtnisrede auf Joh. Lukas Schönlein gehalten am 23.1.1865, dem ersten Jahrestag seines Todes. Berlin, Hirschwald Verlag, 1865.

Am J Nephrol 1994;14:473–476

The Urologic Tradition of Preci

Mario Timio

Department of Nephrology and Dialysis,
Hospital of Foligno, Foligno, Italy

Key Words
Lithotomy
Lithotrity
Surgical instruments
Uroscopy

Abstract
The Preci School was not as well known as those of Salerno and Montpellier, and its members were often confused with quack doctors from nearby Cerretani who begged for alms for medical and religious foundations as a profession. The Preci School surgeons performed lithotomy, phlebotomy and castration, designing and making their own instruments, which were well ahead of their time and used by other surgeons only centuries later. Lithotrity was commonly employed using such tools, before it was known elsewhere. They practised cauterization and disinfection by fire. The Preci School was also familiar with differential diagnosis and uroscopy, which were essential before treating stone disease. The school came to an end after 1751, when a Papal edict declared that only surgeons with a degree could remove stones.

Introduction

Preci is a little Umbrian town in the center of Italy. In Roman times, Preci was part of the Sabina region and was described by Scacchi [1] as: 'Pulchra Sabina Preces alto tenet aggere priscam chirurgis patriam' (Lovely Sabina Preci keeps the old school of surgery in the high castle). This school could probably be classified as both urologic and nephrologic, because the Preci surgeons (also called 'Norcini', as Preci was part of the Norcia (Nursia) district) mainly treated diseases of the bladder and kidneys. The Preci School was not as well known as those of Salerno or Montpellier, even though it enjoyed a widespread reputation in Europe for a long time (14th–18th centuries). The reason for the lack of knowledge about the Preci School is not clear. It could be due to the scanty writings left by the early surgeons, with the exception of the famous surgeon Lanfranco (1306) who mentioned the Norcini in his *Chirurgia Magna et Parva* [2]. The first book was written by Durante Scacchi [1], in 1596, about 4 centuries after the beginning of surgery in Preci, and later a few more writers devoted their attention to the Preci School.

A second, and more important, reason could be the identification of the Norcini with the 'Cerretani' medical activity [3]. The name Cerretani was used in the 13th century to describe those inhabitants of Cerreto, a little town not far from Preci and Nursia, who followed the occupation of 'questores elemosinarum per universum mundum' (beggars all over the world) on behalf of hospitals, leprosariums, monasteries and churches. While the Cerretani begged for money, they dispensed medical aids, e.g. healing herbs, ointments, pain relievers and anthelminthic powders, and sold medical services, e.g. uroscopy, pregnancy diagnosis, tooth extraction and kidney and bladder stone treatment [4]. They were not professionally qualified and had absolutely no authorityto give or to prescribe any medical treatment; they were simply dishonest 'questores' and frauds. Unfortunately, the Norcini, whose history was by contrast clear, honest and professional, were probably associated with this ethical dishonesty. Apart from living in the same area, the Norcini and the Cerretani had nothing else in common.

Professor Mario Timio, MD
Via XX Settembre 22
I–06121 Perugia (Italy)

Kidney Stone Operations and the Origin of the Preci School

The main factors that contributed to the origin and history of the Nephrourologic Preci School were the natural and empiric turn to surgery on animals, mainly pigs, and a great skill in operating on the genitourinary organs. Such surgery was practised by ordinary people as far back as the 6th–7th centuries AC, and with their knowledge of animal anatomy and observation of kidney and bladder stones and cysts of pigs and donkeys, some inhabitants of Preci began operating on other men suffering from the same disease, and soon achieved some success [5].

In addition to its empiric origin, the Preci School was greatly influenced by monastic medicine practised in the Benedictine Abbey of San Eutizio, located near Preci. It is well known that St. Benedict of Nursia included in his *Regola* (534 AD): 'infirmorum cura ante omnia' (first, the care of patients). He himself was a famous healer, and legend ascribes to him the faculty of removing bladder stones. The influence of Benedictine medicine on the Preci School is evident in the writings of Constantinus Africanus, who was a surgeon of the Salerno School of Medicine and who followed in his urologic practice the teachings of both monastic surgery and the Preci School of lithotomy. The Preci School took great advantage of the Abbey of San Eutizio, with its library, its hospital and its surgeon-monks *(monacus infirmorum)*, who were also experts in renal–urologic diseases [6].

The Empirics of Preci and 'Half-Surgery'

The operators of the Preci School can be divided into 2 categories: the empirics and the professionals. The former were the earlier and practised so-called 'half-surgery'; they performed lithotomy, phlebotomy and castration. Gathered in the St. Cosma and Damiano College, they used avant-garde surgical tools for many centuries which were later (15th–16th centuries) described by famous surgeons such as Parè and Santo as new techniques.

The Preci empirics, nicknamed 'Cerusici' or 2nd-class 'Vulnerari', had no medical degrees, even though many were given a certificate of 'half-surgery' until the 18th century. They were excellent lithotomists and were asked to teach in some universities, e.g. Perugia, Bologna and Padua. Above all, however, they were called on by prominent people to relieve the problems caused by kidney and bladder stone disease. For example, Pope Innocent IV (1249),

King Luis I d'Angio and Amedeo VI (1382) had stones removed by Preci lithotomists [1].

The 2nd category of Preci surgeons included the 'Doctors Physici', physicians with a degree in medicine and philosophy from the universities of Perugia, Bologna, Pisa, Parma and Venice, who had specialized in lithotomy. These doctors were usually from the noble families of Preci; they were much sought after to teach in universities as lecturers in anatomy, medicine, surgery and lithotomy and to act as consultants in hospitals. They continued the old traditions of the empirics from the 16th century. When the empirics were no longer allowed to perform lithotomy (1751) according to an *editto* (a law) enacted by Carlo Guattani of Novara, *archiatra* (personal physician) of the Pope, only surgeons with a degree could remove the stones, and so the Preci School came to an end.

Instrumentation of the Preci School

The surgeons of the Preci School, both empirics and doctors, were the forerunners of modern lithotomy, by virtue of the tools they invented and crafted some centuries before the spread of modern surgery. There were many lithotomy techniques, named according to their respective inventors. In his book *Surgery,* Guglielmo Saliceto (1210–1280), a famous physician of Piacenza, did not mention the early methods of Preci, and although his lithotomy technique was adopted by many European surgeons, it had fewer advantages than Preci technology. In fact, Saliceto did not use cauterization, nor fire-disinfected tools. He removed only small bladder stones, because he had no proper instrumentation to break the larger ones; lithotrity was unknown to him. The Preci surgeons were the first to fragment large bladder stones with the *frangitore* (crusher), a peculiar strong pincer which was used early in the history of the School [7]. They removed all fragments of the broken stone with a spherical silver cup; they had already realized that even 1 fragment left in the bladder could be the nucleus for another stone. Although the Preci instruments and technology introduced refinements into the treatment of bladder stones, they were not used by other surgeons for many centuries. Only in the 18th century did some surgeons, e.g. Jean Baseilhac, nicknamed Frère Come (1703–1781), and Civiale (1796–1867), introduce an instrument called *rompipietra* (stone-breaker), which was no different from the early *frangitore* of the Preci School.

When bladder stones were believed to be incurable by bloodless lithotomy, the Preci surgeons attempted to remove the stone by an operation performed by a very modern technique with new instruments, e.g. *culter rasorius* (razor), lancet, scalpel, tenaculum, dilator, *strumentum alfonsium* (dissecting forceps), cautery and blow pipe. In addition, they used *siringa* (catheters) to treat urinary retention; if the difficulty in micturating was due to urethral infection or prostatism, the Preci lithotomists replaced the harmful caustic products with emollient *candelette* made with wax, almond oil and kid fat held on catgut, rabbit skin, lute string, or silver wire.

It is important to emphasize that the Preci lithotomists were used to making a differential diagnosis before inserting a catheter, which was unsuitable for stone and gravel disease and for stenosing lesions of the bladder neck. In this case they tried to relieve the urinary retention by local application of a poultice, warm baths and eventually blood-letting. If these cures were ineffective they used the *candelette.*

They soon realized that it was mandatory to cure urine retention as quickly as possible, as according to Marini:

'The urine starts to regurgitate from ureter to kidney and then mixes with blood, and the patient unavoidably dies' [8].

In other words, they connected renal obstruction with acute renal failure many centuries before the development of modern nephrology.

Uroscopic Diagnosis of Stone Disease

The members of the Preci School attached great importance to stone symptomatology and to urine appearance and formation. This knowledge allowed them to make a preliminary evaluation of patients with stone disease before performing lithotomy. They realized early that treatment of stone disease must be directed towards removal of all the stones, together with relief of obstruction and attempts to restore urinary drainage to as near normal as possible.

By direct experience and from knowledge of the most important writings on urine, e.g. the manuscript *De Urinis* from the Salerno School of Medicine [9], the Preci lithotomists were able to rationalize uroscopic diagnosis. They knew, according to the common belief of the Middle Ages, that urine was indicative of 2 things: disease of the liver and veins or the kidneys and bladder [10]. When urine was examined in a special glass bottle named the *matula,* they realized that light, milky and scanty urine indicated bladder stone; if a sandy sediment persisted for a long time this meant there were stones in the kidney, or that stones would be formed in the future. Sulfurous urine was a sign of a bruise in the bladder; foamy urine in the upper section of the *matula* indicated kidney pain. White urine clear around the central part of the matula indicated pain or stone in the kidney.

When the kidney or ureter stone moved down into the bladder after empiric but effective medical treatment, i.e. 2 loaves of warm bread soaked with olive oil locally applied to the kidney area, they noticed that the urine became reddish and dense with round white and red corpuscles in the bottom of the matula. This was a good sign and indicated progression of the stone into the bladder and an urgent need for lithotomy.

Pale urine with white corpuscles in the lower part of the *matula* indicated kidney pain in males, and genital disorders in females. Milky, thick and scanty urine with a great amount of white sediment meant stones in the urinary tract; if there was no sediment it indicated disorders of micturition. After lithotomy, urine was very cloudy for 7 days; then a white sediment appeared. When the patient passed clear urine with a white sediment, it indicated a good result of the lithotomy [11].

The Preci people first, and the Preci School later, knew of many plants and herbs growing in their area with healing properties. This popular medicine combined with monastic herb prescription was also applied to urinary tract diseases, and the remedies were excellent. Diuretic dog's tooth was used for renal stone; elder was effective in uricemic patients and in a gravel-like appearance of urine. Wall pellitory helped to dissolve bladder stones; fried garlic had antihypertensive properties and betony alleviated dropsy and urinary retention [5]. In addition, the Preci people and doctors treated dropsical patients with foxglove, many centuries before Withering used this drug for cardiac and renal disorders [12].

Preci and Nursia were rich in mineral waters with diuretic and uricosuric properties. These mineral waters were used by Preci laymen and surgeons of the School mainly to alleviate dropsy, to improve urinary retention, to dissolve kidney and bladder stones and to mitigate strangury. This was another application of popular medicine to urinary tract disease, on which it had beneficial effects.

Even though there is only slight evidence of originality in pharmacotherapeutics, the Preci School furnishes an instructive example derived from the wise application of natural healing aids to the needs of renal patients.

Conclusion

The urologic tradition in Preci is considered by some historians of medicine to be the continuance of the Salerno School of Medicine. Based on popular empiricism, it is an example of the type of medicine that developed in Umbria and spread throughout Italy for many centuries. Its importance deserves more fame and appreciation. The urologic tradition expressed great interest in diagnosis, in differential diagnosis, in medical and above all in surgical treatment of kidney and bladder stones. Lithotomy was performed by both bloodless and operative methods. The Preci lithotomists were the first to perform lithotrity; their skill was due to the availability of a large variety of instrumentation, which they had invented, made and used. Today, the modernity of these instruments can be admired in many collections of old Preci and Nursia families and in some national museums, e.g. the Instituto di Storia della Medicina in the University of Rome.

References

1 Scacchi D: Subsidium Medicinae, Urbini, Ragufios, 1596.
2 Lanfranchi G (Lanfranco): Chirurgia Magna et Parva. Venice, 1490. Quoted by Fabbi, see Ref. 5.
3 Sensi M: Cerretani e ciarlatani nel secolo XV. Medicina nei Secoli 1978;15:69–91.
4 Pirri P: I Cerretani. La Civiltà Cattolica 1935; 3:350–365.
5 Fabbi A: La Scuola Chirurgica di Preci. Spoleto, Arti Grafiche Panetta-Petrelli, 1974, p 53.
6 Timio M: La Scuola Chirurgica di Preci e l'arte della litotomia; in La Storia Tecnologica del Guarire. Rome, Borla, 1990, pp 85–90.
7 Sculteti J: Armamentarium Chirurgicum. Venice, Typis Combi and La Nou, 1665.
8 Marini G: Pratica delle Principali Operazioni di Chirurgia che Riguardano il Litotomo ed Oculista. Rome, 1723. Quoted by Fabbi, see Ref. 5.
9 Pantaleoni M, Bernabeo R: Un inedito Tractatus de Urinis Salernitano. Rivista Storia della Medicina 1966;10:126–145.
10 Dal Canton A, Castellano M: Theory of urine formation and uroscopic diagnosis in the Medical School of Salerno. Kidney Int 1989;34:273–277.
11 Leonardi E: Una terra di Medici e di Santi. Atti II° Riunione di Scienze Mediche e Naturali, Venice, 1909 in: Rivista d'Italia e d'America, Venice, 1923.
12 Withering WA: An Account of the Foxglove and Some of its Medical Use. Birmingham, M Swinney, 1795.

The Salerno School of Medicine

Am J Nephrol 1994;14:477

Bernardo D'Onorio

Abbot of Montecassino, Italy

Cultural Links between Salerno and Montecassino

Key Words

Cassiodorus
Abbot Bertario
Codex 97 from Montecassino
Juvenal
Salerno School of Medicine

Abstract

A meeting on the History of Nephrology is an opportunity to discuss the links between science and faith which were split until the 6th century. However, this was changed by Cassiodorus and monasticism. From the times of Abbot Bertario (died 883 AD) in Montecassino, medicine was regarded as an art and a science. Codex 97 from Cassino offers a program of professional deontology, based on sensitivity, discretion, respect and responsiveness to the need of patients.

Talking about the history of nephrology, as in this conference, means touching on an important topic in the history of medicine as a whole, but at the same time it provides an opportunity to consider the issues that link science and faith. One of the great merits of monasticism, in fact, was its contribution to the evolution of the medical sciences by means of both studies and codex transcriptions of *Ars Medica,* thereby developing a solid bridge between the two. Until the 6th century, faith and science were profoundly divided; however, this was changed by Cassiodorus and monasticism, both providing a new stimulus to medicine as an art and a science in the ancient Greek settlements of southern Italy, particularly in Naples. In Montecassino, traces of this can still be found in some of the manuscripts dating to the time of Abbott Bertario (died 883 AD).

Among the texts of Codex 97 from Cassino, it is worthwhile highlighting *Quomodo Visitare Debeas Infirmum,* which became quite popular in southern Italy. This text offers a 'program' of professional deontology – the study of moral obligations and ethics – which reached its apex in the Salerno School of Medicine. Here is the beginning, precise and exemplary: *Non omnem infirmum uniter visites, sed, si integre audire vis, disce* ... The physician has, in a certain sense and at least at a certain stage, to give up his abstract scientific knowledge and learn directly from the experience of physical pain from the patient. It is necessary to be sensitive and responsive to the needs of the patient. Sensitivity and discretion, not without reason, also are the key words of the monastic Benedictine language! The text is followed by a reminder of the way of analyzing the various pathologies: *Mox quo ingredieris ad infirmum, interroga eum si quis forsitan ei dolet ... Postea tenes ei pulsum et vide si febricitat an anon ... et requires ab eo ... et interroga si ... et require ...* (When you see a patient ask him if he has pain, thereafter take the pulse, check the presence of fever, ask him ... enquire ... try to understand ...). It is the sign of empiric attention, based on experience, to man and his illnesses. Medieval medical science did not possess the same certainty as ancient medicine, but it gained from Christianity a sense of respect of the individual and of sensitivity to humanity as a window on the divine. All this for a precise scientific aim: to investigate the causes of diseases and to find adequate cures for them.

A teaching that is still valid nowadays comes to us from medieval science, which did not develop outside the needs of man, but in conjunction with practice, to regain the physical health that ancient culture considered an essential part of spiritual fitness. The aphorism of Juvenal, a Roman lawyer (55–135 AD), underlines this teaching with great clarity: *Mens sana in corpore sano* (a sound mind in a sound body).

Abbot Bernardo D'Onorio
Abbazia di Montecassino
I–03043 Cassino (Italy)

Am J Nephrol 1994;14:478–482

Maria Pasca

Soprintendenza per i Beni Ambientali
Architettonici Artistici e Storici di Salerno e
Avellino, Salerno, Italy

The Salerno School of Medicine

Key Words
Salerno School of Medicine
Uroscopy
Surgery
Medieval medicine

Abstract

The cultural revival in Salerno was linked to Benedictine monasticism, with its main center at Montecassino. Historical evidence of the activity of the Salerno School of Medicine dates back to the 10th century, though the most productive period of the Salerno masters was in the 11th–13th centuries. The school's knowledge was broadened in the 12th century by the work of Constantinus Africanus, who translated many classical texts from Arabic into Latin. *Circa Instans,* a fundamental text on medicinal botany, was also produced by Mattaeus Platearius. Towards the middle of the 12th century, the school gradually became a theoretical center, rather than a primarily practical one, and many commentaries on earlier texts were produced. Uroscopy was pre-eminent in the teachings of Salerno, which was also one of the first medical centers to recognize the contribution of surgery to treatment. The precepts of the school were widely disseminated by the *Regimen Sanitatis Salernitanum*, which contained remedies for every occasion and advice on keeping healthy.

Introduction

The *ars medica* of Salerno stems from the various cultural influences on the city during the Middle Ages. The geographic position of Salerno in the very heart of the Mediterranean, placed the city at the focal point of important exchanges with the East and Africa, promoted by Amalfi and Sicily. The foundation of the School was attributed by legend to four masters: Helinus, Pontus, Adela and Salernus – a Jew, an Arab, a Greek and a Salernitan, respectively, which can be taken to indicate that Jewish, Arabic, Greek and Latin cultures all contributed to the Salernitan *ars medica.*

Early Activity at Salerno

The great cultural revival in Salerno was linked to Benedictine monasticism, which had its main center at Montecassino and was represented in Salerno by the Abbey of St. Benedict, which played an important role in the evolution of scientific study and therapeutic practice. The *ars medica* enriched its store of experimental knowledge both through its charitable, or to be more precise hospital, activities, which were carried out in the infirmaries of the monasteries, and also through the work of lay doctors, sometimes women, who first of all performed their experiments separately, and then together with a more speculative and didactic aim.

Historical evidence of the activities of the School goes back to the 10th century. Among the sources of the *Chronicon Salernitanum is the Historia Inventionis ac Translationis et Miracula Sanctae Trophimenae*, a hagiographic

Maria Pasca
Via G. Vigorito 6
I–84121 Salerno (Italy)

text dating back to the 10th century and edited by an anonymous writer in Minori. Earlier activities are illustrated in the legend of Teodonanda, a young bride who lived with her husband, Mauro, between Minori and Amalfi. One day she fell ill; Mauro was frantic. When the young woman was on her deathbed, her relatives said: 'Let us take her to Salerno, where the great Gerolamo may be able to find a cure'. Gerolamo the doctor, who was famous throughout Salerno, began to consult 'immensa volumina librorum' in the hope of finding some indication relating to the illness. The year was 870 AD. It would seem that already by that time the organizational structure of the School of Medicine was running well.

Another legend illustrates the importance of Salerno in later years. In 946 AD, over 70 years after the Teodonanda episode, Richeiro of Reims tells that at the court of Lotaire, the King of France (who may have been Charles IV), Derault the bishop of Amiens met a doctor from Salerno who had been invited to court by virtue of his skills. Derault, too, was an expert in medicine. By the 10th century the schools of Chartres, Reims and Montpellier had gradually become the transalpine answer to the international reputation of the Salerno School of Medicine. The 2 archiatras sat with the King and Queen Emma to answer to the question put to them. Derault proved to have a very sound scientific background and was able to expound successfully and articulately on matters. The Salerno doctor was unable to display the same theoretic and dialectic grounding, but was outstanding in the sharpness of his wit and the readiness of his mind owing to his experience. This rivalry between 2 colleagues indicates a competitiveness between the 2 separate schools.

The awareness of Salerno's science in French literature was again demonstrated in the 10th century by Hugo de Flavigny (1065–1140) in his *Chronicon* of 984 AD. Hugo traces the voyage to Italy of Adalbèron, the bishop of Verdun. The prelate reached Salerno with his retinue, hoping to find a cure for his many afflictions, and stayed a while at the School of Medicine.

These narratives from Richeiro of Reims and Hugo de Flavigny stress the prominence of the Salerno School of Medicine in a 9th and 10th century world strongly influenced by the mediating role of Monte Cassino.

Salerno in the 11th–13th centuries

The Salerno School of Medicine was only institutionalized in the 13th century in the articles of Federico II, published in Melfi in 1231, in which it was called the only medical school in the Kingdom. In 1280, Carlo I issued its first statute, in which it was recognized as a 'Studium Generale' in medicine. The School continued its activities under changing circumstances until 1811, when Gioacchino Murat reorganized the public education of the Kingdom, and gave Naples University the exclusive right to grant degrees.

The most productive scientific period of the Salerno masters was from the 11th to the 13th centuries. Salerno's literary production in the 11th century stemmed from an understanding of some practical and pharmacologic treatises by Galen, on the doctrine of humors, the works of Pliny, Dioscorides, Celius Aurelianus and others. This reliance on ancient sources and the fact that the treatments were compilations has given rise to certain difficulties in collating and referencing the works, but there emerges in them a greater interest in practical medicine than in its general theoretic problems. Written in the form of manuals useful for teaching purposes, these treatises are based on prescriptions and observations based on the authors' direct experience as well as on tradition. The literary works of 11th century Salerno are exemplified by the works of Gariopontus, Petroncello, Trotula and Alfano I.

The medicine of the Salerno masters in the 11th century was based on Hippocratic–Galenic theories of the humors and their views of disease as an imbalance of the 4 humors within the human body: blood, bile, phlegm (secretion of the nasal fossae, thought to come from the brain) and *strabile* or black bile (thought to come from the spleen). The therapies adopted to restore the humoral balance tended to eliminate or increase the secretions, taking into account the patient's age, the parts of the body in which they were produced, and the seasons of the year in which the illness occurred, as there was held to be a close connection between the constitutive elements of the human body and Nature.

Constantinus Africanus

The School's knowledge broadened in the 12th century, with the availability of the work of Constantinus Africanus, the first Western doctor to popularize Arabic medicine. After a lifetime of study and travels which took him to Persia, Arabia and Arab-ruled Spain, Constantinus went to Monte Cassino in the 2nd half of the 11th century, where he devoted himself to translating numerous classical texts from Arabic into Latin.

In the detailed list of his numerous works supplied by Pietro Diacono in *De Viris Illustribus* are translations of works by Isaac Judaeus on urine, diet and fevers, of the

Isagoge and *De Oculis* by Johannitius, as well as many works including *De Anatomia,* the *Practica,* the *Cyrurgia,* the *Ginecia* and *Gradibus,* over which scholars have long argued whether they consist of his original works or are plagiarisms. Constantinus translated the *Aforismi* and the *Pronostici* by Hippocrates; the work on acute diseases, with comments by Galen, from whom he had translated the *Ars Parva;* and other works.

The material supplied by Constantinus began to be absorbed by the Salerno masters towards the middle of the 12th century, when the texts he translated were adopted as study material. The *Isagoge* by Johannitius and perhaps *Pronostici* by Hippocrates in translation from Arabic became part of the curriculum, later referred to as *Articella.* It was in the pharmaceutic field above all, however, that the School felt the influence of Constantinus. More than half of the prescriptions contained in the Salerno *antidotaria* and previously unheard of stem from *Pantegni,* Constantinus' translations of the treatises of Galen, replete with Aristotelian doctrine.

Other Writers

The 12th century witnessed the greatest development in the Salerno School of Medicine. Literary production was at its peak in this period: writings on fevers, diets, the pulse and other issues specific to medicine were the subject of many studies and treatises. The Salerno masters of the 12th century do not seem to have blindly followed classical sources; their writing, instead, signalled their adoption of a more critical attitude to previous citations and collections. Thus, the step from the *compendium* (a straightforward collection of principles) to the *commentarium,* which instead is a critical elaboration of models enriched by observation and annotation together with revisions dictated by new experience, was taken.

A practical purpose and a didactic aim were always present in the texts. In fact, what still prevails in the writings on therapy and in the *antidotaria* is the empiric observation of the single pathologic forms which were analytically and systematically treated 'a capite ad calcem'.

Many were the authors of writings in this period: Giovanni Afflacio, pupil of Constantinus and his leading promulgator, Cofone il Giovane, Magister Bartolomaeus and Giovanni Plateario II, probably the father of Mattaeus who about 50 years later prepared the glossary to *Antidotarium* by Niccolo and was author of a treatise on herbs, commonly known as the *Circa Instans.*

Circa Instans was the fundamental work of medieval medicinal botany, and took its title from the first words of the prologue: 'Circa instans negotium in simplicibus medicinis nostrum versatur propositum'. Starting with a detailed description of about 500 plants, the author went on to differentiate the various species, identifying some that had been unknown before then and giving the geographic origin, the Greek and Latin names and, in some cases, the popular name of each plant.

Greater attention towards more general theoretic principles was displayed in Practica by Magister Bartolomaeus, who knew Greek and was a meticulous etymologic researcher. *Practica* was one of the most important and widespread works of the time. Other authors of important treatises on therapy were Magister Salernus, Magister Ferrarius, Petroncello and Niccolo Salernitano, author of the *Antidotarium,* a pharmaceutical handbook widely used in the School.

Medical Theory and Teaching in the 12th Century

Towards the middle of the 12th century the Salerno School of Medicine underwent an important transformation, in which it lost the characteristic of a predominantly practical center of medicine and increasingly became a center dedicated above all to theoretic elaboration through its literary output. The works of the Salerno masters now become objects of study and comment: Mattaeus Platearius annotated the *Antidotarium* by Niccolo; 4 masters (Archimattaeus, Petroncello, Platearius and Ferrarius) commented on the *Surgery* of Rolando da Parma and Ruggero da Frugardo. The affirmation of this literary form and its progressive substitution for the simple collection of prescriptions and antidotes are evidence of a new kind of teaching, centered on the reading and commenting on authoritative texts that became characteristic in subsequent centuries.

The Salerno School of Medicine developed its own teaching curriculum based on the study of a group of classical texts made up of *Isagoge* by Johannitius, translated by Constantinus Africanus, the *Aforismi* and *Pronostici* of Hippocrates, *De Urinis* by Theophilus, *De Pulsibus* by Philaretes and *Ars Parva* by Galen. The last does not appear in any of the manuscripts of the commentaries on the *Articella,* but was added towards the end of the century, probably in Constantinus' translation.

During the 13th century the body of work, printed in the 15th and 16th centuries with the title *Articella,* also came to include the *De Regimine Acutorum* by Hippocrates, translated from Arabic by Gerard of Cremona. In the 13th century it came to be used as a text in Salerno, Naples and Paris, and constituted the basis of the study of medicine until the 18th century.

Uroscopy in Salerno

In the Salerno School of Medicine, the use of uroscopy had a semiologic value. No diagnosis, in fact, was carried out without urine examination. The color, quantity and sediments of urine were observed for many illnesses and the particulars of each case were listed. Many doctors in Salerno used uroscopy, e.g. Alfano, Platearius, Giovanni Afflacio, but distinguished among these were Magister Maurus, Urso of Calabria and the Frenchman Gilles de Corbeil, all authors of texts devoted specifically to this subject, which came to be essential and widespread reading matter.

Maurus' *Tractatus de Urinis* came to be considered a fundamental text. In *De Laudibus et Virtutibus Compositorum Medicaminum*, Gilles de Corbeil praised the work of Maurus and declared that he had obtained all available knowledge on urine. In his treatise, Maurus gave directions for correct uroscopic examination. It is interesting to note that apart from the observation of color and sediment, it was also necessary to examine the level of the urine in which the sediment was deposited. He subdivided it into 4 strata, each of which referred to a part of the body: if the urine appeared cloudy in the upper stratum, the illness affected the head; if the 2nd stratum was cloudy, the heart and lungs were diseased; a disease of the internal organs was shown by cloudiness in the 3rd stratum; while the 4th stratum indicated whether the genital organs and the bladder were unhealthy. Maurus took up the argument dealt with in *De Urinis* once more in *Regulae Urinarum*. In the text already cited, Gilles de Corbeil also acknowledged Urso of Calabria, author of the treatise *De Urinis*, describing him as: 'Strenuus ambiguous causarum solvere nodos'. Urso must be considered as a central figure in the cultural panorama of the 12th century in Salerno.

Gilles de Corbeil also spread the Salernitan doctrine on urine abroad; having studied at the Salerno School of medicine and then established himself in Paris, he described the dictates and teachings of this school in his poem *De Urinis*, which became a classic of uroscopy and was adopted as a text until the 18th century in European medical schools.

Surgery in Salerno

A very interesting aspect of the Salerno School of Medicine was the presence in some treatises, e.g. *Practica* by Petroncello and *De Mulierum Passionibus* by Trocta, of elements of surgery, at a time when it was not considered a branch of medicine, but merely an offshoot activity with no scientific connotations. Surgery in Salerno, therefore, came to be within the doctor's compass, and not something simply entrusted to unqualified persons.

As early as Petroncello there was talk of sutures and the binding of blood vessels in case of heavy hemorrhage, but not until the time of Ruggero da Frugardo was a systematic codification of the fundamental principles of surgical teaching undertaken, which was commented on by 4 Salerno masters. Ruggero's *Rogerina*, known also as *Post Mundi Fabricam*, was very widely circulated; it was known and commented on in Europe, and for almost a century it was considered to be the surgical text *par excellence*.

The most important rework of *Chirurgia* was that of Roland of Parma, who in 1250 produced a new edition of it, in which Ruggero's work was enriched with additions based on Roland's own practical experiences. Roland showed himself to be independent of the master, correcting him in some cases and proposing some new operations.

In the 12th century, Gerard of Cremona translated *Chirurgia* by Albucasis, a Spanish Arab of the 11th century, and thus contributed notably to the development of knowledge in the surgical field. Western surgical practice was influenced by these new teachings. In *Chirurgia Magna* by Bruno da Longobucco, a Calabrian doctor, can be found an example of this mixture of classical knowledge and Arabic innovation.

Medieval surgery reached its culmination with Guglielmo da Saliceto, who in his *Chirurgia* expressed his concept of surgery thus:

'... it is one of the various sciences included in medicine'.

Regimen Sanitatis Salernitanum

The hygienic precepts dictated by the Salerno School of Medicine were widely disseminated by means of a treatise called *Regimen Sanitatis Salernitanum*. There were many editions of the manuscript and prints of the *Regimen*, which spread the Salernitan teachings throughout Italy and abroad.

No information is available about the original version of the *Regimen*, which over the centuries was enlarged by various additions by anonymous authors, so much so that the original 362 verses of the first printed edition in 1479 increased to about 3,520 in its last edition. The origin of the *Regimen* is also not well established, but it seems to have been a collective work, the fruit of popular custom, gathered together and commented on in the 13th century by the Spanish doctor Arnaldo da Villanova and then expanded over the years.

The *Regimen Sanitatis* was written in leonine verse so that it could be easily remembered. Even though it was not a true medical treatise, it was used for centuries as a medical text and contains remedies for every occasion and advice on keeping healthy. The *summa* of Salernitan teachings, however, are condensed in the first few verses, which suggest a hygienic and highly peaceful way of life. This was constantly reaffirmed in subsequent additions.

Maintaining the equilibrium of the 4 humors of body was fundamental for preserving good health, and this required a sober and peaceful way of life.

'Si vis incolumen, si vis te vivere sanum,
curas tolle graves, irasci crede profanum.
Parce mero coenato parum; non sit tibi vanum
surgere post epulas somnum fuge meridianum;
ne mictum retine ne comprime fortiter anum.'

Further Reading

De Renzi S: Storia Documentata della Scuola Medica Salernitana, 2nd ed. Naples, 1857.

De Renzi S: Collectio Salernitana. Naples, 1852–1859.

Westelberg U (ed): Chronicon Salernitanum. Stockholm, 1956.

Historia Inventionum ac Translationis ac Miracula Sanctae Trophimenae, in Acta Sanctorum, Iul. 5, II. Antenurpiae, 1731, pp 233–240.

Giacosa P: Magistri Salernitani Nondum Editi. Catalogo Ragionato della Esposizione di Storia della Medicina Aperta in Torino nel 1838. Turin, 1901.

Kristeller PO: La Scuola Medica di Salerno Secondo Ricerche e Scoperte Recenti. Salerno, 1980.

Kristeller PO: Studi sulla Scuola Medica Salernitana. Naples, 1986.

Sinno A: Regimen Sanitatis, Flos Medicinae Scholae Salerni, Traduzione e Note di Andrea Sinno, Presentazione di S. Visco. Salerno, 1979.

Pazzini A: Ruggero di Giovanni Frugardo Maestro di Chirurgia a Parma e l'Opera Sua. Rome, 1966.

Tabanelli M: La Chirurgia Italiana nell'Alto Medioevo. Florence, 1965.

Pasca M: La Scuola Medica Salernitana, Storia, Immagini, Manoscritti dall'XI al XII Secolo. Naples, 1987.

Am J Nephrol 1994;14:483–487

Massimo Oldoni

Faculte di Lettere, University of Salerno,
Department of Latinity and Middle Ages,
Fisciano, Salerno, Italy

Uroscopy in the Salerno School of Medicine

Key Words
Uroscopy
Salerno School of Medicine
Treatment of women

Abstract

Uroscopy was one of the basic diagnostic tests of the Salerno School of Medicine. The *De Urinis* of Magister Maurus was the work to which all urologic knowledge of the 12th and 13th centuries referred. His urologic doctrine was organized according to the theory of the 4 strata, and represented the extreme opposite from that of Cofone, according to whom the vital stream of urine expressed the depurative needs of the organs themselves. Salerno was also interesting in that it devoted as much attention to urology in women as in men, recognizing their fundamental role in the survival of the species. Unfortunately, much of the original work has become obscured by the many additions to the works of the masters and the spurious texts of lesser physicians.

Introduction

Uroscopy in the Hippocratic age had much in common with the store of medico-semiologic experience of the Salerno School of Medicine. Urine testing was one of the basic diagnostic tests of the School, and the color, quantity, sediments and concretions were recorded together with a classification of the different types of urine present in various diseases, urologic or otherwise. Following the heritage of the treatise *De Urinis* by Cornelius Celsus and Galen, which put to good use knowledge of the subject that had its roots in Arabic culture, the Salerno doctors founded a true tradition of study. Proof of this tradition is to be found in the works of Alfano, Giovanni Plateario and Giovanni Afflacio, and in particular in the work of Magister Maurus, Urso of Calabria and the Frenchman Egide de Corbeil, who were considered the best-known exponents of this branch of medical knowledge.

Writers and Writings of Salerno

The *De Urinis* of Maurus is perhaps the apex of this type of scientific writing, to which all urologic knowledge of the 12th and 13th centuries referred, and which Egide de Corbeil praised in *De Laudibus et Virtutibus Compositorum Medicaminum.*

Maurus devotes particular attention in his diagnostic texts to what he called 'the strata' of urine, each of which could be related to a particular zone of the human body (fig. 1). If the urine appeared turbid in the upper stratum of the sediment, the illness affected the head; if it was turbid in the 2nd stratum, the parts affected were the heart and the lungs; the 3rd stratum related to intestinal infections, while turbidity in the 4th stratum of the urine indicated concretions due to heaviness and density, implying genital disease or adisease of the bladder. Maurus returned to this topic in *Regulae Urinarum,* which together

Prof. Massimo Oldoni
Faculte di Lettere
University of Salerno
Department of Latinity and Middle Ages
I-84084 Fisciano, Salerno (Italy)

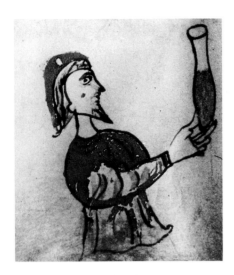

Fig. 1. Maurus, *Glosulae.* National Library, Paris, Codex Lat. 18499, F 144v.

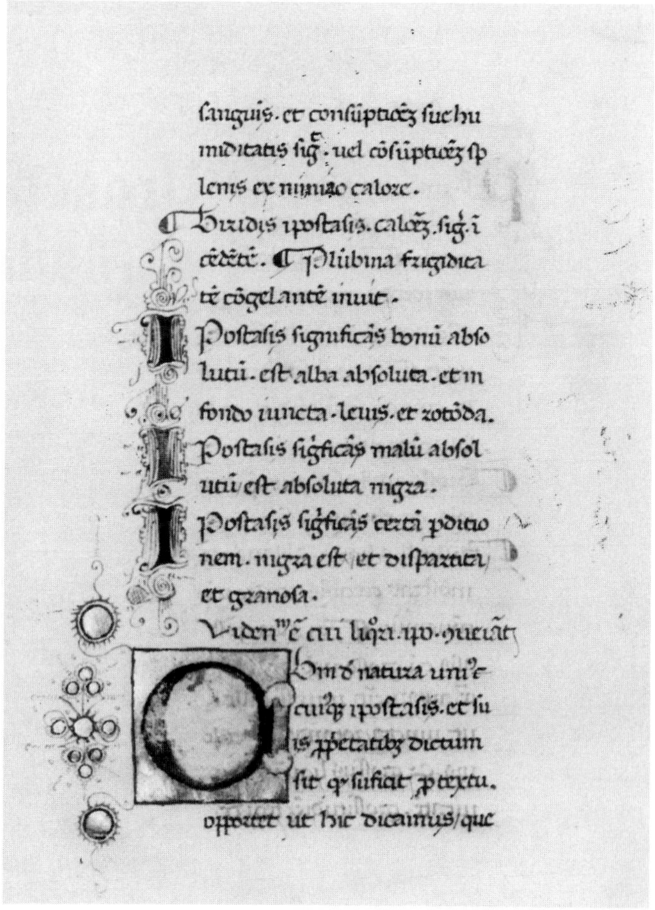

Fig. 2. Urso, *De Urinis.* National Library, Rome, Ms. Vittorio Emanuele 839 (15th century), F 3.

with studies on phlebotomy and febrile states constituted an authentic Salerno urologic *corpus.*

Urso of Calabria was also highly esteemed for his ability to cure cases of renal calculus, defined in the literature of the times as *strenuus ambiguos causarum solvere nodos.* The role of Urso is also notable because in his *De Urinis* (fig. 2, 3) he was clearly influenced by Aristotle's natural philosophy. Coming after Maurus and Urso, Egide de Corbeil was the driving force of uroscopic knowledge from Salerno that dominated the European medical culture until the end of the 18th century. Egide added to the pathologic case histories and succeeded in classifying at least 20 types of urine in which color was considered to be connected to various diseases. Thus, reddish urine implied hepatic ailments, while greenish urine indicated the presence of icterus; when it appeared yellow and very dense this was most likely due to renal problems and the formation of crystals.

Comparing the first draft of *Flos Medicinae Scholae Salerni,* written at the end of the 10th century, with the far more ample later version written at the end of the 13th century by the great Spanish scientist Arnaldo of Villanova, it can be seen that the original meager 64 lines become in Arnaldo's version no less than 29 articles of the 23rd chapter of the 6th part of the work. Apart from confirming the continuity of the *Regimen Sanitatis,* the chapter on urine, translated by Constantinus Africanus (figs. 4, 5) from the Arabic work *Pantegni* by Ali-ibn-Abbas, does not provide much enlightenment regarding

the practice of uroscopy, despite the significance of the original work and the numerous citations from the (at times generic) scientific treatise by Alfano I of Salerno. Instead, it was the doctors of the period from the mid-11th century until the end of the 12th century who provided the outstanding variety of texts and contributions on the urologic-uroscopic theme. Listed below are those manuscripts that most certainly originated in Salerno:

(1) *De Modo Medendi* by Cofone the Elder; (2) *De Urinis et Earumdem Significationibus;* (3) *Anatomia Porci* by Cofone the Younger; (4) *De Urinis* by a pupil of Cofone the Younger; (5) *Liber Urinarum* (or *Regulae Urinarum*) by Giovanni Afflacio; (6) *Tractatus Urinarum* by Bartolomeo of Salerno; (7) *Regulae Urinarum* by Giovanni Plateario; (8) *De Urinis* by Matteo d'Episcopo; (9) *Regulae Urinarum* by Maurus.

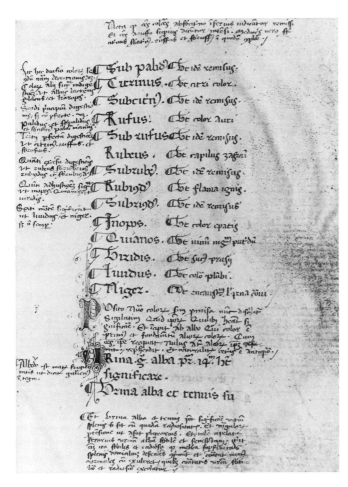

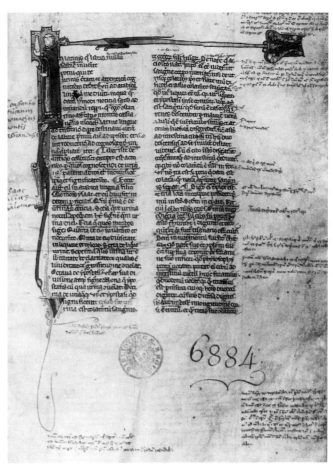

Fig. 3. Urso, *De Urinis.* National Library, Rome, Ms. Vittorio Emanuele (15th century), F 43.

Fig. 5. Isaaci Salomonis Filii, *Liber de Urinis ex Arabico in Latinum Translatus a Constantino Afro, Monacho Cassinensi.* National Library, Paris, Ms. Lat. 6884 (13th century), F 1.

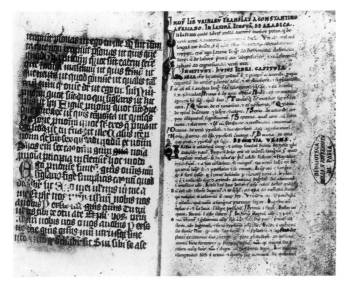

Fig. 4. Ishap ibn Suleiman, *Liber Urinarum.* Translated by Constantinus Africanus. University Library, Pavia, Ms. 449 (12th century), F 1.

Female Urology in Salerno

The most interesting aspect common to all of the texts cited here is that, contrary to common belief, urology in Salerno did not only consider the male aspect of the question, and a similar amount of material is devoted to the female *matrix* and indicates its importance and social role in connection with procreation and the survival of the species. In this typically medieval attention to the perpetuation of the female *matrix* in the continuation of the family line, female urology acquires so much importance that in the work of Cofone, great attention is directed towards the structure of the *matrix.* This is described as being formed in such a way that the sperm are not lost and the process of gestation of the fetus can be initiated. This is considered an authentic gift of nature to the privileged physiology of women.

On the basis of the anatomy of the pig, the solid parts of the body, called *membra,* were classified according to qualities that established their physiology. Thus, there were animal *membra,* active in sensations and movements; spiritual *membra,* which allowed the circulation of the active forces of vitality, and finally natural *membra,* which included the agents of nutrition and of procreation. In the *Demonstratio Anatomica,* an important role was ascribed to the genitals due to their generative faculties. This explained why nature had endowed them with particular protection (the scrotum and external vestibules), while the penis and *matrix* had subordinate roles, closely dependent on the circulation of blood that, in the doctrine of Cofone, influenced their effectiveness. It is necessary therefore to fully understand the Salernitan view of blood flow. The large artery that descends from the heart along the spinal column was believed to divide itself at the level of the kidneys where the vital spirit was transmitted to the testicles, present in both men and women, and with a function believed to be a determining factor for procreation. Equally, through the inferior vena cava, the blood descended along the sides of the spinal column.

From the *Pantegni* of Ali-ibn-Abbas were taken the notions of sperm ducts protected in a *folliculum,* a small sac formed under the skin at the height of the peritoneum, similar to a small hernia protected by membranes. Postmortem observation of the pig did not, however, help those who carried out dissection in order to compare these characteristics with human physiology, in which the penis was described as an authentic force of nature and for this reason the *caro nervosa* extended the organ when desire was felt. In this movement Cofone recognized an element much neglected in the later treatise: the sense of pleasure:

'Per vasa sua in vulvam prosiliat sperma, unde virga fit nervosa ut in spermatis emissione et tali actione turpissima per nimia sensibilitate magna fiat delectatio.'

The *actio turpissima* seemed to annul the reward constituted by pleasure, so much so that the following description of the *matrix* was very precise in specifying that the 2 orifices, the external one called *collum matricis* and the internal one called *os matricis,* had their own sensitivity only so long as their contact with the male organ stimulated it to erection and forceful ejaculation. Some sensitivity transpired in the brief *meditatio* ascribed to the *collum matricis,* which varied according to age, epoch and nature. In adolescent girls and old women this organ was smaller than in adult women and was wider in passionate women than in less ardent ones.

A text that descends directly from this analysis is the *Anatomia Nicolai Physici,* in which the author narrated the disapprobation of Christians towards the dissection of cadavers, rejecting the criterion of the similarity between man and animals. Despite this, the *Anatomia Nicolai* is an advancement of the typical Cofonian observations in *Anatomia Porci,* adding to it the notion of *didymus,* superior sperm canals where sperm material was formed and developed. The notable application of Galenic observation still seems much present in the description used by the texts.

Uroscopic Doctrines

The *Liber de Urinis et earumdem significationibus,* perhaps written by one of Cofone's pupils, offers some further points of interest in its distinction between 'color' and 'substance' in urinary science. In this *substantia* the author describes 3 characteristics: *tenuitas, pinguedo* and *mediocritas.* While the color of the liquid comes directly from the 'humoral' characteristics of the individual, according to the fundamental division into 4 temperaments (choleric, melancholic, sanguine and phlegmatic), the application of the concept of 'substance' is more original. The *De Urinis* thus classifies *urina tenuis* as the liquid that is most difficult to study. 'Light' urine, in healthy subjects, implies *nimia intensio siccitatis*; in the unhealthy, it implies instead a *constrictio* and a *mortificatio materiae.* Light urine often has an *albus* color and a rather cool temperature. In illness, its *mortificatio* renders it, after about 7 days, *spissa,* prolonging the fever for at least 20 days; the internal decay of the *membra* of the organism made the liquid dense. In Cofone's opinion, there is nothing like *dissolutivi* remedies, based on herbs such as scammony, hellebore and euphorbium. Spissa urine, nevertheless, was also characteristic of some ages, e.g. *pueritia,* which was *calida et humida*; whereas in women the 'density' of the urine was proof that it was formed due to too much food and bulimia. In the age of *iuventus* light urine must be *rubea procalore dominante*; in old age it must be *pallida* and *albissima.*

Cofone's urologic theory and that of his school differed from the other great theory of some decades later, developed by Magister Maurus and his school. Maurus organized his doctrine according to the theory of the 4 strata. In this geology of analysis, Maurus differed profoundly from the hydrology of Cofone, according to whom the vital stream of urine expressed the same depurative needs that the organs have in themselves. Moreover, Cofone understood well the *quatuor complexiones,* but does not seem to have given them the fundamental importance typical of the other, more simplistic Salerno clinicians. Cofone and Maurus can be considered as the two poles of a theory of observation.

The *De Urinis et earumdem significationibus* also provides a precise list of the relationships existing between the *urina tenuis* and the disease process. If there is *rubea* and *multum spissa* on the surface, there is pleurisy. If the urine is *alba* and with a very frequent desire to urinate, hydropsy is present, but if it remains *alba* in women over the age of 14 years, it means retention due to menstruation. An arthritic man can also be recognized by 'light' urine that appears *alba* and contains small round bodies in suspension; when a *phreneticus* shows abundant urination it means that its *phrenesis* has been dissolved, but if the light liquid becomes dark the indications are even worse: jaundice without remedy, a difficult fever. Finally, when the urine is red but very scanty and accompanied by thirst, absence of sweating, or the skin burns, and there is also a constant flow of liquid from the belly, the person is close to death. All things considered, the equilibrium much theorized on by the Salerno tradition seems to be somehow present in the school of Cofone, where the humidity of the body and the sweat of the limbs seem to reflect the importance of the liquid temperament of human physiology.

Conclusions

The quantity of empiric observations and the variety of cases examined make the urologic tradition of Salerno a vast container of scientific principles and convictions, which often in the space of a generation contradict themselves. In the author's opinion, it is essential to compare the etiology of certain diagnoses and the precision of some classifications proposed by some of the authors. It is necessary to be able to distinguish within the different schools (of Cofone, Maurus and Plateario) the main currents of the urologic research. From this need was born the 'systemization' of Arnaldo of Villanova, and the original few verses of the first *Regimen* became the *Semioticae Urinae* in 29 articles. Salerno urologic semiotics is therefore necessary and helpful in identifying the many confusions that some unworthy doctors of the School perpetuated in the fund of urologic knowledge. At the end of this examination very few coherent contributions will be found that are scientifically based on the Salerno masters, as opposed to numerous, none-too-cultured tutors who at times undeservedly included themselves in the hall of fame of the great physicians.

Further Reading

De Renzi S: Collectio Salernitana. Bologna, Forni Editore, 1967 (facsimile reproduction of the original printed in Naples in 1852–1859).

De Renzi S: Storia Documentata della Scuola Medica di Salerno. Milan, Fierro Edizioni, 1967 (facsimile reproduction of the original printed in Naples in 1857).

Beccaria A: I Codici della Medicina del Periodo Presalernitano (IX–X Century). Rome, Edizioni Scuola e Letteratura, 1956.

Kristeller PO: Studi sulla Scuola Medica Salernitana. Naples, Istituto Italiano Studi Filosofici, 1986.

Oldoni M: Un medioevo senza santi: la Scuola Medica di Salerno dalle origini al XIII secolo; in Pasca M (ed): La Scuola Medica Salernitana. Storia Immagini e Manoscritti dall'XI al XIII Secolo. Naples, Electa, 1988, 13–29.

Oldoni M: La cultura latina; in Pugliese Carratelli G (ed): Storia e Civiltà della Campania, vol 2, Medioevo. Naples, Electa, 1992, pp 295–401.

Am J Nephrol 1994;14:488–493

Translated from latin by
Albert Coward, Garabed Eknoyan,
Natale Gaspare De Santo

Naples/Houston, Tex.

Codices on the Art of Medicine in the Montecassino Archives

....

Key Words
Works of Alcuin
Anonymous medical excerpts
Medical works of Galen
Works of Hippocrates and Pseudo-Hippocrates
Constantinus Africanus

....

Introduction

At the conclusion of the International Conference on History of Nephrology on October 30, 1993 in the Abbazia of Montecassino, the participants had the privilege to visit a very special exhibition of codices. Father Faustino Avagliano, Curator of the Archivio di Montecassino, selected 8 codices from the IX to the XIV Century and prepared a Latin catalogue [1].

The codices exhibited were:
- *3KK* (ext. 3; int 655):
  Alcuini opera nonnulla, astronomica et alia complura. (Saec. IX)
- *69 V* (ext. 69 et 157):
  Anonymi varia excerpta medica. (Saec. IX)
- *97 V* (ext. 97 et 88):
  Galeni, Hippocratis, Ps.-Hipp., ac aliorum opera medica. (Saec. X)
- *225 V* (ext 225 et 304; int. 709):
  Iohannitii Isagog. liber; *Antidotaria, Medica complura.* (Saec. XI)
- *200 V* (ext. 200 et 394; int. 661):
  Constantini Africani et Iohannis Saraceni Particula IX libri secundi Pantegni. (Saec. XII)
- *70 V* (ext. 70 et 84; int. 956):
  Galeni opera nonnulla latine

Following are the translations of the excerpts taken from the Catalogue of Montecassino (Descriptiones codicum excerptae sunt ex 'Codicum Casinensium manuscriptorum catalogus' Montis Casini 1915 ss).

9th Century

3 KK (ext. 3; int 655): Some Works of Alcuin, Astronomy and Many Others
1 (pp 1–11). Several works of astronomy (Flor. Casin., pp 57–65 from this codex).
2 Some works of B. Alcuin. (pp 12–83) *Concerning the Faith of the Holy Trinity.* Books I–III, some chapters, preceded by a dedicatory letter, which are extant at the Migne publishers in printed form, and following the Invocation to the Holy Trinity and the Symbol of Faith. (M 101, 11–58. Ending: 'The blessing and glory of all the saints'). (pp 83–90) Questions I–XXVIII regarding the Trinity. (M 59–64. In the ms the title is missing with I Interrogation). (pp 90–109). Book about the reasoning of the mind. (M 639–650. In the ms the title is likewise missing. Ending: 'So may He shine for His sacred deserts, like a pious maid').
3 (pp 109–114). On the 6 ages of the world, (Flor. Casin., pp 65–69 of this codex in which the title reads *De Etes*

Natale Gaspare De Santo
Chair of Nephrology, Department of Pediatrics
Second University of Naples
Via Pansini, 5
I–80131 Naples (Italy)

(sic) *Mundi.* Cf. also among the works of Hieronymus and Bede. M 29, 915–918; 94, 1173–1177).

4 (pp 114–130). Many works of astronomy (Flor. Casin., pp 69–76 of this codex) among which we read (p 118), beginning: *Concerning the Eclipse of the Sun.* Beginning: 'The eclipse of the sun occurs almost at the ninth hour in the year of the incarnation of our Lord 7th October Seventy Six.' Ending: 'Likewise, in the year of our Lord, September 78 on the Lord's day' (cf. Art de vérifier les dates. Chronol. des Eclipses, p 66). (pp 126–127) The second problem concerning the moon's phases (M 101, 986–990). (pp 128, 129) Pseudo-Bede's *On Various Matters* (M 90, 724–725).

5 (pp 131–140) 'Pseudo-Bede's Nineteen circles from no.1 to no. 28' (cf. M 90, 832–835). In the margins of these tables appear notes added by someone else's hand, which you may read in Bibl. Casin., 1, pp 92–93.

6 Pseudo-Bede: (pp 141–143). Tables in which are found *Calculation Regarding the Behaviour of Embolisms* (Flor. Casin., pp 77–79 of this codex). (pp 144–147). *On the Behaviour of the Calculus* (M 90, 677–680). A numerical table tt(?) is contained in the codex in which the calculus does not proceed to the fractionings of the whole unit, but, omitting 16, passes on to 19, 28 and 30.

7 (p 148) Without a title, The Word of the Lord arranged in verse, is to be read herein (Flor. Casin., p 80 of this codex).

8 (pp 148–153) Some works of astronomy (Flor. Casin., pp 80–83 of this codex).

9 (pp 153–156) Here begins the calculation of how many working days of the week are needed in 14 years for Easter. (Beginning: 'The first year of the cycle,' M 90, 710, lines 19–711, line 16. Among the spurious works of the Venerable Bede).

10 (pp 155–165) Several works of astronomy, (Flor. Casin., pp 83–89 of this codex), among which (p 158): 'Lines on the same matter', i.e. concerning the fixing of the Easter period (cf. M 90, 708 among the spurious and dubious works of the Venerable Bede).

11 (pp 16–167) *Concerning the Calculation or Language of the Fingers* (i.e. sign language), preface missing (Flor. Casin., pp 90–91 of this codex. See also M 90, 689ff among the works of the Pseudo-Bede).

12 (pp 168–171). Some lines. *Lines on Individual Months.* Lines of Ausonius. Ending: 'The month is overcast, so December is a-coming' (Riese A: Anthologia Latina, Fasc. II, no. 639, Leipzig, 1870; and Flor. Casin., p 91 of this codex). Likewise, lines about individual months, beginning: 'The harsh gates of the temple of the Roman god Janus remain open in wartime. Whence comes December beloved by genial winter.' Ending: 'The entire species of the sun is dry under the implacable force of Scorpion.' (Riese A: op. cit., Fasc.I, no. 394, Leipzig, 1869; and Flor. Casin., p 91 of this codex). Authentic calendar about individual months. Lines about the twelve signs. (Riese A: no. 395; and Flor. Casin., pp 91–92 of this codex). Among the dubious poems of the Venerable Bede (M 94, 637; Flor. Casin., p 93 of this codex). Likewise, lines about the twelve signs. In chapter XVI (M 90, 358). In Bede's *About Reasoning of the Times,* lines on the yearly cycle, extant among the spurious and dubious works of Bede.

13 (pp 172–176) Beginning from the birth and death of the Fathers (Flor. Casin., pp 93–96 of this codex. cf. also M 29, 915; 94, 1173 among the works of Hieronymus and Bede).

14 (pp 177–192) Pseudo-Bede's pamphlet *On the Signs of the sky.* (cf. M 90, 945–948. Beginning: 'The greater Helix will ward off ... (?), ending: 'that which is almost opposite to the dog constellation'). Descriptions of the signs of a figure accompany this work which is artistically and neatly outlined. A few works precede the aforementioned booklet (p 193): 'Concerning the five stars which are called planets and also wandering stars because they have their own motion' (Flor. Casin., p 96 of this codex).

15 (p 194) A few works under the titles: 'when Pliny the Younger in Book 13 discussed astrology, they discussed these two stars,' as a little earlier in the same book: 'About the course of the sun and moon through signs.' (Flor. Casin., p 96 of this codex. cf. Plinii Secundi Natur. Hist., published by Mayhoff, Leipzig, 1892, vol 3, lib. XVIII, p 241, p 221). Some works on astronomy which are contained in this codex, and which are also published in the Flor. Casin. may also be read in the Cod. Vat. Lat. 645 as follows: 38, 39, 45v, 54v, 55, 69v, 72v, 77v. (cf. Vatasso M, Franchi de Cavalieri P: Cod. Vatic. Latini, tome 1 Rome, 1902).

Parchment, 310 × 210 mm, 194 pp, 9th century, Beneventine script (874–892 AD, cf. Loew: *The Beneventine Script,* p 314). The codex is neatly written, partly in double columns, partly on full page, titles in inch-size lettering, in minium and adorned in capitals and written in Beneventine script. Initial letters are decorated in gold, red, yellow and green colors. The early pages are worm-eaten, but are not completely ruined.

P 17, a letter of Desiderius the Abbot to Peter Damianus written in Carolingian script by a later hand is to be found published several times (cf. Bibl. Casin., I, p 87) is included.

Seven lines written by the same hand, now badly worn away, precede the letter P 1 in the lower margin, a more recent hand has added the title *Alcuin on the Trinity*. In the outer margin some names occur (cf. Bibl. Casin. p 96). Cf. Montf., L 217, 220; Car., i 29–30, 42; ii 17; Beth., XII, 498; bibl. Casin., I, XXXIV; Thiele: *Antike Himmelsbilder*, 161; ROD., 326, 330; Loew: *Die ältesten Kalendarien aus Monte Cassino*, 8; Reusens: *Eléments de Paléographie*, 64; Thompson: *Handbook of Greek and Latin Palaeography* 220 and *Introduction to Greek and Latin Palaeography*, Oxford, 1912, p 348, 350; Loew: *The Beneventine Script*, 124, 179, 200, 208, 216, 243, 247, 275, 290, 296, 314, 341. Specimen of writing in Pal. Cass. Long., tab. XXXVI, XXXVII; bibl. Casin., I, tab. II; Thompson: op. cit., tab. 120; Loew: Script. Benev., tab. 24.

69 V (ext. 69 and 157): Various Anonymous Medical Excerpts

1 (pp 1–6) Acephalous codex begins: 'Wherefore each liquid that resides in the head – place (?) in the nostrils and you will drive away sleep.' Some sheets appear to be missing among these pages.

2 (pp 7–260). A collection of medical prescriptions taken from various medical treatises, preceded by 42 chapters (cf. Bibl. Casin., II, pp 220–224).

3 (pp 261–524). Antidotes begin here. A series of 86 chapter headings preface the *Antidotarium* (cf. Bibl. Casin., ibid. pp 224–227).

4 (pp 524–527). Galen's book on the Substitutes (cf. Diels: *Die Handschriften der Antiken Ärzte in Abhandlung der Königl Preuss Akad der Wissenschaften*. Berlin, 1906, I, p 114. In ms: beginning: 'Ante. Apollominas Galieni).'

5 (pp 527–536). Here begins the names of the herbs. Bitumen, i.e. anthracite, or better bitumen. Ending: incomprehensible: Ramnus, i.e. whitethorn (?). (Flor. Casin., II, pp 14–19 of this codex).

6 (pp 537–544). On weights, measures and their signs. Acephalous, beginning: 'Semobolus seliqua (?). I.' There follows written by another hand: 'a purulent ointment for all ills.'

7 (pp 545–551) In the name of Our Lord Jesus Christ. Here begins the Book. On medical urines of the Philosopher Hermogenes. Beginning: 'He has spoken on urines'. Ending: 'signifies disease'.

8 (pp 551–562) Here begins. The signs of fever from urines and pulsations according to the precepts of Dionysius. Beginning: 'While it was difficult in reasoning.' Ending: 'a certain density containing milk.'

9 (pp 562–565) The Pseudo-Hippocrates' *Concerning the Ivory Capsule* (cf. Diels, op. cit. I, p 55 and Cod. Casin. 97, p 1ff, and Rose V: *Lateinische Handsch. der Königl. Bibl. zu Berlin*, Erster Band, p 373).

10 (pp 565–570). Here begins concerning acute fevers. It is to be understood why (?) they grow on the fourth day. Ending: 'he is thinking mostly for man.'

11 (pp 565–570) This begins with regard to the times they should abstain for individual months. The month of February about the thumb for the hands. Ending: 'And so many are cured.'

12 (pp 570–571) 'The Pseudo-Hippocrates' Prognostics'. Cf. Diels: op. cit. I, p 15 and Cod. Casin., 97, p 3).

13 (p 571–581) About citizens and many other matters whose titles you will find in De Renzi: *Storia Docum. della Scuola Medica di Salerno*, 2nd ed, Naples, 1857: *Documenti*, p VIII–IX and Bibl. Casin., II, pp 229–230.

Parchment 370 × 265 mm, 582 pp, Beneventine script, 9th century. The codex is written in double columns, with the headings adorned in red lead/minium. The initial letters are painted in yellow and red. Some sheets are missing. In the lower margins of the first part of the codex more 'Antidotes' have been added by a more recent hand. P 682 erased. Between the columns of p 574 a well-known hand of the 14th century has added these notes: 'Liber Ecclesie Casinensis muatus (sic) Eustasii Barberii de Sancto Germano.' The last page is not attached in its right place. Cf. Montf., I, 221; De Renzi: op. cit., 56ff; Car., I, 42, 101; II, 20; Giocosa: *Magistri Salernitani* (unpublished), Turin, p 31; Loew: *The Beneventine Script* 19, tab. VI; Loew: *Script. Benev.*

10th Century

97V (ext. 97 and 88): Medical Works of Galen, Hippocrates, Pseudo-Hippocrates and Others

1 Pseudo-Hippocrates' work: (pp 1–3) *On the Ivory Receptacle* (cf. Diels, op. cit. in Cod. 69, I, p 6, 55; Cod. Casin., 69, p 562); (pp 3–4). Prognostics (cf. Diels: I, p 45; Cod. Casin., 69, p 570). Acephalous codex begins (They precede Ps. Hippocrates treatises (p I)): 'Nor may you ask the years – they are not cured at all.' About cataracts. Cataracts cured – and the healthy person is produced.

2 (p 4) How you must examine the patient (cf. De Renzi: *Collectio Salernitana*, II, p. 73 of this codex).

3 Vindicianus' (pp 4–6) letter to Pentadius. (Galen's works published in Venice, 1550, p 41); (pp 6–8) *Gynaecia* (cf Rose V: *Theodori Prisciani Euporiston*. Leipzig, 1894, pp 427–462, where, among other things, it presents a reading of our codex).

4 (pp 8–10) Letter of Hippocrates on phlebotomy (cf. Diels, I, p 552).

5 (p 10) On measuring blood to be drawn according to the extent of sickness, and the strength of virtue. Beginning: 'The first is the contemplation of phlebotomy.' Ending: 'the cause of blood is deduced (?).'

6 (pp 10–12) Problems of Aristotle. (cf. Diels, II, p 19).

7 (pp 12–13) Beginning: 'On human bones. Regarding how many bones in man VIIII. Likewise, about bones from which liquid diseases arise. Human bones from treatment – that he may make an abortion (?).'

8 (pp 13–26) Various letters attributed to Hippocrates (cf. Diels, I, pp 51, 53) the first of which is of St. Isidorus of Spain. chapters I–XII, book IV Etymology (M 82, 183–196).

9 Certain Latin works of Galen's: (pp 26–33) cf. Diels, I, pp 128–132); (pp 89–109) On urines and pulsations. To Glaucon on methods of treatment. Book I–II (cf. p 127). In the codex works numbers 2 and 3 are marked under a single title: 'Galen's .... about different types of fever, are given.'

10 (pp 109–131). Works of Aurelius on acute suffering. (cf Daremberg C: in Ianus, II, Bresl., 1847).

11 (pp 131–199) Here begins the book of Scolapius the Physician (published among the works of Guarimpotus of Salerno and under his own name).

12 (pp 199–282) Books I–VII regarding a presentation of Hippocrates' aphorisms, with preceding prologue (prologue edited De Renzi: op. cit., I, p 87).

13 (pp 282–466) Books I–III of Alexander Theosophista. Books I–III (cf. Diels, II, p 11, among the works of Alexander Trallianus. In the codex the work is attributed to Alexander Trosphista).

14 (pp 466–476). Pseudo-Galen's *On Simple Medicines to Paterianus*. (Galienus' works edited cit. cf. Diels: I, p 142ff and p 545 of this codex.

15 (pp 475–476). Fragments of Herlarius, acephalous, beginning: 'Remedy of tablets as a health aid.' Ending: 'Dropsy (edema) is cured with a dry fig.'

16 (p 476) Begins another work from the book of Dioscorides. These are excerpts from Pseudo- Dioscorides (cf. Diels, II, p 34).

17 (pp 479–523) The Herbarium of Apuleius Platonicus. Acephalous, beginning with Chapter XXI. Name of herb – herobulbus (?) (cf. Edit. Basle, 1528).

18 (pp 523–532) Another herbarium which is equally acephalous, beginning: 'The seed itself which is in oil.'

19 (pp 532–545) Begins on quadrupeds (cf. Tosti, I, 388).

20 (pp 545–552) Pseudo-Galen's. About simple medicines to Paterianus (cf. p 466 of this codex). The selected works numbers 9–14 are preceded by chapter headings (cf. Bibl. Casin., II, pp 367–384). The titles of all the treatises and all the works which are read in the codex are likewise published (pp 366–391).

Figures of plants and animals painted in black and red ink accompany the works which are indicated as numbers 16, 17 and 19.

Parchment 415 × 295 mm, 552 pp Beneventine script written in double columns, the greater number of the initial letters of the codex are crudely colored. In some parts the sheets are spoiled through dampness, with consequent conjecture about what is written. The headings are painted in red lead. In the lower margin p 552 a more recent hand has been at work: 'I, brother Transmundus introduced these 4 pages concerning offering, and likewise Iohannes presented another 4 concerning the good son' (cf. Montf., I, 222; Caillau, 9; Puccinotti F: *Storia della Medicina*, Livorno, 1855, II, pp 294, 350, 353; De Renzi, op. et l.c.: *Storia Docum. della Scuola Medica di Salerno* 2nd ed, Naples, 1857, p 56ff; Car., I, 43; Beth., XII, 500; Tosti, 1, cit.; Giacosa, op. cit. in codex 69, p 21ff, 353; Loew, *The Beneventine Script* 19, 134, 178, 200, 224, 295, 343. Specimen of writing in De Renzi, op. cit., p 59; Bibl. Casin., II, tab. XII; Loew, *Script. Benev.*, tab. 36.

11th Century

225 V (ext. 225 and 304; int. 709). The Book of Johannitius Isagogus; Lists of Antidotes; Some Medicines

1 (pp 1–3) The letter of Pseudo-Hippocrates (in the manuscript. Here begins the letter of Hippocrates and others. Beginning: 'There are four winds.' Ending: 'for 30 women.' (cf. De Renzi: *Storia Documentaria della Scuola Medica di Salerno*, Naples, 1857, p 6; Car., II, 53).

2 (pp 3–16) Etymology. 4 books of St. Isodorus of Hispal.: (pp 3–15) chapters I–XI with some omissions; (pp 15–16) chapter XIII (publ. De Renzi: op. cit., App., p 8, no. 5); (pp 16–17) chapter XII, no. 7–11 (M 82, 183–198).

3 (pp 17–20) Vindecianus' letter to Pentadius his grandson. Beginning: 'Vindecianus sends his wishes of good health to his grandchild. You may wish to know, my dearest grandchild, you who are versed in Greek literature.' Ending: 'I, your grandfather, duly gave you these in memory of me, that you may know more.' Ed. Rose V: *Theodori Prisciani Euporiston* Leipzig, 1894, pp 485–492. (cf. Cod. Casin., 97, p 4 in Cod. Casin. Catal. vol. 1, p 97).

4 (pp 20–26). The Pseudo-Galen's *On the Limbs of Men*. Title missing, beginning: 'Exposition of limbs in what order and with what joints.' Ending: 'Thus the teeth are pulled from the head' (cf. the works of Galen published in Venice by Juntae, 1573, I, p 43).

5 (pp 26–30). About Interrogations. Beginning: 'Wherefore, if the lower wind, it drains and desiccates those parts which are around the stomach (?).' Ending: 'it bites the members or, being frightened by nature, suffers rigour/cold.'

6 (pp 31–33). About the 4 elements of the body. Beginning: 'Nor any doctor not knowing the nature (?) of the organ of the stomach or intestines on applying inappropriate medicine.' Ending: 'that which may make cold before heat.'

7 (pp 33–34). On the types of cleansing/catharsis. There are 3 types of catharsis: 1 drawing (cholagogue), another evacuating and a 3rd purging. Ending: 'to pull out the root from three seeds (?).'

8 (pp 34–35) Galenus' letter to Glaucon (cf. Diels: *Die Handschriften der Ärzte*. Berlin, 1906, I, cf. also Cod. Casin., 97, p 33).

9 (pp 35–36) *On the Nature of Waters*. Beginning: 'The physician should know the benefits of water.' Ending: 'If in the lawful days as the disease matures it causes diseases (?).'

10 (pp 36–128) *List of Antidotes*. (pp 36–80) In the name of the Lord here begins the List of Antidotes. Among the first, Adrianum, beginning: 'adrianum is the best antidote which is effective for all despairs of death – Melaticum which suffices.' Ending: 'the antidote Misterion is interpreted as full of benefits or causal. Misterion cures all fevers – You are to administer it on an empty stomach with moderation and with hot water.' The first particular is explained. (pp 58–81) Here begins the second section: among the first the antidote of Galeopsis. It is indicated as a Conqueror. The name is taken from the author Galienus. The very strong antidote is made with pincers and is used against stomache ache. It receives those of Aprotanus IIII. Ending: 'and cures strangury' (titles of individual antidotes will be found in Bibl. Casin., IV, pp 213–215). (pp 81–128) In the name of Christ here begins the list of antidotes, beginning: 'A better antidote which is beneficial for many weaknesses. Zuccari lib ...' Ending: 'a potion approved for constraining love. The skin of a pear – so drink it warm' (the titles of the antidotes are to be found in Bibl. Casin., IV, pp 215–217).

11 (pp 129–146) Here begins the book of the introductions *(isagoges)* (cf. Johannitius' introduction to Galen's modest art. With regard to publication cf. Neuburger-Pagel, I, p 596).

12 (pp 146–148) 'Certain medical prescriptions'. Editor Car., II, pp 54–56).

Parchment 250 × 155 mm, 148 pp, Beneventine lettering, written in full lines. Headings in red lead. Initial letters in red lead and colors, capital letters in red (cf. Montf., I, 224; Car., 179, II, 53; De Renzi, op. cit., p 60; Puccinotti F: *Storia della Medicina*. Leghorn, 1855, II, p 351; Tosti, II, 337; Giacosa P: *Unpublished Masters of Salerno*, Turin, 1901, pp 21, 23; Loew, *The Beneventine Script* 19, 346ff. Specimen of writing in Bibl. Casin., IV, tab. XIX, no. 3.

12th Century

200 V (ext. 200 and 394; int. 661). IX Particulars of Constantinus Africanus and John Saracenus of the 2nd Book of Pantegnus

The title written in 13th Century Gothic script (p 1) heads the series of chapters. Of the book of Pantegnus containing 110 chapters, 43 chapters are translated by a certain Constantine/Constantinus, the others by a certain Saracen.

There follows (pp 1–8) a series of chapters: (I) In the first concerning a manual operation and its division ... (XLII) About a wound made in the stomach where the intestine comes out translated hitherto by Constantinus and before then by a certain 'Sarracenus'. (XLIV) About the wound whence the pus issues. About the dissolution of ruptures and wounds. (CIX) A series of chapters of Constantinus' translation includes 42 chapters (but not 43), another 66 of John's (not 67), but in the text of the codex there are the 67 chapters. John's translation (pp 8–175) is prefaced by the following note, written in Gothic script on scratched parchment: 'Hitherto the nine principles in sections is called Surgery and have been translated by Constantinus. Prior to this, the source of the same section was translated by a certain Saracen.' Beginning: 'About the wound where the pus issues forth.' (XLVIII) If the wound had gone into the stomach where the pus and the intestine may come out and the wound made an abscess and it swelled in its course. Ending: 'They may be cured and the wounds healed.' The 9th section explains concerning the second book of Pantegnus (cf. the works of Constantine publ. at Basle, 1539, by Henricus Petri. Cf. also cod. 898 in Rose V: *Verzeichnis der Latein. Handschr. der Königl. Bibl. zu Berlin*, II, 3, Berlin, 1905, p 1061ff. In this codex the signature is wrongly held by some to be that of Constantinus. There is no written authority of his, except for the series of chapters 1–42, mentioned above). Certain medical precepts are added: (pp 175–177) About boils which occur between the finger-nails. Beginning: 'Sometimes in the circle of the finger nails.' (pp 177–178) Should the nail regrow twisted it may develop painfully. Beginning: 'on which wounds it is applied. Great basil as an ointment. It is useful for wounds.' Ending: 'as much as suffices.' (p 178) Lesser basil as an ointment. Pitch resin. Ending: 'Why a bad bruise lingers on.' (p 179) Almansor-Al Mansur (?). Book VII in the chapter about those things that are to come out are ruptured, so it is necessary to treat with irons. Thistle and pitch honey and may be kept for use. For inducing sleep. Remedy: a well-beated white of an egg will induce sleep.

Parchment 235 × 160 mm, 180 pages, Carolingian-Gothic lettering, full-lined, annotated by an unskilled hand. The initial letters and headings written in scarlet. Page 179 written by another hand.

Page 180 white. In the lower margin p 1, the title, written in 16th century hand, we read: 'a treatise on surgery by Constantinus the African, a monk of Montecassino.' Cf. Montf., I, 223; Grossi G: *La Scuola e la Bibliografia Cassinese*, Naples, 1820, p 80; De Renzi: *Storia Documentaria della Scuola Medica di Salerno*, Naples, 1857, p 58ff., 222; in *Collectio Salernitana*, I, Naples, 1852, p 171 (where Chapter LVII of Pantegnus – concerning abscesses on the vulva. Published in this codex); Puccinotti F: *Storia della Medicina*, II, Leghorn, 1855, pp 294, 351–352; Car., 284; Beth., XII, 501. Specimen of writing in De Renzi: Storia etc., p 59; Bibl. Casin., IV, tab. XI; Pal. Casin. Lat., tab. LX.

14th Century

70 V (ext. 70 and 84; int. 956). Some of Galen's works in Latin

The works of Galen translated into Latin which follow are contained in the codex.

1 (pp 1–50). *On Accidents and Disease*. Books I–VI.

2 (pp 51–90). *On Days of Dying*. Books I–III.

3 (pp 90–147). *On Crises*. Books I–III, which are followed by a few works from book I, *About Natural Virtues* (cf. 251 of this codex).

4 (pp 148–154). *On the Use of Pulses, with Mark of Toledo as Commentator*.

5 (pp 154–163) *On Pulses with Argundio of Pisa as Commentator*.

6 (pp 163–249) *On Afflicted Areas*. Books 1–6.

7 (pp 251–290) *On Natural Virtues*. Books 1–3.

8 (pp 291–398). *Methods of Practising Medicine*. Books 7–14. Mutilated codex: without previous phlegmon.

All these works are to be found in the Juntine edition of Galen (Venice, 1550), but the version differs. The titles of the treatises that can be read in the codex and those that are found in individual chapters are contained in Bibl. Casin., II, pp 231–542).

Regarding works numbers 1–4, 6, 8, cf. Diels H: op. cit. in previous codex. I, pp 136, 91, 90, 74, 85 and 92.

Parchment 425 × 260 mm, 398 pages in 14th century Gothic character, written in double columns. The codex presents initial letters of individual works showing various figures painted elegantly in colors. Other initial letters are painted alternately in red and blue and are adorned with lines of the same colors. Titles are red. The codex is filled with marginal notes of the same age. At the top margin of its pages the book titles are colored in red lead. P 250 is completely empty. Cf. Montf., 221; Car., I, 366. An example of the characters in Bibl. Casin., II, tab. VI.

Reference

1 Codices artis medicae qui in tabulario casinensi asservantur. I Symposium Historiae Nephrologicae Neapoly. Montis Casini XXX Octobris MCMXCIII.

Am J Nephrol 1994;14:494–495

Codex Casinensis 69: Anonymi Varia Excerpta Medica (Saec. IX)

Edited by
Father Faustino Avagliano

Archivio di Montecassino, Italy

Key Words

Hippocrates recommendations
Codex Casinensis 69
Bloody urine
Urinary stones
Bladder lesions
Micturition

Abstract

This is a transcription of page no. 570 and 571 of Codex Casinensis 69 which includes the Beginning of Recommendations of Hippocrates on Disease.

Pag. 570: Incipiunt indicia valitudinum Yppogratis

I. Si tinnitum aurium fuerit vel sonitum inanitas capitis modestia exquilias humores vacantur, ut in oculos festinent.

II. Si ante oculorum visum musculae vel nigre inanes vagantes videantur, liptisim alleu comata habiturum significat.

III. Si palpebra oculorum prorigo grandis invaserit suriniones habit, qui vermis palpebras incidit, ex quibus adulteri pili, palpebre nascuntur significat.

IIII. Si capite pars dimidias doluerit vel tempora sepius emigraniu significat.

V. Si in ore salibam infinita assidue creverit, vessice querella ex perfrictione est, quoniam cauculum ex perfrictione vessice nascitur.

VI. Si pavor hominis sepius fuerit, ex eo pulsus cordis nascitur.

VII. Si faucis nimium tumuerit, aut stumas aut periculum significat.

VIII. Si vomitus infinitum manaverit, equali coli querella est.

VIIII. Si inflactio stomachi fuerit, ut suspirare vix possi ex pulmonibus querella est.

X. Si prorigo multa fuerit, ita ut scabie exeant, habundantia sanguinis dicit esse.

XI. Si flegma fuerit in putridine versa, ex pulmonis et ulceratione continget.

XII. Si prorigo fuerit gravis ut scabias non exeant, felix (*sic, per* felis) querella est.

XIII. Si colore aureo facies, si rufo fuerit, idem felis querella est nimia.

XIIII. Si pectines doluerit, vessice perfrictio est.

XV. Si urina cum dolore fecerit, cauculum indicium ostenditur.

XVI. Si a vissica sepius proditur, vermiculi nati sunt, qui hoc faciunt, ex hoc fistuli nasci solent.

XVII. Si vertebre coxe doluerit, scia (tica) significat.

XVIII. Si genucula hominis frigida fuerit, sive nasus, et sudor sepius emittatur, emithritheum significat.

XVIIII. Si suffraginis seu genucula doluerit, dolum art[r]iticum significat.

XX. Si pollice pedum in nudis eiusdem punctionis sepius dederit, indicium podagre significat.

XXI. Si plante nimis pruriantur, perniones habiturum significat.

Translated by A. Perna, L. Gallo, G. Eknoyan,
N.G. De Santo, Naples/Houston, Tex.

Father Faustino Avagliano
Archivio di Montecassino
I–03043 Cassino (Italy)

© 1994 S. Karger AG, Basel
0250–8095/94/0146–0494
$8.00/0

XXII. Si nervi ad pedum in articulis contrahuntur, articulaginem significat.

XXIII. Si nares sepius pruritum habuerit, ex pulmonibus laborantem significat.

XXIIII. Si ani pondus fuerit, ita ut disinteria salvari ex perfrictione est, caldamentis et potionibus subvenies.

XXV. Si vulnus fuerit et cottidie medicamina inposita non eruit, vermiculi habentem dicit.

XXVI. Si confrictio stomachi sepius emanaverit, colum significat.

XXVII. Si urina sanguinea mingerit infinitam sive incarnatam, perfrictio vessice insistit, quod si tarde remediatum fuerit, maximum periculum evenit.

XXVIII. Si urina cum dolore venerit, confrictio vessice est, ex quo cauculum generatur.

Page 570: Beginning of the Recommendations of Hippocrates on Disease

I. If on a modest head rotation you have tinnitus or thundering noises develop, that is because of lack of free humors shunted towards the eyes.

II. If you see flies or fluctuating light black spots in front of the eyes, it is a sign that you will get another eyelid infection.

III. If a diffuse itch affects the eyelid, you have an inflammation of the eyelid, from which lascivious hair grow.

IIII. If the area at the top of the head aches, or more commonly it does at the temples, it is a sign of migraine.

V. If saliva from the mouth flows uninterruptedly, the illness arises from bladder excoriation, because the stone starts from bladder excoriation.

VI. If fright in a man becomes frequent, from this will originate heart palpitation.

VII. If the throat will be swollen, it is a sign that there is danger of glandular swelling.

VIII. If vomit will flow with no limits, the colon will suffer as well.

VIIII. If you have so much stomach swelling that you breath with difficulty, then it is a sign that you have lung disease.

X. If itch will be so diffuse that sand comes out, you will say that there is abundance of blood.

XI. If mucus changes to gangrene, this means there is lung ulceration.

XII. If itch will be unbearable until sand will not flow, there is reason to suffer.

XIII. If your face looks of a golden color or reddish, the same will be reason of excessive suffering.

XIIII. If there is lower abdominal pain, there will be urinary bladder excoriation.

XV. If urine will be eliminated with pain, it is a sign of stones.

XVI. If urine will be emitted rather frequently from the bladder, from this small worms will come forth, that will give rise to fistulas.

XVII. If the hip joint will hurt, it means that there is sciatica.

XVIII. If the knees and the nose will be cold and you will have sweat emission rather frequently, it means that there is tertiary fever.

XVIIII. If the ankles or knees will cause pain, it means that there is arthritic pain.

XX. If in the big toe and in the skin around it there will be acute and frequent pains, it is a symptom of gout.

XXI. If the soles of the feet itch very much, it is a sign that chilblains are advancing.

XXII. If the foot nerves contract in the joints, it is a sign of limb disease.

XXIII. If the nostrils itch rather frequently, it means that there is lung disease.

XXIIII. If there will be heaviness of the anus so that dysentery is cured with coldness, you will cure it with hot wrappings and beverages.

XXV. If there is a wound and even with ointments applied every day there is no discharge, it means that he has small worms.

XXVI. If the tickling of the colon is rather frequent and diffuse, it is a sign of colic.

XXVII. If bloody urine will cause a micturition that is abundant and meat-like, beware of bladder lesion, because if the remedy will be administered late, great danger will issue.

XXVIII. If urine will be discharged with pain, there is bladder lesion, and from this stones will be generated.

Author Index

Subject Index